Advanced Surgical Techniques for Rural Surgeons

Amy L. Halverson • David C. Borgstrom

Editors

Advanced Surgical Techniques for Rural Surgeons

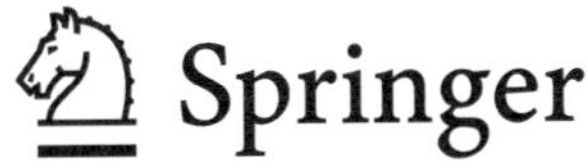

Springer

Editors
Amy L. Halverson, M.D., F.A.C.S., F.A.S.C.R.S.
Department of Surgery
Northwestern University Feinberg School
   of Medicine
Chicago, IL, USA

David C. Borgstrom, M.D., F.A.C.S.
Department of Surgery
Mithoefer Center for Rural Surgery
Cooperstown, NY, USA

ISBN 978-1-4939-4823-9   ISBN 978-1-4939-1495-1 (eBook)
DOI 10.1007/978-1-4939-1495-1
Springer New York Heidelberg Dordrecht London

Advanced Surgical Techniques for Rural Surgeons is a textbook that is vitally needed for the twenty-first century rural surgeon. In the previous century, the surgical world transmuted from essentially untrained surgeons to the golden age of general surgery when surgeons taught by Halsted, Wagenstein, Moyer, and others who populated the landscape with scientifically trained surgeons. From those classic traditions sprang the post-World War II explosion of surgeons who concentrated on specific problems now approachable by the coinciding explosion in technology. The result was the specialist surgeon increasingly dominated the field of surgery while the general surgeon became ill defined and more obscure. Despite these changes, in the rural parts of the USA and in the world in general, a need for the broad-based, well-trained "omni-surgeon" remains. *Advanced Surgical Techniques for Rural Surgeons* is an effort to address that need, to reinvigorate the specialty of rural general surgery, and to support rural surgeons in their practices. *Advanced Surgical Techniques for Rural Surgeons* will quickly become a valuable reference for rural surgeons who, not only must maintain their operative skills, but who must also keep pace with a rapidly changing environment. Today's surgeons are challenged by advancing technologies at a much greater pace than in the past. *Advanced Surgical Techniques for Rural Surgeons* will form the basis to meet those demands.

Urban and rural surgeons offer identical general surgical procedures, such as cholecystectomy, hernia repair, bowel resection, and breast operations. However, rural surgeons are often required to perform additional types of procedures such as gynecologic, urologic, ENT, and orthopedic operations, Cesarean sections, and endoscopies, all of which are performed only by subspecialists in urban areas. Because many surgeons usually select and perform only the operations that have been taught to them, there is a rising gap between training and the operations *required* for a specific, rural population.

Subspecialty surgeons may not be available in rural settings, but rural residents prefer to receive surgical services in their local environments. It is estimated that more than 60 million people live in rural areas in North America. These citizens are confronted by many obstacles, such as the long travel distances and geographic isolation. Rural patients, much like inner-city urban populations, can have limited financial resources. These patients tend to be older, sicker, and are often underfunded for health care. Surgeons who practice in rural locations must address these issues. A rural surgeon must be capable of performing many operative procedures with high skill and quality despite low volumes. All of this practice must occur while the surgeon is truly integrated into the community.

Fewer surgeons are choosing to practice in rural locations, which already have low surgeon to population ratios. The exposure to rural practice is variable and in most instances severely limited. Although providing surgery residents with a dedicated and significant experience in a rural setting increases the likelihood that a resident will decide to practice in a rural area, years will pass before training is modified by rural fellowships and rural residencies produce another generation of "omni-surgeons." In the interim, for those surgeons who are recently trained and who select rural surgical practices, *Advanced Surgical Techniques for Rural Surgeons* will be a valuable reference. The skilled rural surgeon of the future will not supplant subspecialty care, but complement it by offering and performing uncomplicated, routine specialty procedures in order to allow subspecialists to truly specialized and advanced cases. Rural citizens will also be served by obtaining high quality care at home. These benefits have been validated. An unsuccessful experiment in Ireland demonstrated the futility of having all subspecialty work, regardless of complexity, sent to referral centers. The effort was made in the name of improved quality. All breast cases were mandatorily referred to specialty centers. As a consequence of this mandate, these centers became inundated with benign breast disease, and delays in the treatment of complicated breast diseases, including malignancies, resulted. Benign disease could have been easily treated on a local level, and the more advanced pathologies would have been more efficiently managed at the referral centers. *Advanced Surgical Techniques for Rural Surgeons* will give rural surgeons the techniques in order to provide the best practices for routine procedures, which are only offered by subspecialists in urban centers.

Advanced Surgical Techniques for Rural Surgeons is a textbook written by rural surgeons who clearly understand the demands of rural practice. The challenges and potential limitations of rural practice are considered by the authors. Chapters cover gastrointestinal surgery, abdominal wall procedures, surgical oncology, head and neck operations, thoracic surgery, vascular surgery, trauma, obstetrics and gynecology, urology, orthopedics, and pediatric surgery. Each chapter is comprehensively written to include indications for any procedure and the preoperative preparation that is required. Operative strategies and techniques are detailed. Potential pitfalls are clearly pointed out. Postoperative care is described; common complications and the potential need for rehabilitation are discussed. Every chapter concludes by addressing transfer needs for patients who may require specialized care. Selected readings are included for rural surgeons who want additional documentation and information on every subject.

Besides possessing common sense, commitment, compassion, and communication skills, rural surgeons must demonstrate superior competence. Competency must cover practice elements not routinely part of today's surgical training. *Advanced Surgical Techniques for Rural Surgeons* addresses the requirements that come from all the aspects of a rural surgical practice. A broadly trained general surgeon, practicing general surgery in a rural setting, has a varied, interesting, and stimulating career. This textbook will be an integral part of that career.

Tyler G. Hughes
Philip R. Caropreso

Preface

Surgeons in rural practice encounter a wider range of conditions requiring surgical intervention compared to their urban counterparts. The majority of the cases they perform include endoscopic procedures, cholecystectomy, hernia repair, appendectomy, and colon resection. Due to limited availability of surgical subspecialists, rural surgeons are also called upon to address various issues that would otherwise be referred to urologists, plastic surgeons, surgical oncologists, etc. This expanded scope of practice may also include the care of pediatric and obstetric patients. Our aim was to provide rural surgeons with a resource that corresponded to their expanded scope of practice.

Much discussion and deliberation went into choosing which topics to include. There were numerous conversations with surgeons in rural practice and with surgical subspecialists. The list of chapters was revised repeatedly. The topics that we ultimately choose consisted of urgent surgical issues requiring immediate intervention and elective subspecialty procedures that were unlikely to be included in other general surgery references. We also included topics addressing recent updates in relatively common procedures such as polypectomy and central line insertion. Although central venous catheter insertion is a relatively basic procedure, we thought that the insight of a surgeon who has such vast experience with this procedure would be of value. Most surgeons in rural practice were trained long before ultrasound was used as a routine adjunct to central venous catheter insertion.

The authors were chosen based on their expertise in a given specialty. Most authors have either direct experience working in rural areas or experience caring for patients transferred to regional centers from outlying rural areas. We are extremely grateful to the authors for the many thoughtful discussions about what topics are appropriate for this book. We appreciate their efforts to share information that is most supportive to surgeons who will likely encounter many of these procedures only rarely.

We worked under the assumption that our audience would have a solid foundation of knowledge regarding surgical principles in general. We choose the format of a narrative atlas to provide surgeons an accessible guide to various procedures. Each chapter discusses the indications for a particular procedure. The overall operative strategy is summarized, and a step-by-step description of the procedure is accompanied by exquisite illustrations. Common complications and postoperative care are also explained. Unique to this book is a discussion about prudent limitations of care and when to transfer a patient to a specialist.

The determination of appropriateness of surgical intervention should be based on the surgeon's comfort with the procedure and the resources of the local hospital. Surgical emergencies such as massive gastrointestinal hemorrhage, testicular torsion, and obstetric emergencies require urgent intervention even if subsequent transfer is planned. In some cases transfer may be warranted, but not possible due to weather or transportation limitations. Another consideration regarding transfer to a regional center is the additional burden on the patient and the patient's family in terms of travel costs and time away from work.

We would like to acknowledge the editors at Springer who supported our vision for this book. We are grateful to our working editor, Joni Fraser, who endured countless revisions to the table of contents and cheerfully kept us and the authors on track. Finally, we are thrilled with the numerous, outstanding illustrations created by the Springer Art Department.

Chicago, IL

Amy L. Halverson

Cooperstown, NY

David C. Borgstrom

Part VIII Urology

Part IX Pediatric Surgery

Contributors

Mohammed Alghoul, M.D. Division of Plastic and Reconstructive Surgery, Northwestern University, Chicago, IL, USA

Krista M. Bannon, M.D. General Surgery, Providence Hospital and Medical Centers, Southfield, MI, USA

Carlos E. Bermejo, M.D. Department of Surgery, Bassett Medical Center, Cooperstown, NY, USA

David C. Borgstrom, M.D., F.A.C.S. Department of Surgery, Bassett Medical Center, Cooperstown, NY, USA

Ervin B. Brown, M.D., F.A.C.S. Department of Surgical Oncology, University of Texas M.D. Anderson Cancer Center, Houston, TX, USA

Philip R. Caropreso, M.D., F.A.C.S. Department of Surgery, Surgery University of Iowa Hospitals and Clinics, Keokuk, IA, USA

Charles Carroll IV, M.D. Orthopedic Surgery, Northwestern University Feinberg School of Medicine, NOI NorthShore Orthopedics, Chicago, IL, USA

Jennifer E. Cheesborough, M.D. Division of Plastic and Reconstructive Surgery, Northwestern University, Chicago, IL, USA

Christine E. Van Cott, M.D., F.A.C.S. Frank H. Netter MD School of Medicine, Quinnipiac University, North Haven, CT, USA

St. Vincent's Medical Center, Bridgeport, CT, USA

Gene B. Duremdes, M.D., M.B.A., F.A.C.S. Princeton Surgical Group, Inc., Princeton, WV, USA

Ronald A. Gagliano Jr., M.D., F.A.S.C.R.S. Department of Surgery, General Surgery Service, Tripler Army Medical Center, Honolulu, HI, USA

Michael Gart, M.D. Division of Plastic and Reconstructive Surgery, Northwestern University, Chicago, IL, USA

Amy L. Halverson, M.D., F.A.S.C.R.S. Department of Surgery, Northwestern University Feinberg School of Medicine, Chicago, IL, USA

Siobhan Hayden, M.D. Obstetrics and Gynecology, Bassett Medical Center, Cooperstown, NY, USA

Brett Howard, M.D. Department of Surgery, Mercer University School of Medicine, Medical Center of Central Georgia, Macon, GA, USA

Tyler G. Hughes, M.D., F.A.C.S. Department of Surgery, McPherson Hospital, McPherson, KS, USA

Eric S. Hungness, M.D., F.A.C.S. Department of Surgery, Northwestern University Feinberg School of Medicine, Chicago, IL, USA

W. Thomas Huntsman, M.D. Division of Plastic Surgery, Bassett Medical Center, Cooperstown, NY, USA

Patrick R. Kenny, D.O. Division of Gastroenterology, Department of Medicine, Tripler Army Medical Center, Honolulu, HI, USA

Kent Lam, M.D. Department of Otolaryngology, Northwestern University Feinberg School of Medicine, Chicago, IL, USA

Anouk R. Lambers, M.D. Obstetrics and Gynecology, Bassett Medical Center, Cooperstown, NY, USA

Gary H. Lipscomb, M.D., F.A.C.S. Department of Family Medicine, University of Tennessee Health Science Center, Memphis, TN, USA

Gary H. Lipscomb, M.D., F.A.C.S. Department of Obstetrics and Gynecology, University of Tennessee Health Science Center, Memphis, TN, USA

David H. Livingston, M.D., F.A.C.S. Department of Surgery, Rutgers-New Jersey Medical School, University Hospital M234, Newark, NJ, USA

Jennifer J. Lucas, M.D. Department of Surgery, Bassett Medical Center, Cooperstown, NY, USA

Wallace F. Martin, M.D., F.A.C.S. General Surgery, Gwinnett Surgical Associates, Lawrenceville, GA, USA

Alan J. Micev, M.D. Department of Orthopedic Surgery, Northwestern University Feinberg School of Medicine, Chicago, IL, USA

Kyle R. Miller, M.D., M.B.A. Department of Surgery, Northwestern University, Feinberg School of Medicine, Chicago, IL, USA

Mary J. Milroy, M.D., F.A.C.S. Department of Surgery, Yankton Medical Clinic, Yankton, SD, USA

Robert Moglia, M.D., F.A.C.S. Bassett Hospital, Cooperstown, NY, USA

William H. Montano, M.D., D.D.S., F.A.C.S. William Montano, MD, Inc., Fairbanks, AK, USA

Eric K. Mooney, M.D. Department of Surgery, Bassett Healthcare, Cooperstown, NY, USA

Don K. Nakayama, M.D., M.B.A., F.A.C.S. Department of Surgery, West Virginia University School of Medicine, Morgantown, WV, USA

Tracy L. Nolan, M.D. Department of Surgery, Mercer University School of Medicine, Medical Center of Central Georgia, Macon, GA, USA

Emily A. Norris, M.D. General Surgery, Naval Medical Center Portsmouth, Portsmouth, VA, USA

William F. Nowlin, M.D., F.A.S.C.R.S. Porter Regional Hospital, Valparaiso, ID, USA

Guy J. Petruzzelli, M.D., Ph.D., F.A.C.S. Department of Surgery, Mercer University School of Medicine—Savannah Campus, Savannah, GA, USA

Danny R. Robinette, M.D., F.A.C.S. Department of Surgery, University of Washington, Fairbanks, AK, USA

Michael D. Sarap, M.D., F.A.C.S. SE Ohio Physicians Inc., Cambridge, OH, USA

Mark Thomas Savarise, M.D., F.A.C.S. Department of Surgery, University of Utah, Salt Lake City, UT, USA

David R. Schmidt, M.D., F.A.C.S. Gwinnett Surgical Associates, Lawrenceville, GA, USA

Tim Schwartz, D.O. Department of Surgery, Rutgers-New Jersey Medical School, University Hospital M234, Newark, NJ, USA

Douglas M. Sidle, M.D., F.A.C.S. Department of Otolaryngology, Northwestern University, Chicago, IL, USA

Lauren Smithson, M.Phil., M.D. Department of Surgery, Providence Hospital and Medical Centers, Southfield, MI, USA

Ezra N. Teitelbaum, M.D. Department of Surgery, Northwestern University Feinberg School of Medicine, Chicago, IL, USA

Daniel J. Vargo, M.D., F.A.C.S. Department of Surgery, University of Utah School of Medicine, Salt Lake City, UT, USA

Jeffrey D. Wayne, M.D., F.A.C.S. Department of Surgery, Northwestern University, Feinberg School of Medicine, Chicago, IL, USA

Timothy Whitaker, B.S., M.D., F.A.C.S. Department of General Surgery, Bassett Healthcare, Cooperstown, NY, USA

Brent C. White, M.D., F.A.C.S. Geisel School of Medicine, Dartmouth-Hitchcock Medical Center, Lebanon, NH, USA

John Williamson, M.D., F.A.C.O.G. Department of OB/GYN, Clinical Medicine, Lincoln Memorial University, Harrogate, TN, USA

Robert J. Wilmoth, M.D., F.A.C.S. Department of Surgery, Clinical Medicine, Lincoln Memorial University, Harrogate, TN, USA

Rachel D. Wooldridge, M.D. Division of Surgical Oncology, UT Southwestern Medical Center, Dallas, TX, USA

Randall S. Zuckerman, M.D., F.A.C.S. St. Vincent's Medical Center, Bridgeport, CT, USA

Endoscopic Control of Upper GI Bleeding

Michael D. Sarap

Indications

Upper gastrointestinal bleeding (UGIB) is a common potentially life-threatening emergency. This condition results in over 300,000 hospital admissions annually in the USA. The incidence of UGIB is approximately 80–100 cases per 100,000 population with mortality rates historically reported from 7.5 to 10 %. Recent studies have documented a decrease in inpatient UGIB mortality rates from 4.6 % in 1989 to 2.13 % in 2009. During the same period the percentage of combined endoscopic procedures, diagnostic and therapeutic, rose from 69 to 85 %. The rise in therapeutic procedures was 2–27 % in the same time period. The nearly 50 % drop in death rates may likely be a result of the wider use of diagnostic and therapeutic inpatient endoscopies and improved specific medical treatment of UGIB.

The most common etiologies for UGIB include peptic ulcer disease (20–50 %), gastric or duodenal erosions (8–15 %), esophagitis (5–15 %), varices (5–20 %), Mallory–Weiss tears (8–15 %), vascular malformations (5 %), and neoplasm (3 %). The remaining causes of UGIB involve other more uncommon conditions including anastomotic ulcers, polyps, submucosal lesions, hemobilia, foreign bodies, and postprocedural bleeding.

Comorbid illnesses, rather than actual bleeding, are the major cause of death in patients with UGIB. One or more comorbid illnesses are noted in 98 % of deaths from UGIB with 72 % listing the comorbid illness as the cause of the death. The increase in percutaneous coronary interventions (PCI) in recent years, utilizing the use of multiple combinations of anticoagulants, significantly increases the risk of major GI bleeding in this patient population. Major GI bleeding rates after PCI have been reported from 0.2 to 2.3 %. Dual therapy with aspirin and clopidogrel results in a fourfold increase in the risk of major bleeding. The inability to quickly reverse the effects of some of these medications and the cardiac risks of withdrawing the medications complicates the treatment of these patients with UGIB.

Preoperative Preparation

Patients with acute UGIB require prompt evaluation and resuscitation prior to any endoscopic procedures. Patients with suspected acute bleeding should be evaluated in the Emergency Department or Intensive Care Unit. As with any acutely ill patient, a thorough patient history and physical exam should be completed. Important information relating to UGIB includes a history of liver disease, alcoholism, malignancies, prior bleeding episodes and use of anticoagulants and NSAIDS. Evaluation of adequacy of the airway and potential hypovolemia is critical. Venous access via two large bore peripheral IVs should be established in hemodynamically unstable patients. Consideration for urinary catheter placement and endotracheal intubation early in the resuscitation of hypotensive patients is advisable. Blood should be drawn for hemoglobin and hematocrit, platelet count, coagulation profiles and blood typing and cross matching. Patient vital signs including blood pressure, pulse, urine output, oxygen saturation, and orthostatic changes must be closely monitored.

Resuscitation for the hypotensive patient is begun with crystalloid fluids to maintain adequate blood pressure but patients with ongoing blood loss may need blood products including packed red blood cells, platelets, fresh frozen plasma, and coagulation factors. The availability of six units of PRBCs, FFP, and platelets within 1 h of patient arrival with a significant UGIB is no less crucial than in the treatment of a major trauma patient. Reversal of anticoagulants should be considered if feasible. In addition to the usual initial assessment of possible hemodynamic instability, airway compromise, coagulopathy, and other organ dysfunction, the rural surgeon must quickly evaluate each surgical emergency

M.D. Sarap, M.D., F.A.C.S. (✉)
SE Ohio Physicians Inc., 100 Clark Court, Cambridge,
OH 43725, USA
e-mail: msarap@msn.com

A.L. Halverson and D.C. Borgstrom (eds.), *Advanced Surgical Techniques for Rural Surgeons*,
DOI 10.1007/978-1-4939-1495-1_1, © Springer Science+Business Media New York 2015

in respect to available resources. Acute variceal hemorrhage and aorto-enteric fistula are examples of UGIB conditions that can quickly deplete the entire resources of a small hospital ancillary staff and blood bank. In these instances, it is much more efficient and efficacious to consider an early transfer to a tertiary center than to try and definitively treat the patient in the rural facility with limited resources. Emergency measures can be instituted to begin resuscitation and stabilization while transfer arrangements are being made. Familiarity and open communication between rural surgeons and their tertiary colleagues facilitates a more seamless and effective transfer between facilities and improved patient outcomes.

Certain factors help predict the need for immediate endoscopic evaluation. These include a history of cirrhosis or malignancy, hematemesis, and signs of hypovolemia (hypotension, tachycardia, shock, and hemoglobin less than 8 g/dL). Placement of a nasogastric tube is sometimes considered in patients with UGIB to assess for active hemorrhage or in patients presenting with significant bleeding from the rectum and an unclear etiology. The absence of blood in a gastric aspirate however, does not exclude an active UGIB. The presence of bile without blood in the NG tube however significantly decreases the chance of a bleeding source within reach of the UGI endoscope. The use of proton pump inhibitor (PPI) therapy is recommended for patients suspected of presenting with acute UGIB. Intravenous PPI given before endoscopic procedures significantly reduces rates of high-risk stigmata identified on endoscopy and reduces the need for endoscopic therapeutic maneuvers. The routine use of prokinetic agents (intravenous erythromycin and metoclopramide) in UGIB is not recommended but their use may result in a higher diagnostic yield at endoscopy in patients with fresh blood in the stomach.

Operative Strategy

Esophago-gastro-duodenoscopy (EGD) is the main diagnostic and therapeutic procedure for UGIB. The endoscopist can locate the source of the bleeding in the majority of cases and perform therapeutic maneuvers to control active hemorrhage. Preparation prior to initiating the procedure is crucial. The ability to perform the procedure in the Emergency Department or ICU by the use of a mobile endoscopy unit is very beneficial in cases of unstable or critically ill patients. A fully stocked endoscopy cart and dedicated endoscopy staff familiar with all equipment, devices, and medications that might be utilized for therapeutic procedures is mandatory. In an emergency situation, laminated index cards attached to the endoscopy cart can be very helpful in prompting the endoscopy staff on the appropriate settings for coagulation devices and instructions for mixing saline/epi or other injections. Surgeons working in rural areas need to be very

knowledgeable in therapeutic endoscopic maneuvers and constantly strive to advance these skills.

Treatment of Specific Causes of UGIB

Peptic Ulcer Disease and Stigmata of Hemorrhage

Peptic ulcer disease is the most common cause of UGIB. Predisposing factors include acid, *H. pylori* infection, NSAID use, and anticoagulation therapy. Clinical trials have documented the effectiveness of injection, ablative, and mechanical therapies depending on the specific appearance and location of the lesion.

Endoscopic features of the bleeding source are important prognostic indicators of recent or potential hemorrhage. Multiple classification systems, including the Forrest system (Fig. 1.1), attempt to identify and stratify the stigmata of recent hemorrhage (SRH) to help determine which lesions have a high risk of rebleeding if not actively treated. Critical SRH requiring mandatory treatment include lesions with active bleeding (Aa, Ab) or a nonbleeding lesion with a visible vessel (Ba), defined as an elevation within an ulcer base that is pigmented. Less concerning SRH include an adherent clot on an ulcer (Bb) or a pigmented flat spot on an ulcer base (Bc). Simple clean-based ulcers (C) with no oozing, no adherent clot, no visible vessel, and no pigmented spots lack SRH. With medical therapy alone, major SRH have a greater than 50 % risk of continued bleeding or rebleeding with low SRH lesions having a much lower risk of these complications.

Controversy exists regarding how aggressive the endoscopist should be in attempting to dislodge an adherent clot from a nonbleeding ulcer.

Esophageal Varices Associated with Portal Hypertension (Fig. 1.2)

Early endoscopy with confirmation of a variceal source of bleeding and therapeutic banding of bleeding varices should be carried out in those institutions with skilled endoscopic support. Smaller institutions with limited resources should consider early transfer to a tertiary center with advanced endoscopic and radiologic support, unlimited resources, and capabilities for emergent portal-systemic shunting (TIPS). Specific measures can be utilized to better stabilize the patient whether the patient is treated locally or while arrangements are being made for transfer to a tertiary center.

Specific measures include:
- Intravenous fluid resuscitation.
- Early endotracheal intubation to prevent aspiration and respiratory compromise.
- Blood component therapy to correct anemia and coagulopathy.

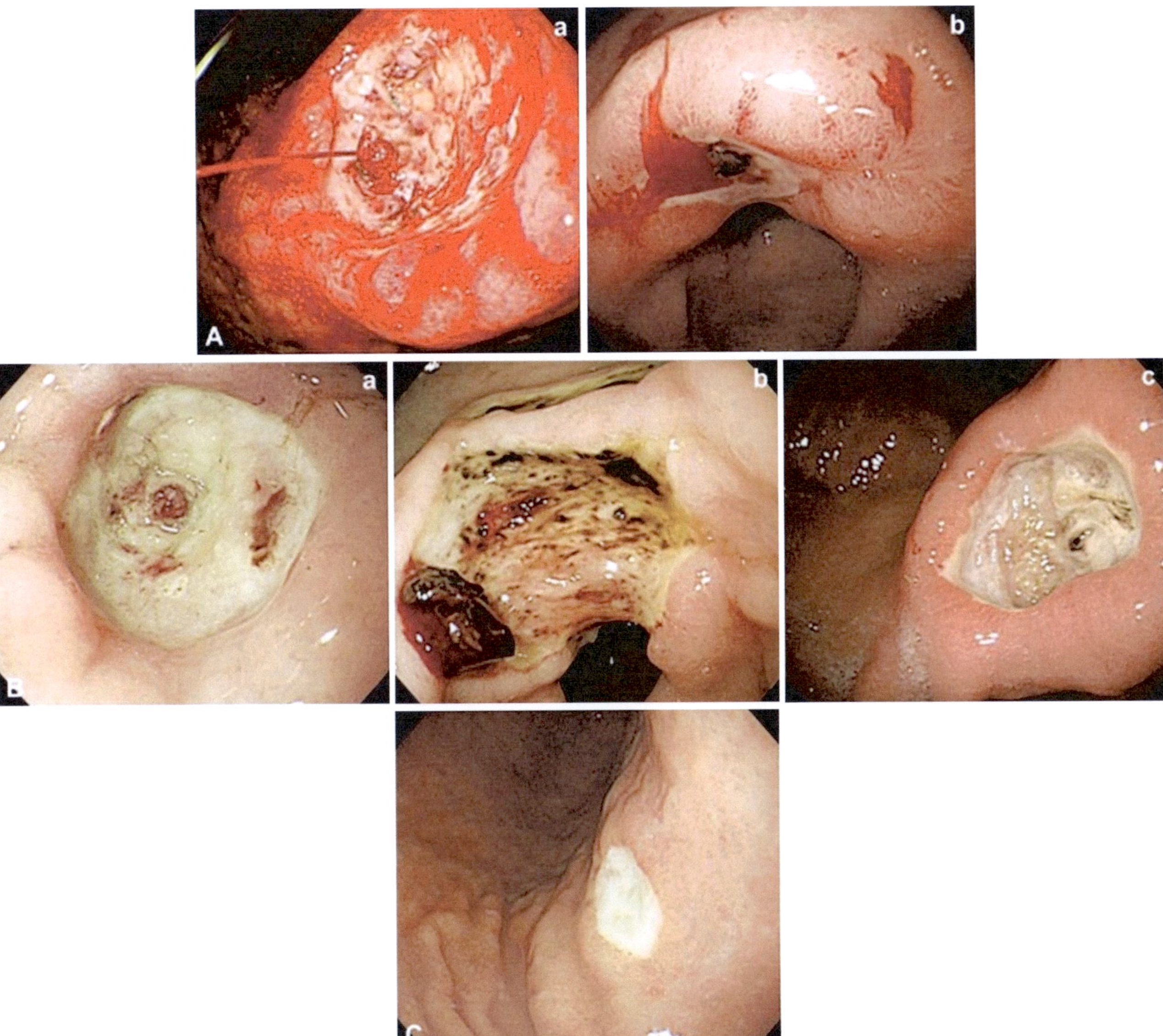

Fig. 1.1 Forrest classification can be summarized as grade: (**Aa**) Arterial hemorrhage ("spurting"). (**Ab**) Diffuse hemorrhage ("oozing"). (**Ba**) Non-bleeding visible vessel. (**Bb**) Adherent clot. (**Bc**) Flat pigmented spot. (**C**) Ulcer without recent stigmata of bleeding ("clean base"). From Seung Young Kim, Jong Jin Hyun, Sung Woo Jung, and Sang Woo Lee, Management of Non-Variceal Upper Gastrointestinal Bleeding, Clin Endosc. 2012 September; 45(3): 220–223

– Octreotide infusion (50 μg bolus then 50 μg/h infusion) to increase splanchnic vascular resistance and decrease bleeding. Octreotide has been shown to be equally as effective as vasopressin in reducing or stopping variceal bleeding and avoids the cardiac and mesenteric vascular complications of vasopressin.

– Mechanical compression of bleeding varices with a Sengstaken–Blakemore tube or one of its variants.

Mallory–Weiss Tears (Fig. 1.3)

Mallory–Weiss tears are lacerations in the region of the esophago-gastric junction that account for 5–15 % of cases of UGIB. Vomiting is the usual cause for the tear. Bleeding is self-limited in 80–90 % of cases with a very low incidence of rebleeding. Supportive therapy is usually all that is indicated although if necessary, endoscopic therapy with electrotherapy, heater probes, clipping, and injections are all effective (Fig. 1.4).

Dieulafoy's Lesion

This lesion was first described in 1896. It consists of an abnormally large submucosal artery protruding through a minute mucosal defect. Dieulafoy's lesion can cause significant bleeding and are often difficult to diagnose especially if there is not active bleeding present during endoscopy. The lesions occur twice as often in men than in women and

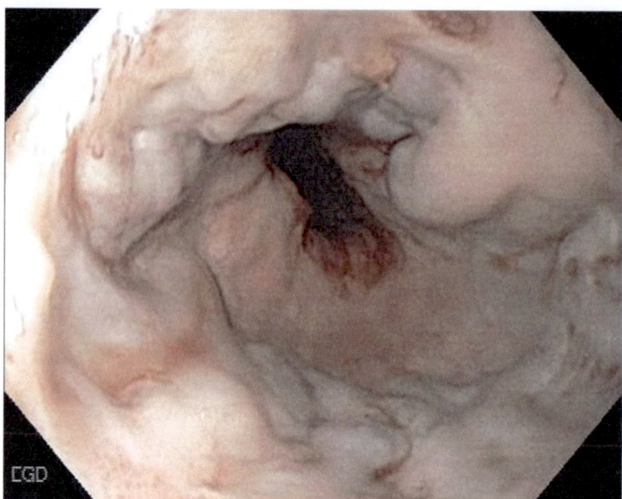

Fig. 1.2 Esophageal varices

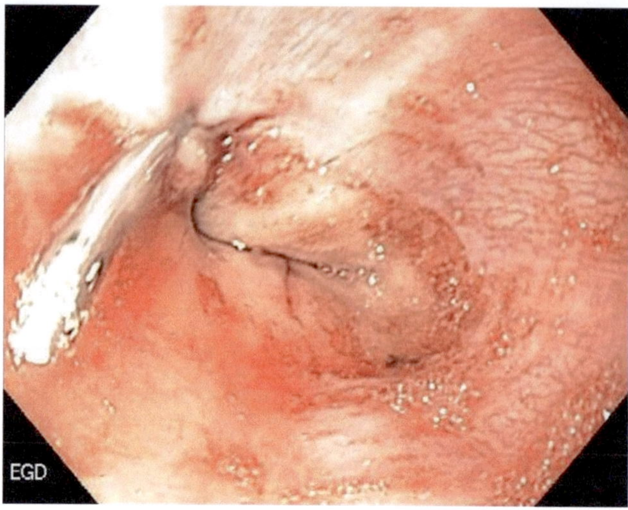

Fig. 1.4 Mallory–Weiss tear treated with injection and clipping

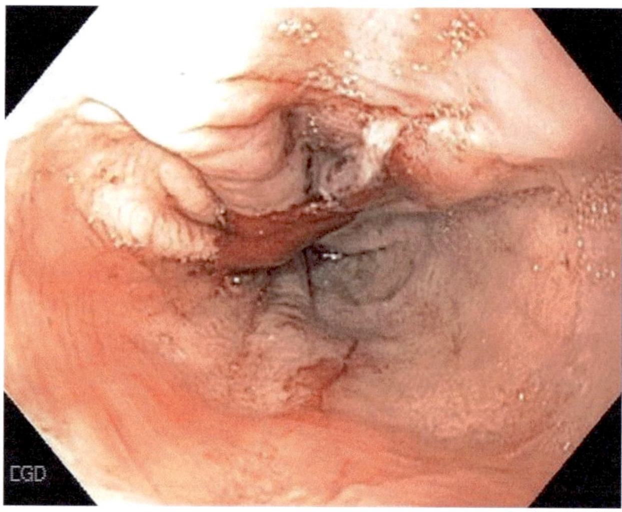

Fig. 1.3 Mallory–Weiss tear at GE junction

usually in patients with multiple comorbidities. The lesions are found in the upper part of the stomach in 75 % of cases usually on the lesser curve within 6 cm of the GE junction. Combination endoscopic therapy (injection/clipping or injection/coagulation) is exceedingly effective in arresting the hemorrhage and preventing rebleeding when the lesion is identified and treated (Fig. 1.5).

Congestive Gastropathy

This is a condition related to portal hypertension that causes chronic blood loss in cirrhotic patients. It mimics gastritis on endoscopy and microscopically reveals dilated submucosal veins and vascular ectasia in the muscle layer. The primary therapy is reduction of portal venous pressure and not endoscopic therapy.

Vascular Conditions

Angiodysplasia accounts for 5–7 % of UGIB. It can be associated with advanced age, chronic renal failure, hereditary hemorrhagic telangiectasia, and prior radiation therapy. Individual lesions can be treated with mechanical clipping or ablation techniques but patients with multiple diffuse lesions are problematic from an endoscopic approach.

Gastric antral vascular ectasia (GAVES) or "watermelon stomach" is an uncommon vascular malformation of unknown etiology. The lesion presents endoscopically as wide stripes of erythematous friable mucosa in the gastric antrum resembling a watermelon rind (Fig. 1.6). Argon plasma coagulation (APC) and radiofrequency ablation have been described to treat this condition.

Aorto-Enteric Fistula

Fistulae between the aorta and bowel can occur after Dacron graft replacement of the aorta. Atherosclerotic plaque or mycotic aneurysm can less commonly result in a fistula. The lesion involves the third or fourth portion of the duodenum and in many cases the graft can be visualized protruding through the back wall of the duodenum (Fig. 1.7). A CT scan with IV contrast can also make the diagnosis. Patients have an initial "herald bleed" which can abate on its own to be followed by a massive exsanguinating event hours, days, or weeks later. Endoscopy can make the diagnosis but there is no role for endoscopic therapy for this life-threatening condition. Even with immediate transfer and surgical therapy there is a very significant rate of morbidity and mortality with this condition.

Neoplasms

Malignant lesions of the upper GI tract are uncommon causes of UGIB and usually self-limited. Endoscopy plays a limited role in therapy.

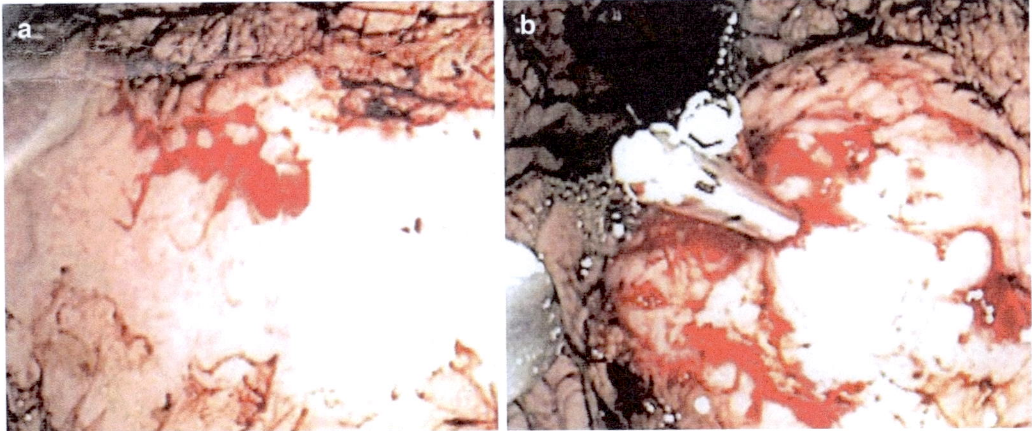

Fig. 1.5 Bleeding Dieulafoy's lesion (**a**) with injection/clip application (**b**)

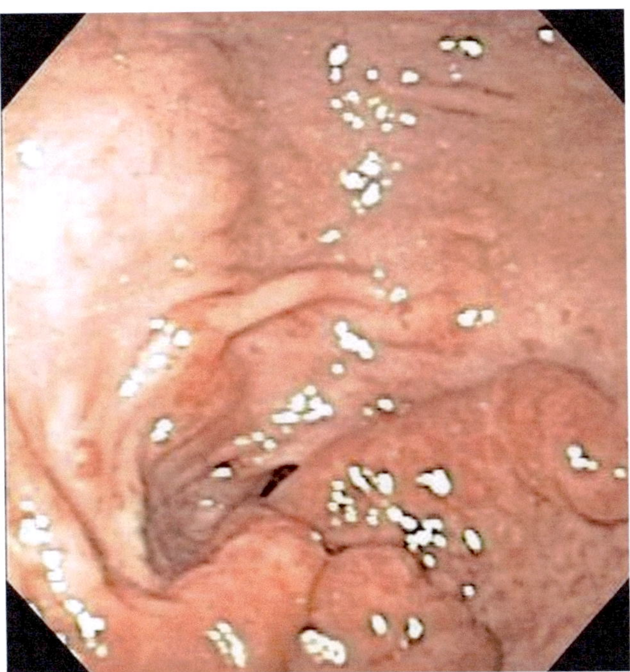

Fig. 1.6 Gastric antral vascular ectasia (GAVES)

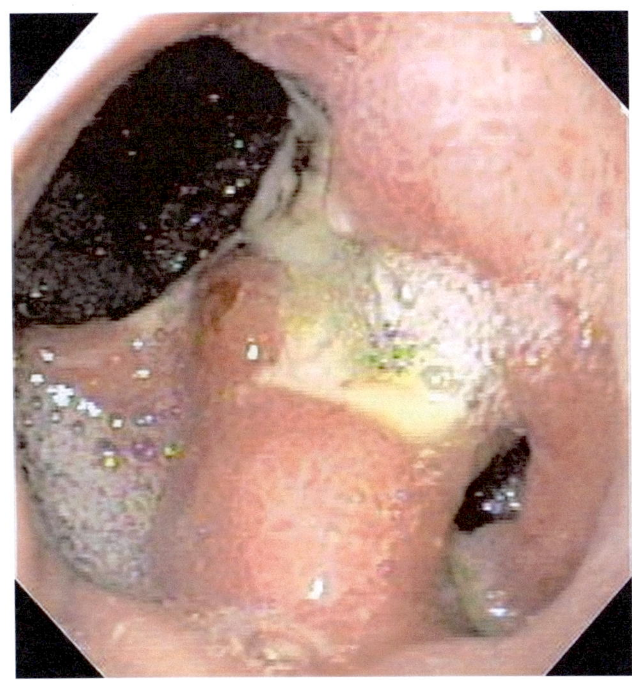

Fig. 1.8 Anastomotic ulcer

Anastomotic Ulcers (Fig. 1.8)

Anastomotic ulcers, also termed marginal or stomal ulcers, occur in 0.6–16 % of bariatric patients treated with laparoscopic rou-en-y gastric bypass. Nonsurgical approaches are successful in healing the lesions in 68–88 % of the cases. Up to 1/3 of patients may ultimately need surgical revision and even in these re-operated cases up to 10 % may have a recurrence. Bleeding lesions are treated in the same fashion as peptic ulcers.

Operative Technique

A plethora of injections, devices, and tools are available to the endoscopist treating patients with UGIB. The availability of certain therapies in smaller institutions may be limited by

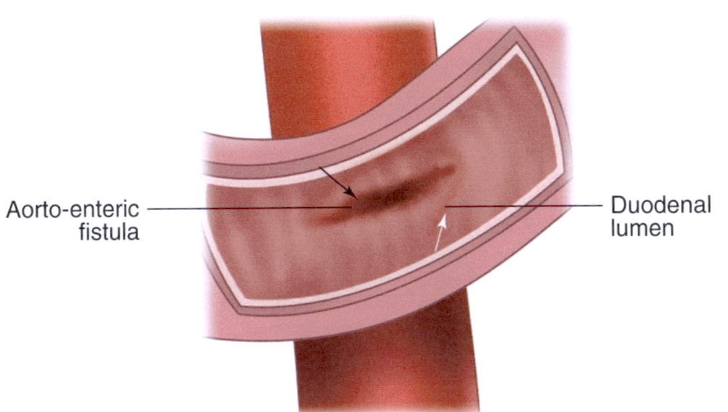

Fig. 1.7 Aorto-enteric fistula, endoscopic view. *White arrow*—duodenal lumen; *black arrow*—aorto-enteric fistula

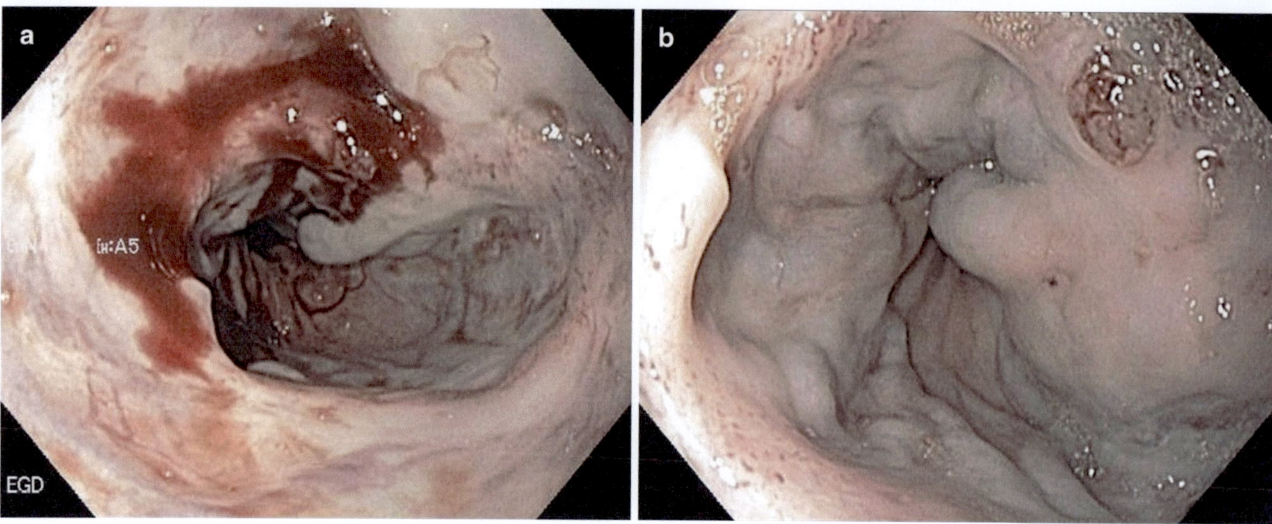

Fig. 1.9 (**a**) Bleeding esophageal varix; (**b**) esophageal varix after saline/epi injection

financial constraints but most cases of UGIB can be treated with many different single and combination modalities. Each endoscopist must become comfortable and familiar with the available devices in their individual institution. Obviously, the rural surgical endoscopist must be knowledgeable and confident in their ability to perform standard open surgical therapy to control hemorrhage when endoscopic therapy fails to stabilize the patient. The timing, surgical approach, and resources required should be considered even as the initial endoscopy is being carried out.

A partial list of available modalities includes:

- Injection therapy:
  - Normal or concentrated saline injection
  - Epinephrine (adrenaline)
  - Sclerosants (ethanol, ethanolamine, polidocanal)
  - Thrombin
  - Fibrin
  - Cyanoacrylate glues
- Cautery devices:
  - Heat probes
  - Neodymium-yttrium aluminum garnet lasers (YAG)
  - Argon plasma coagulation (APC)
  - Electrocautery probes (BICAP, GOLD Probe)
  - Radiofrequency ablation devices
- Mechanical therapy:
  - Endoscopic clips
  - Endoscopic Band Ligation devices
- Future modalities undergoing clinical testing
  - Endoscopic nanopowder spray
  - Endoscopic suture methods

Therapeutic Endoscopic Techniques

Injection Therapy
Saline With/Without Epinephrine
Injections with concentrated saline solutions containing diluted epinephrine are widely utilized because of its ease of use and beneficial effects. A standard retractable 25-gauge sclerotherapy needle is used to inject a solution of 1:10,000 epinephrine and saline into and around the bleeding point. Injection of 1.0 mL aliquots into the submucosal space promotes hemostasis by local tamponade, by promoting vasospasm and causing thrombosis (Fig. 1.9). Rebleeding occurs in 15–20 % of lesions treated by injection alone. Application of a second hemostatic technique (ablative or mechanical), in addition to injection, can provide a more permanent hemostasis. Limiting the volume of epinephrine solution to 12 mL or less reduces potential toxic cardiac effects including angina, tachycardia, arrhythmias, and hypertension. To further decrease the cardiac risks in at-risk patients, concentrated saline without epinephrine can also be effective.

The technique of using concentrated saline alone for sclerotherapy involves mixing together 17.4 mL of Sterile Water and 2.6 mL of 23.4 % NaCl (4 mEq/mL). This makes 20 mL of 3 % saline for injection. Sclerotherapy with saline and epinephrine is accomplished by adding 2.5 mL of Epinephrine 1:10,000 to each 20 mL syringe of 3 % saline.

Sclerosants
Sclerosants are substances that cause local tissue inflammation and edema which compresses and tamponades the bleeding lesion and promotes clotting. Resultant necrosis and fibrosis occurs which can cause ulcers, strictures, and perforation. Examples of these agents include sodium tetradecyl sulfate, polidocanol, ethanolamine, and absolute alcohol.

Thrombin, fibrin glue, and cyanoacrylate glue have all been described for use in UGIB but are less effective, less practical, or more expensive than other injection therapies.

Ablative Therapy
Devices that deliver intense energy to the bleeding lesion to promote hemostasis are termed ablative therapies. The energy causes coagulation of tissue proteins that results in edema, vasoconstriction, thrombocoagulation, and tissue

Fig. 1.10 Rimming technique for contact ablative therapy

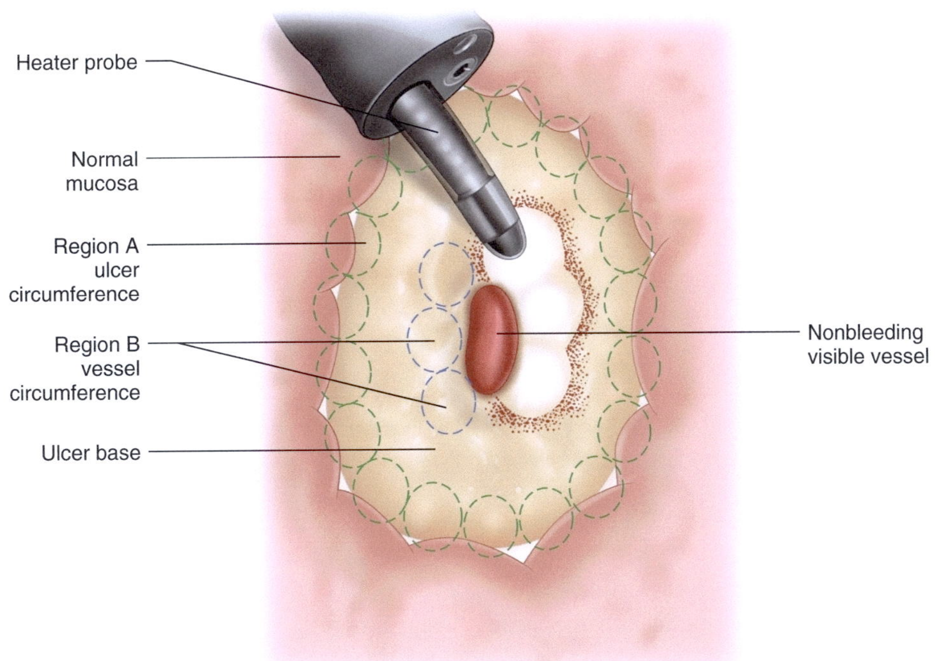

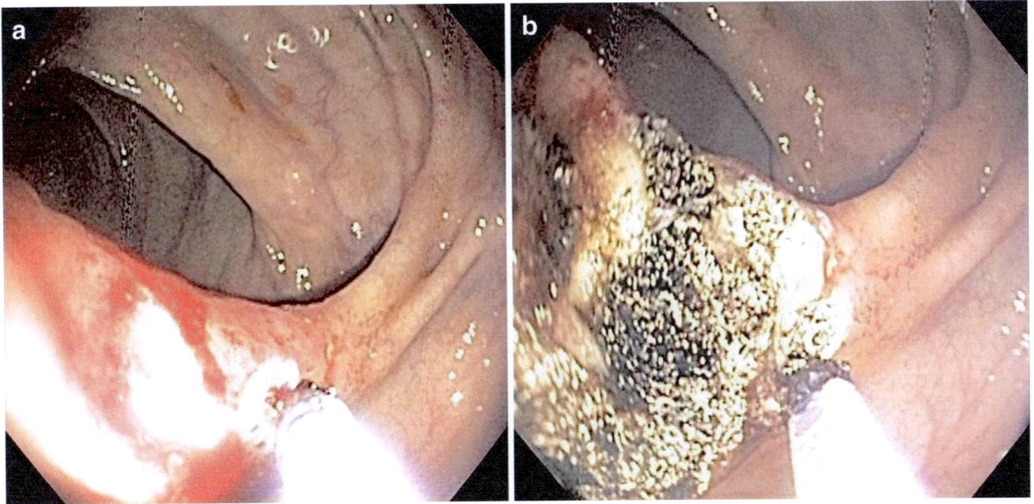

Fig. 1.11 Bleeding lesion (**a**) treated with argon plasma coagulation (**b**)

destruction. Thermocoagulation (Heater Probe) uses heat, electrocoagulation (BICAP, Gold Probe) uses electricity, radiofrequency uses high frequency alternating current, and APC uses excited electrons to achieve the desired beneficial results. Electrocoagulation, thermocoagulation, and radiofrequency ablation require the probe or catheter to contact the tissue for delivery of the energy. Compression of an exposed vessel by the probe reduces blood flow in the vessel making the energy more efficient. A rimming technique is used to treat the area immediately around a visible or bleeding vessel before applying the device to the actual bleeding site

(Fig. 1.10). The end result is to fuse or weld the two sides of the vessel together for hemostasis. Water irrigation during probe removal helps prevent pulling tissue away from the site which may cause rebleeding.

APC is a noncontact technique for UGIB. Monopolar electrocoagulation is used to ionize argon gas into a plasma that coagulates tissue (Fig. 1.11). Various sizes of catheters are available as well as a choice of devices that deliver the plasma beam from the tip or the side of the catheter. The thick-walled stomach is well suited to use of the APC where there is much less risk of perforation (<0.5 %) than other

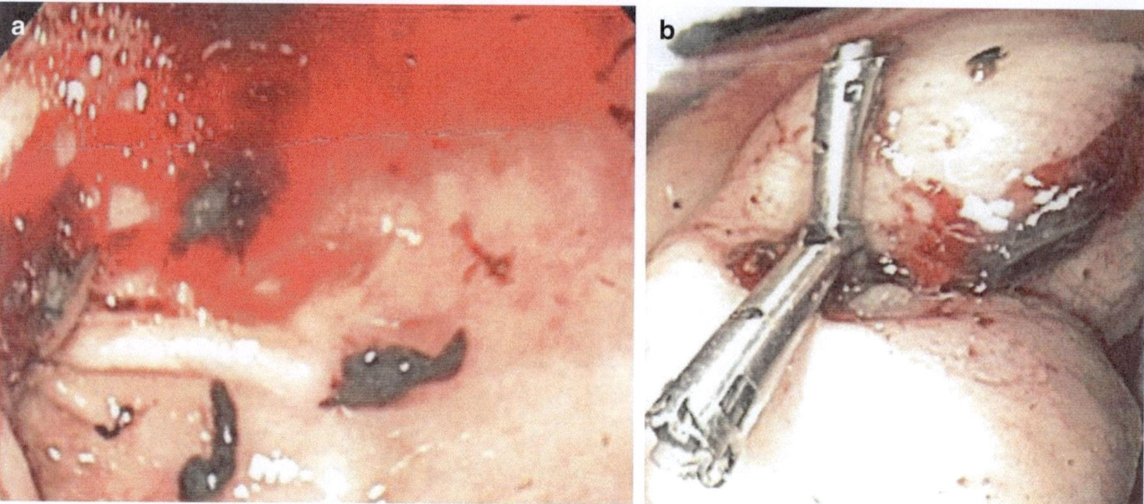

Fig. 1.12 Bleeding gastric ulcer (**a**) with clip application (**b**)

areas of the GI tract, particularly the cecum. A benefit of the APC is that the gas displaces fresh blood from the bleeding site aiding in visualization during application of the energy. Argon gas accumulates in the lumen of the bowel during the treatment and needs to be periodically suctioned to prevent distention or perforation of the GI tract. The normal settings for the APC application for esophagus, stomach, and small intestine are 60–80 W of power with single shot duration of 1–3 s. A secondary benefit of the availability of APC technology in a rural facility is its use to control liver bed bleeding during laparoscopic cholecystectomy and to treat splenic capsular injuries.

The Nd:YAG laser deeply penetrates and injures tissue and therefore has a perforation rate of approximately 3 %. Studies show a lower rate of hemostasis than other ablative therapies and it has high initial and ongoing maintenance costs.

Radiofrequency ablation has been utilized for ablative procedures in the fields of cardiology, invasive radiology, venous surgery, pain management, and for Barrett's esophagitis. The device has been used to treat large bleeding areas such as occur in GAVES and other vascular malformations in the GI tract.

Mechanical Therapy

This class of therapy mechanically compresses the bleeding point to achieve hemostasis (Fig. 1.12).

Hemoclips presently are the most commonly used mechanical therapy. Accurate placement can sometimes be challenging but they are very effective in controlling bleeding in the right circumstance. Fibrosis and acute inflammation can be problematic in approximating and compressing the tissue. Three brands of endoscopic hemostatic clips are currently available, each having different capabilities in terms of size, rotation, and reversibility.

Endoscopic band ligation (EBL) is a technique usually reserved for esophageal varices. They can be utilized for primary hemostasis in acutely bleeding varices, ones deemed to have bled recently and for prophylaxis in high-risk nonbleeding varices. The bands are preloaded onto a delivery device at the end of the endoscope. The varices are suctioned into the cap of the device and the band is fired onto the varix. Successful deployment results in the treated varix having a dusky pedunculated appearance with the band visualized at the neck (Fig. 1.13). EBL has been described for use in peptic ulcers, Mallory–Weiss tears, and Dieulafoy's lesions.

Combination Therapy

Significant improvement in rebleeding rates can be achieved by combining epinephrine injection with ablative or mechanical therapies. The specific combination varies with the endoscopist, the specific bleeding lesion and the available resources.

Insertion of Sengstaken–Blakemore Tube

A Sengstaken–Blakemore tube is a device inserted through the nose or mouth for management of UGIB secondary to esophageal or gastric varices in patients with portal hypertension. Use of the tube was originally described in 1950 and the device can be used as adjunctive therapy in cases of massive bleeding to stabilize patients until resuscitation, endoscopic therapy, or transfers are carried out. The device consists of a flexible plastic tube containing several channels and two inflatable balloons (Fig. 1.14a). More modern versions, termed Minnesota tubes, have channels for suction at the gastric tip and in the upper esophagus section. The two inflatable balloons are used to compress areas of varices in the proximal stomach and distal esophagus. Due to the high risk of aspiration in these patients, endotracheal intubation is usually indicated before placement of the S–B tube.

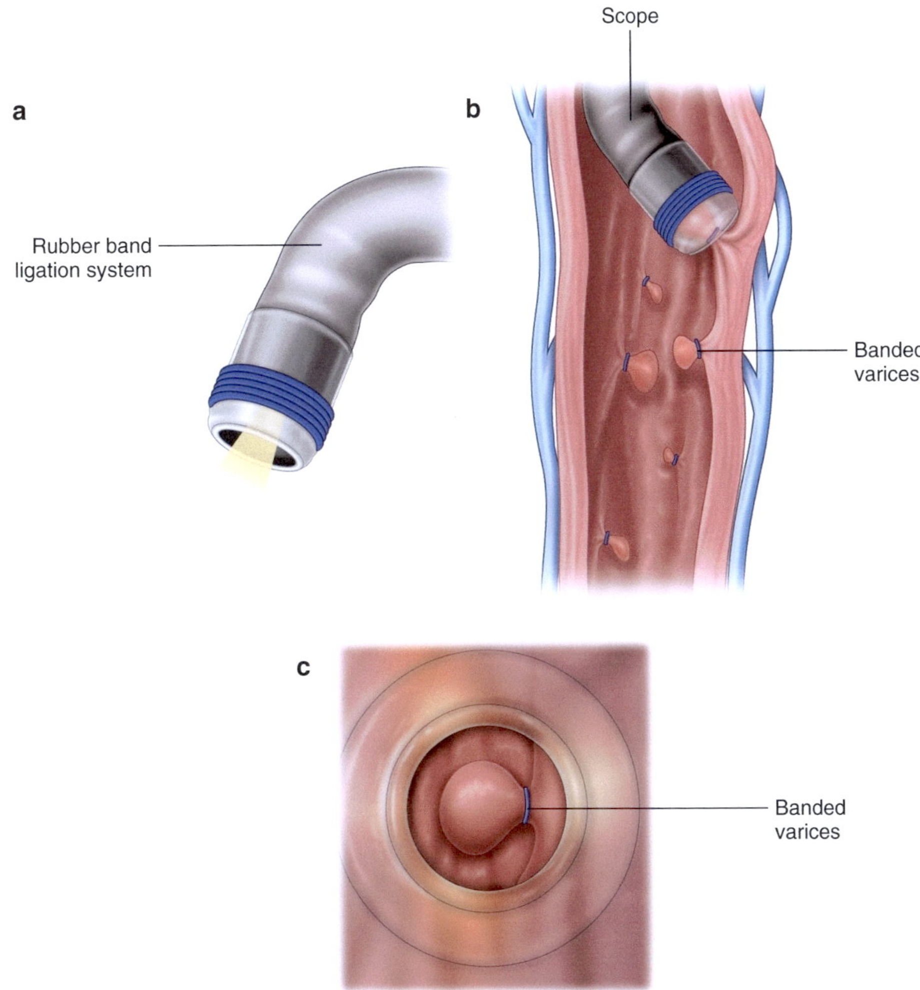

Fig. 1.13 Endoscopic band ligation of esophageal varices

The tube is usually inserted via the mouth and into the stomach (Fig. 1.14b). Confirmation of position on CXR or fluoroscopy will prevent inflation of the gastric balloon in the esophagus, which can cause perforation and death. The gastric balloon is inflated using 50 mL increments of air up to 250–300 mL for S–B tubes (450–500 mL for Minnesota tubes). Manometry can be used to measure the pressure in the gastric balloon with specific volumes of air before insertion. If the pressure during insertion is >15 mmHg more than the pre-insertion pressure at the same pre-insertion volume then the gastric balloon may be in the esophagus and needs to be re-positioned. Using a pulley system and a 500 cm³ bag of IV fluid, traction is placed on the tube to cause compression of the gastric fundus. If bleeding continues, the esophagus balloon can also be inflated to 40 mmHg. Deflation of the balloons should be attempted every 6–12 h to prevent necrosis and then re-inflated if there is continued bleeding.

Potential Pitfalls

Complications of endoscopic therapy for UGIB include the inability to arrest the hemorrhage, rebleeding after treatment, and perforation. Multiple studies document rates for successful control of bleeding, rebleeding and perforation for each type of bleeding lesion and the different therapies utilized in their treatment (Table 1.1).

Rural facilities with smaller caseloads and limited financial resources must make sound decisions regarding technology acquisition for the treatment of patients with UGIB. Cost, efficacy, and adaptability for multiple uses (endoscopic and surgical) are important considerations. Table 1.2 lists the approximate relative costs of the various modalities used to control UGIB. Each individual facility and vendor will obviously have varying pricing depending on purchasing groups, agreements, and contracts.

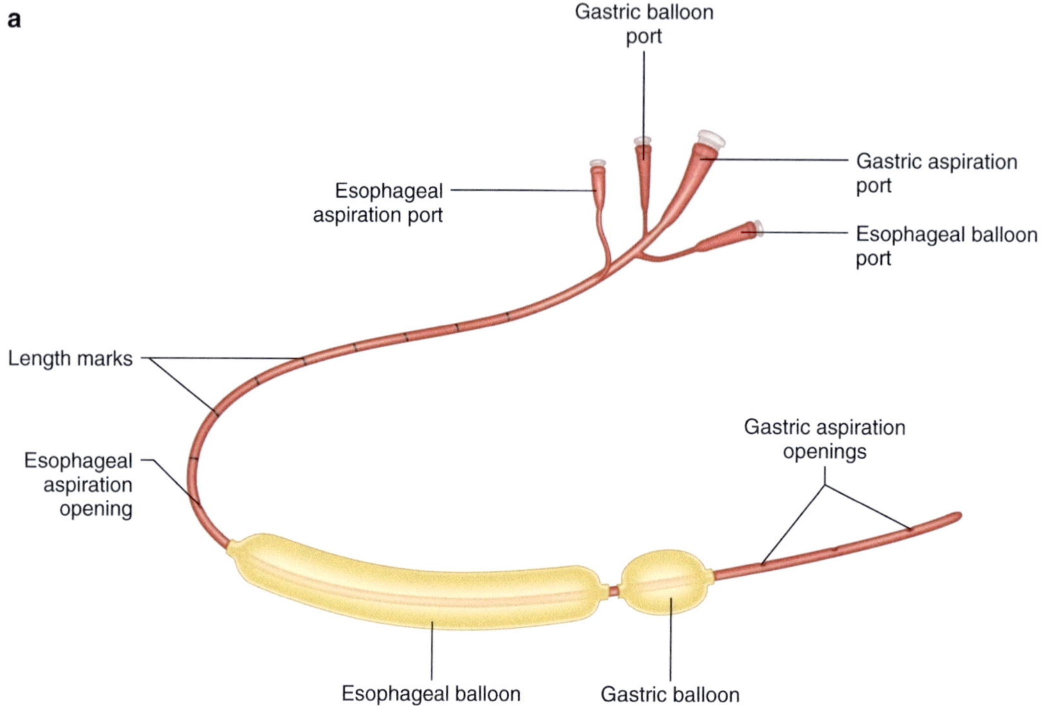

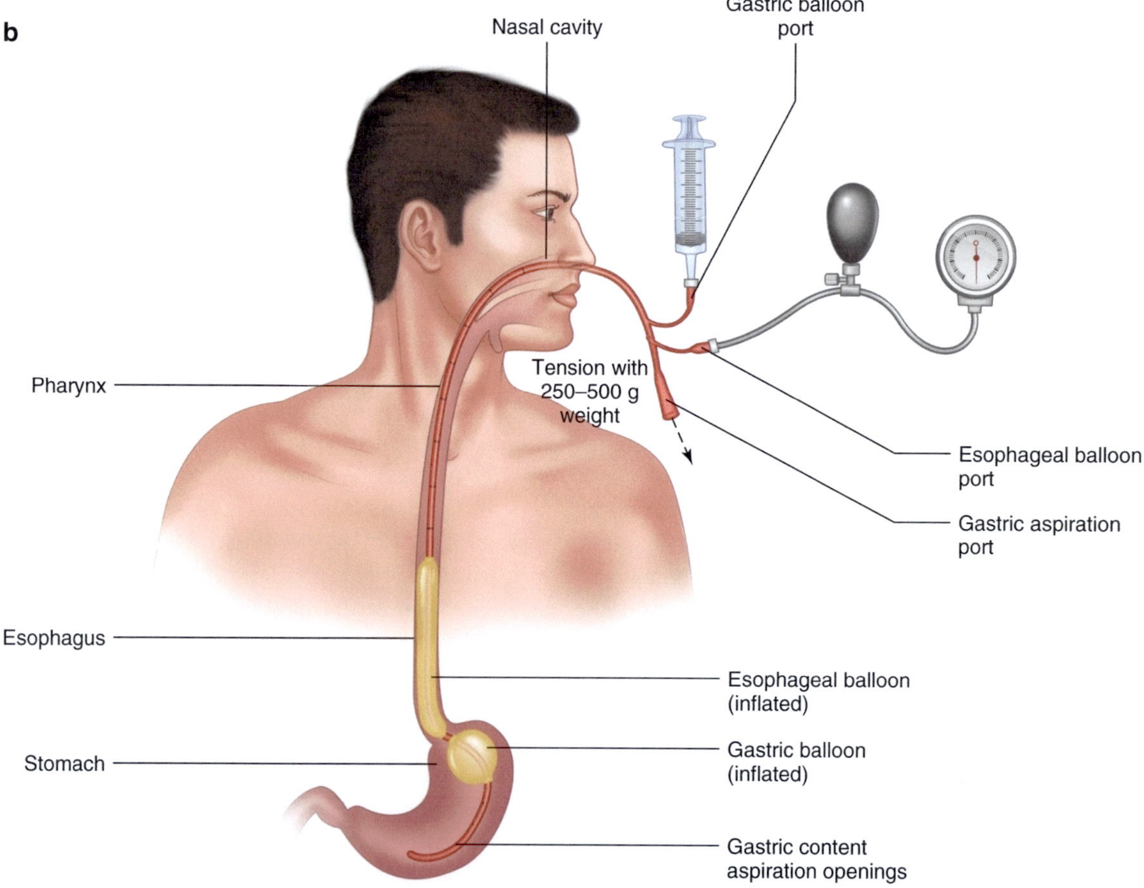

Fig. 1.14 (**a**) Sengstaken–Blakemore tube; (**b**) proper insertion of S–B tube

Table 1.1 Various therapeutic modalities for active UGI bleeding

Therapy	Rebleeding rate (%)	Complications
Medical therapy	>50	
Therapeutic endoscopy (all modalities)		Aspiration
		Arrhythmia
		1.0 % Perforation
Therapeutic endoscopy (repeat procedure)		3.0 % Perforation
Epi/saline alone	20–30	Cardiac toxicity (epi)
Epi plus heater probe	6.5	Cardiac toxicity (epi)
Epi plus clipping	3.8	Cardiac toxicity (epi)
Clipping	18	
Heater Probe	0–10	
BICAP/Gold Probe	10–20	
APC	14	<0.5 % Perforation
		Bowel distention
		Pneumomediastinum
		Pneumoperitoneum
Nd:YAG	22	3.0 % Perforation
Thrombin	14.6	
Polidocanal	9.1	
Fibrin glue	15	

Table 1.2 Relative costs (approximate) of UGIB therapeutic drugs and devices

Therapy	Approximate cost ($)
Sclerotherapy catheter	46.00
Saline/Epi	40.00
Endoscopic clips	185.00
Endoscopic band ligator	200.00
Heater probe unit	9,000.00
Heater probes (reusable)	500.00
Electrocautery unit	11,000.00–23,000.00
Electrocautery probes (BICAP, GOLD)	250.00–350.00
Argon plasma with electrocautery unit	16,000.00–26,000.00
Argon plasma with probes (singe use)	170.00–240.00
Radiofrequency ablation unit	13,000.00–35,000.00
Radiofrequency probes	900.00–1,600.00
Sengstaken–Blakemore tube	350.00

When to Transfer

The rural surgical endoscopist must be aware of the limits of the resources available in their individual institution. Significant UGIB can rapidly deplete a small hospital blood bank. Rural surgeons need to have established affiliations with gastroenterologists and surgeons at the nearest tertiary centers to help with the care of these complicated patients. Improved communication and cooperation between rural and tertiary providers results in better patient outcomes. Early transfer must be considered even prior to the initial endoscopy in cases of suspected massive hemorrhage as can occur with esophageal varices and aorto-enteric fistula.

Suggested Reading

Abougergi M, Saltzman J. The inpatient mortality rate for UGI Hemorrhage is decreasing in the US: a nationwide analysis over two decades. American College of Gastroenterology 2012 Meeting (abstract 2).

Bauer J, Kreel I, Kark A. The use of the Sengstaken-Blakemore tube for immediate control of bleeding esophageal varices. Ann Surg. 1974;179(3):273.

Cappell M. Therapeutic endoscopy for acute upper GI bleeding. Nat Rev Gastroenterol Hepatol. 2010;7(4):214–29.

Cappell M, Friedel D. Initial management of acute UGI bleeding from initial evaluation up to gastrointestinal endoscopy. Med Clin North Am. 2008;92:491.

Chung I. How can we maximize skills for non-variceal UGI bleeding: injection, clipping, burning or others? Clin Endosc. 2012;45(3):230–4.

Chung I, et al. Bleeding Dieulafoy's lesions and the choice of endoscopic method: comparing the hemostatic efficacy of mechanical and injection methods. Gastrointest Endosc. 2000;52(6):721.

Hsu Y, Chung C, Wang H. Application of endoscopy in improving survival of cirrhotic patients with acute variceal hemorrhage. Int J Hepatol. 2011;2011:893973.

Hwang J, et al. The role of endoscopy in the management of acute non-variceal GI bleeding. Gastrointest Endosc. 2012;75:6.

Kellici I, Kraja B, Mone I, Prift S. Role of intravenous omeprazole on non-variceal UGI bleeding after endoscopic treatment: a comparative study. Med Arh. 2010;64(6):324.

Ki E, Lau J. New endoscopic hemostasis methods. Clin Endosc. 2012;45:224.

Kim S, Hyun J, Jung S, Lee S. Management of non-variceal upper GI bleeding. Clin Endosc. 2012;45(3):220.

Liou T, Lin S, Wang H, Chang W. Optimal injection volume of epinephrine for endoscopic treatment of peptic ulcer bleeding. World J Gastroenterol. 2006;12(19):3108.

Martins N, Wassef W. Upper gastrointestinal bleeding. Curr Opin Gastroenterol. 2006;22(6):612.

Robotis J, Sechopoulos P, Rokkas T. Argon plasma coagulation: clinical applications in gastroenterology. Ann Gastroenterol. 2003;16(2):131.

Rodriguez S, et al. Review of mucosal ablation devices. Gastrointest Endosc. 2008;68(6):1031.

Sengstaken R, Blakemore A. Balloon tamponage for the control of hemorrhage from esophageal varices. Ann Surg. 1950;131(5):781.

Wallace M, Rankin J, Forbes G. Acute GI bleeding after percutaneous intervention. Expert Rev Gastroenterol Hepatol. 2012;6(2):211.

Wolfe M. Therapy of digestive disorders. 2nd ed. Philadelphia: Elsevier; 2006.

Endoscopic and Laparoscopic Techniques for Enteral Access

Brent C. White

Indications

Long-term (>30 days) enteral feeding in cases of inability to maintain nutrition, e.g., post-stroke, prior to chemo-XRT for advanced Head/Neck Malignancy, ALS.

Decompression, e.g., gastroparesis, malignant bowel obstruction not amenable to surgery or stent.

Preoperative Preparation

Understand prior surgical and medical history, including any relative contraindications (massive ascites, peritoneal dialysis catheter, coagulopathy).

Decide upon the optimal point of access, pre- or post-pyloric, using appropriate tube: G-tube, GJ tube, or J-tube (Fig. 2.1); consider possible alternatives or fallback plans.

Administer prophylactic broad spectrum antibiotics prior to the procedure.

Decompress the stomach of contents prior to decompressive enteral tube placement to minimize aspiration risk.

Potential Pitfalls

Aspiration during an endoscopic procedure.
Visceral Injury with percutaneous endoscopic technique.
Bleeding along the newly established enteral access tract.

B.C. White, M.D., F.A.C.S. (✉)
Geisel School of Medicine, Dartmouth-Hitchcock Medical Center,
One Medical Center Drive, Lebanon, NH 03756, USA
e-mail: brent.c.white@hitchcock.org

Operative Strategy

Prior to providing long-term enteral access, the surgeon must have a clear understanding of whether pre-pyloric or post-pyloric feeding is appropriate. In most instances, a percutaneous endoscopic approach with good technique can provide safe long-term enteral access to meet a patient's needs with morbidity and discomfort less than that associated with open or even laparoscopic surgery. Nevertheless, alternative surgical techniques are sometimes needed. In certain cases, it may even be appropriate to have multiple different plans available for a single operative encounter to provide a feeding tube for a given patient, e.g., PEG (Plan A), possible laparoscopic assisted PEG or a laparoscopic G-tube (Plan B), or even an open G-tube placement (Plan C). It is therefore crucial to be familiar with a number of different techniques as well as different types of feeding tubes. It is also of paramount importance that appropriate feeding tubes and equipment are available for these procedures and the facility's staff is familiar with their use and maintenance prior to performing a given procedure.

In general, the only two conditions that will preclude a percutaneous endoscopic approach to providing long-term enteral access include the inability to access the gastrointestinal tract with an endoscope (e.g., obstructing oropharyngeal mass or trauma, esophageal obstructing tumor) and the inability to establish a safe window for percutaneous tube placement. In this context, a safe window is a site where the feeding tube can be passed percutaneously through subcutaneous tissues, abdominal wall musculature, and gastric or jejunal wall with minimal chance of inadvertently damaging adjacent visceral structures. In these two situations—no endoscopic access or no safe window, a laparoscopic approach to feeding tube placement can generally be utilized as a viable alternative procedure.

A.L. Halverson and D.C. Borgstrom (eds.), *Advanced Surgical Techniques for Rural Surgeons*,
DOI 10.1007/978-1-4939-1495-1_2, © Springer Science+Business Media New York 2015

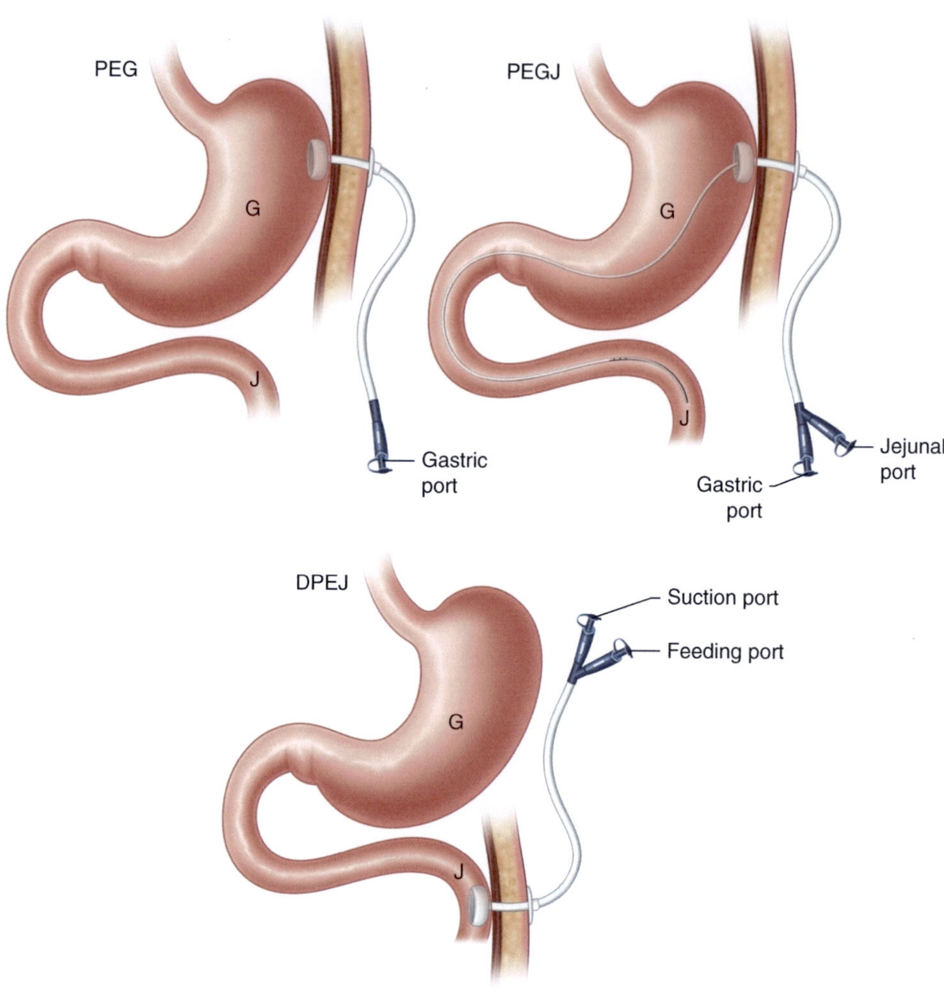

Fig. 2.1 Three different types of percutaneously placed endoscopic enteral tubes: (**a**) typical PEG with inner and outer flange, single port, (**b**) PEG with jejunal tube extension, double port for gastric aspiration, distal jejunal feeding, (**c**) direct percutaneously placed endoscopic jejunostomy

Operative Technique

Endoscopic Techniques

PEG

The pull technique for PEG placement can be performed using a one operator and one nurse/technician assistant approach. The patient should be positioned supine with supplemental oxygen and monitoring devices in place. A diagram of patient, operator, and assistant positioning is presented (Fig. 2.2). The abdomen should be generously prepped and draped as the safe window of PEG placement is not always strictly in the left upper quadrant—it can be epigastric and rarely even just to right of the patient's midline. The PEG kit and associated equipment should then be opened and ready. Many commercial vendors provide different versions of these kits and not every kit will have everything needed. If the kit is anticipated to provide for everything including an endoscopic snare, scissors, etc., then this must

be checked and ensured prior to starting the procedure. After the appropriate administration of conscious sedation or monitored anesthesia care, the operator introduces a flexible upper endoscope into the esophagus and a brief, standard EGD examination is performed. After ensuring no unexpected pathology, insufflation of the gastric body is provided sufficient to efface the rugal folds.

At this point, the crux of the procedure is finding the safe window for tube placement. There are three evaluations which should routinely be conducted to ensure such a safe window is found prior to PEG placement.

1. The operator can use the back of the plunger of a syringe of anesthetic (e.g., 1 % Lidocaine) to carefully palpate with this sterile instrument thereby finding a site with good 1:1 ratio of palpation that is discrete in appearance (Fig. 2.3).
2. The endoscope is then driven up to approach the greater curve, placing the tip of the scope on the anterior gastric wall. This will then achieve transillumination, casting a warm/orange glow across the abdominal wall seen at the

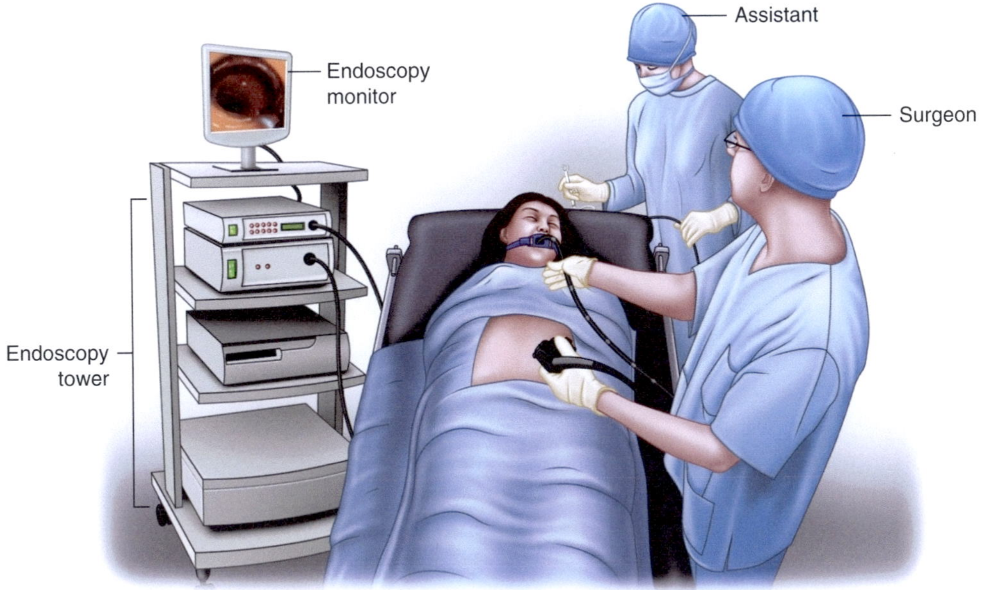

Fig. 2.2 A surgeon using this setup can perform both the endoscopic component and abdominal placement component of the procedure while an assistant (RN or GI Technician) assists by activating the transillumination feature and running the endoscopic snare

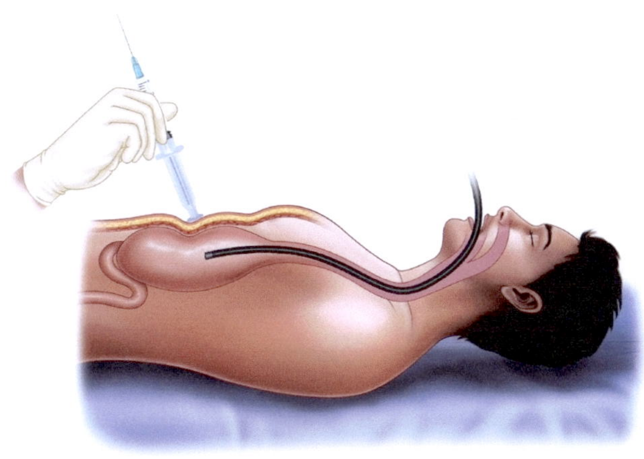

Fig. 2.3 The surgeon/endoscopist palpates the abdominal wall using the back of the plunger so as to maintain sterility of the field even as she runs the endoscope. This demonstrates discrete, 1:1 palpation at site of potential PEG placement, aiding in establishing a safe window for percutaneous placement

level of skin at the site of anticipated PEG placement. In morbidly obese patients, the assistant may need to press/deploy the transilluminate button so as to provide sufficient intensity of lighting to transilluminate a truly long abdominal wall distance. This button/feature is not generally needed in patients of normal body habitus.

3. The needle of the syringe of anesthetic is then passed into the lumen of the stomach at the site of 1:1 palpation and transillumination. While passing this needle through the subcutaneous, abdominal wall, and visceral tissues, the syringe is aspirated to ensure no bubbles are found until the needle enters the hollow gastric lumen visualized endoscopically. If no bubbles are seen until the needle enters the stomach lumen, this is deemed a "safe track" for PEG tube placement. If bubbles or gas is aspirated prior to entry into the stomach, this track is not safe and either another track should be found or the PEG procedure potentially aborted (Fig. 2.4). In performing the safe track aspiration, it is very helpful to ensure that the operator watches the screen to ensure passage of the syringe into the gastric lumen even as the assistant watches the syringe to notify the team when bubbles are first observed within the syringe."

Authorities have traditionally used the lack of transillumination during this procedure as a contraindication for completing the PEG procedure as planned. If however there is good 1:1 palpation and the safe track is negative for any bubbles prior to entry into the gastric lumen at the site, there are series which have demonstrated the safety of completing the procedure as planned in this setting. Thus at least two of these three criteria must be found to establish the safe window for PEG placement.

An endoscopic snare is then passed through the endoscope and is left waiting in the gastric lumen. With this done, a 1 cm incision is made through skin at the selected site. A catheter is passed through the incision along the same trajectory as the 1:1 palpation and aspiration anesthetic needle into the stomach lumen. The snare is used to encircle the catheter thus securing it. The operator passes the looped wire through the catheter into the gastric lumen, taking care to

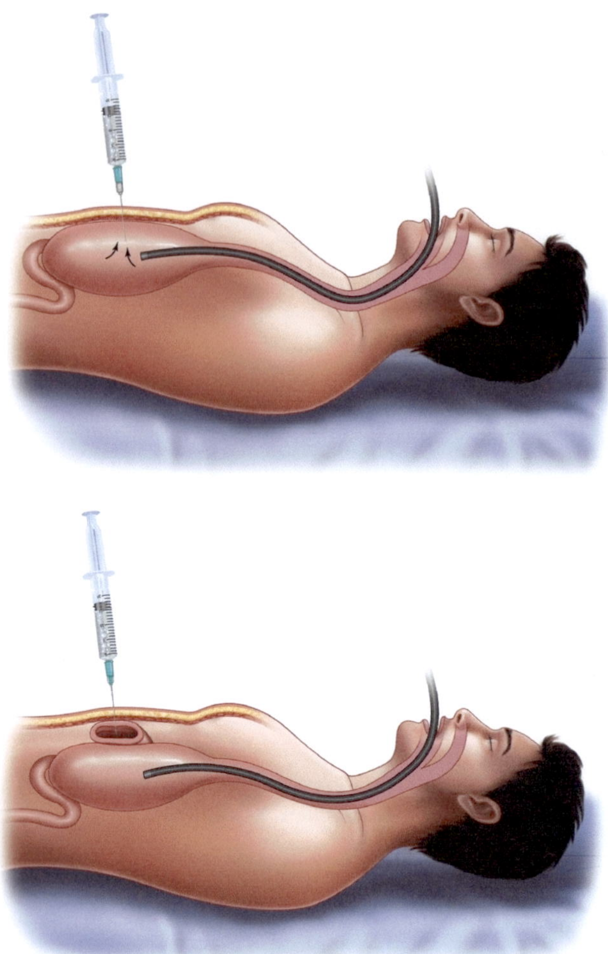

Fig. 2.4 (**a**) This demonstrates a negative safe track aspiration with the anesthetic/sounding needle, helping to assure a safe window for percutaneous placement of a PEG even as (**b**) demonstrates a positive safe track aspiration suggesting viscera between the stomach and abdominal wall, potentially despite apparent 1:1 palpation

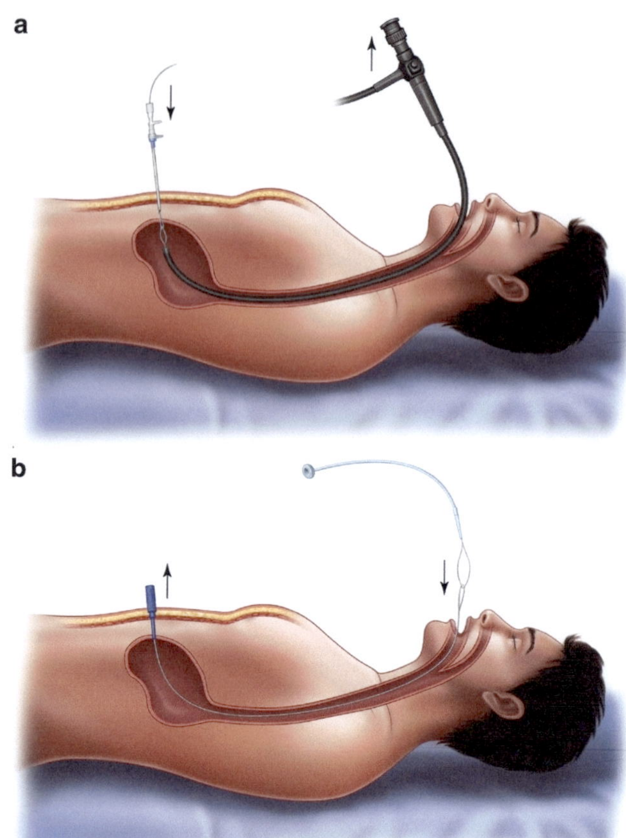

Fig. 2.5 (**a**) This sagittally depicts the endoscopic snaring of the transabdominal, trans-gastric wire which has been passed through a catheter. This wire, snare, and endoscope are then pulled back out of the oropharynx. (**b**) This depicts the pulling of the wire, now secured to the PEG tube, back out and across the abdominal wall until the inner flange is felt to abut the gastric and abdominal wall

orient it properly. The snare is then moved from where it is secured on the catheter to the wire. Once the snare is securely around the wire, the entire endoscope along with snare and wire are removed from the patient's mouth. The wire is then freed from the endoscope channel and secured to the tip of the PEG tube. The wire is then pulled (thus PULL technique) at the level of the abdominal wall, bringing the wire and the now secured tip of the PEG tube completely out of the patient until gentle traction or resistance is felt as the inner flange abuts the gastric wall (Fig. 2.5). Once positioned, an outer flange is placed down the tube (typically resting at 2–4 cm on the skin of a normal body habitus patient), the wire and some of the excess length of tubing is cut free and the cap is applied. At this point, a repeat endoscopic evaluation may be performed to ensure the inner flange is sitting without undue tension and no bleeding is visualized.

When completed, the outer flange of the PEG should rest snugly upon skin but not so snugly as to excessively dimple the skin.

Tension between the skin and outer flange is mirrored in the form of tension between the gastric mucosa/wall and the inner flange—excessive tension can lead to eventual necrosis of skin, abdominal wall, and even gastric tissue. This in turn can lead to gastric erosion, leakage/infection, or a buried bumper syndrome.

PEG-J

The PEG-J is placed as a PEG tube with a J-tube extension nested within its lumen. Therefore, the first part of the procedure is conducted just at the PEG tube is with the following caveats. The size of a nested J-tube is dictated by the diameter of the PEG tube that is selected. Therefore in order to have a larger diameter J-tube, a larger diameter PEG tube must be used. With commercially available BARD kits, a 9 Fr J tube can be nested within a 20 Fr PEG even as a 12 Fr J tube can be nested within a 28 Fr PEG. J-tubes themselves can be selected with different elements: (1) different diameters: 9, 12 Fr, (2) single port for jejunal feeding only versus dual port allowing for both gastric decompression as well as jejunal feeding, and (3) a prefabricated loop on the end for pull placement versus no such loop for guidewire push placement (Fig. 2.6). In order to minimize clogging issues with medications as well as certain enteral formulations, use of a 28 Fr PEG with a 12 Fr J-tube ideally with two ports should be used. Additionally, the use of a pediatric colonoscopy, with its longer length, has the advantage of more readily allowing for proximal jejunal intubation and should generally be used for the PEG-J procedure.

Following the establishment of the PEG using the previous technique description, the pediatric colonoscope is used to re-intubate the stomach and an endoscopic clip is passed into the gastric lumen. A 12 Fr J-tube is passed through the

PEG tube into the gastric lumen where its distal tip loop is then grasped with an endoscopic clip (Fig. 2.7). The endoscopic clip with loop in tow is then pulled into the instrument channel of the colonoscope so that it is no longer visible endoscopically. The scope is then driven out into the duodenum and as far as possible, ideally into the proximal jejunum—the endoscopic clip holding the loop at the tip of the j-tube ensures that the tube is in tow. C-arm fluoroscopy can be used adjunctively to ensure that reasonable depth of intubation is achieved. Once the proper depth of intubation is achieved, the endoscopic clip is used to secure the loop onto the small bowel mucosa (Fig. 2.8). The scope is then withdrawn. The endoscopic clip ensures that j-tube extension migration is minimized both with scope withdrawal as well as in the postoperative period.

DPEJ

The use of a direct percutaneous endoscopically placed jejunostomy tube using a modification of the Pull PEG technique can be technically difficult in an anatomically intact upper gastrointestinal tract. So much so, that some authorities have advocated using double balloon enteroscopy technique to facilitate reaching an appropriate loop of jejunum and stabilizing it against the abdominal wall. Without resorting to these more complex endoscopic approaches, the DPEJ approach is therefore most likely to be successful in patients who have already undergone previous esophageal or gastric resection (e.g., a Billroth II).

Bearing this in mind, the procedure requires a setup and sedation or MAC as in the previous percutaneous endoscopic procedures. A pediatric colonoscope is advanced into the jejunum—C-arm fluoroscopy may prove helpful adjunctively in some cases. As in the PEG technique, a safe window must be obtained for purposes of DPEJ placement. This therefore requires: (1) careful palpation with 1:1 movement

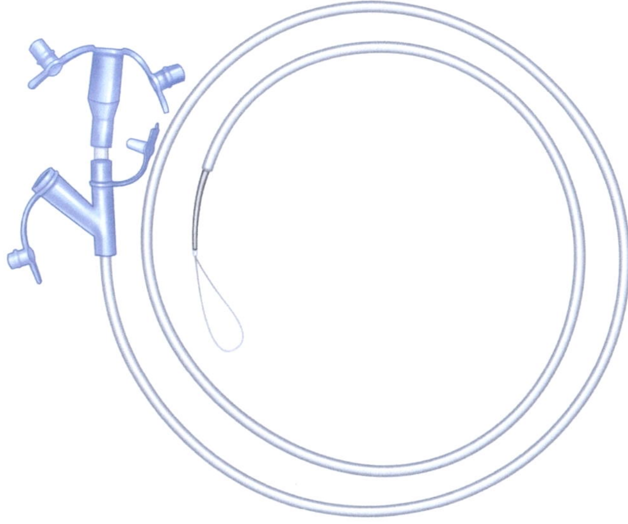

Fig. 2.6 This is a 12 Fr J-tube which can be placed in a nested fashion within the lumen of a 28 Fr PEG tube. Notice there are two ports—a proximal gastric decompression and distal jejunal feeding port. Also there is a distal tip suture/loop provided for endoscopic placement distally

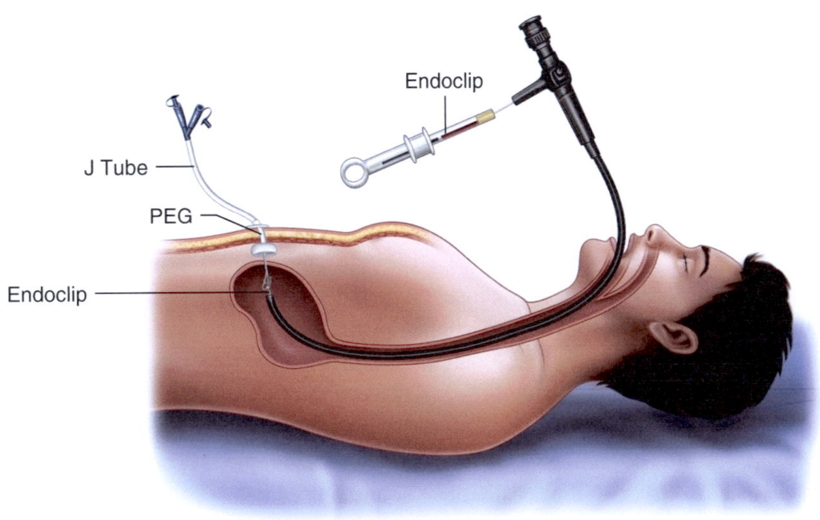

Fig. 2.7 This sagittal figure demonstrates the jejunostomy tube being threaded through the lumen of the previously placed PEG tube. A pediatric colonoscope grabs the loop on the distal tip of the jejunostomy tube with an endoscopic clip

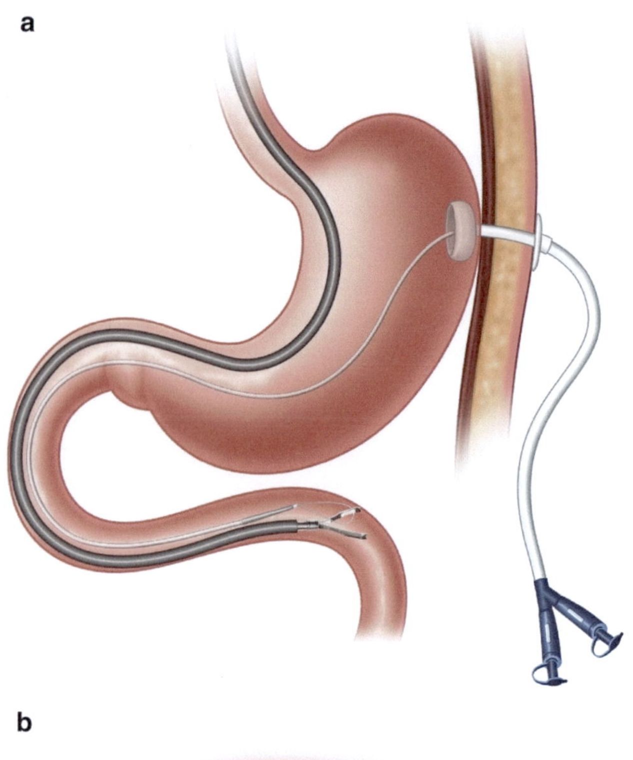

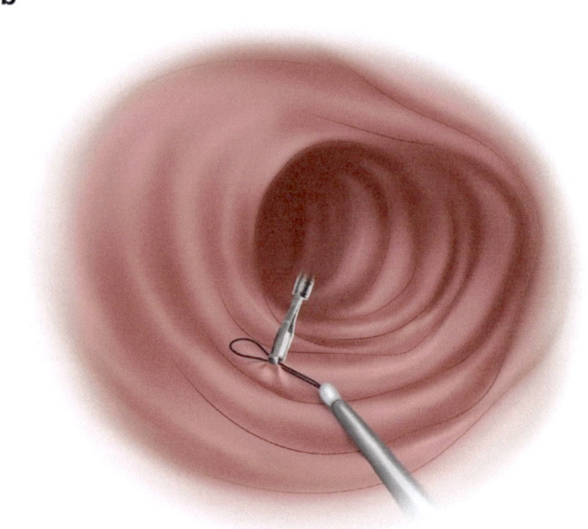

Fig. 2.8 (**a**) A pediatric colonoscope is used to drag the jejunostomy extending tube distally to the proximal jejunum with the use of an endoscopic clip. (**b**) This same clip is then used to secure the loop to the mucosa of the small bowel at this point, reducing likelihood of proximal migration

transabdominally and a discrete endoscopic "indention," (2) transillumination—this can conceivably be almost anywhere in the abdomen unlike the PEG location and thus the abdomen must be widely prepped, and (3) a Safe Track aspiration which is free of bubbles/gas until entering the lumen endoscopically. At this point in contrast with the PEG technique, it is advisable to LEAVE the anesthetic or sounding needle in place and secure it with the endoscopic snare so as to avoid

movement or shifting of the loop of jejunum and loss of apposition of the small bowel loop to the abdominal wall. With this needle secured in place for bowel fixation, a catheter is placed into the lumen of the bowel alongside the snared needle. The snare is then removed from the sounding needle and used to snare the catheter. A looped wire is then passed through the catheter and ensnared in the jejunal lumen. Again, the entire endoscope, snare, and ensnared wire are then removed as a unit orally. The wire is then freed from the endoscope channel and secured to the tip of a typically 16–18 Fr PEG type tube. The wire is then pulled (thus PULL technique) at the level of the abdominal wall, bringing the wire and the now secured tip of the DPEJ tube completely out of the patient until gentle traction or resistance is felt as the inner flange abuts the jejunal wall (Fig. 2.9). Once positioned, an outer flange is placed down the tube, typically resting at 2–3 cm on the skin of a normal body habitus patient, the wire and some of the excess length of tubing is cut free and the cap is applied. At this point, a repeat endoscopic evaluation may be performed to ensure the inner flange is sitting without undue tension and no bleeding is visualized.

Laparoscopic Approaches

Laparoscopic-Assisted PEG

Either due to a patient's morbid obesity or some other factor a safe window for conventional PEG placement occasionally cannot be demonstrated and the procedure is aborted. This is an opportunity for using a laparoscopic-assisted PEG approach. As well as requiring general anesthetic, this requires someone operating the endoscope as well as someone using the laparoscope and cannulating the stomach—a potential setup is diagrammed (Fig. 2.10). The patient's abdomen is sterilely prepped and draped in usual fashion and a trocar is placed peri-umbilically for direct laparoscopic visualization of the abdominal contents. After insufflation with CO_2, the abdomen is surveyed to ensure no unexpected pathology or abnormalities. An endoscope is then passed orally and the stomach insufflated. With direct laparoscopic visualization, an appropriate location is selected along the abdominal wall and a catheter passed directly into the stomach under combined laparoscopic/endoscopic visualization. If needed, an additional trocar can be placed so a grasper can bring the gastric wall—typically along the anterior aspect of the greater curve—closer to the catheter to allow gastric cannulation (Fig. 2.11). Once the intragastric wire is ensnared by the endoscope, the remainder of the procedure is performed in a manner similar to conventional PEG placement. The laparoscope can be used to demonstrate the inner flange sitting against the gastric wall with no undue trauma or bleeding. The tube once brought out through the abdominal

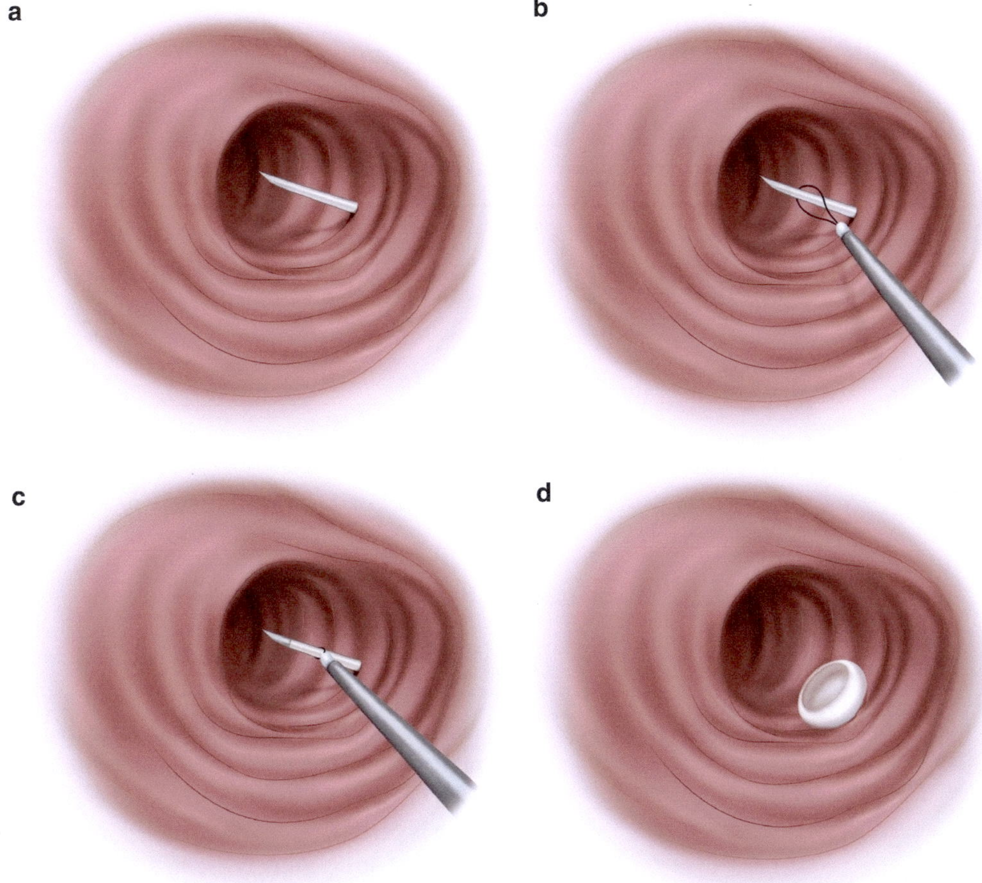

Fig. 2.9 (**a**) An anesthetic needle is introduced into the jejunal lumen. (**b**) This needle is ensnared to prevent jejunal loop migration or movement and loss of apposition to the abdominal wall. (**c**) The snare is transferred to the angiocatheter once this is introduced alongside the anesthetic needle. (**d**) A 16 or 18 Fr PEG type tube is secured in a manner similar to gastric PEG placement with inner flange securing the tube to the abdominal wall

Fig. 2.10 The typical setup for a surgeon on the patient's left performing laparoscopy even the endoscopist assists while standing at the patient's head

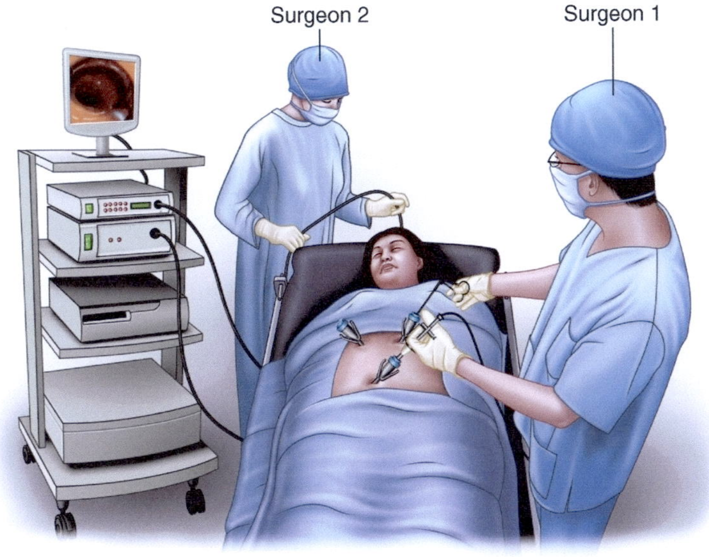

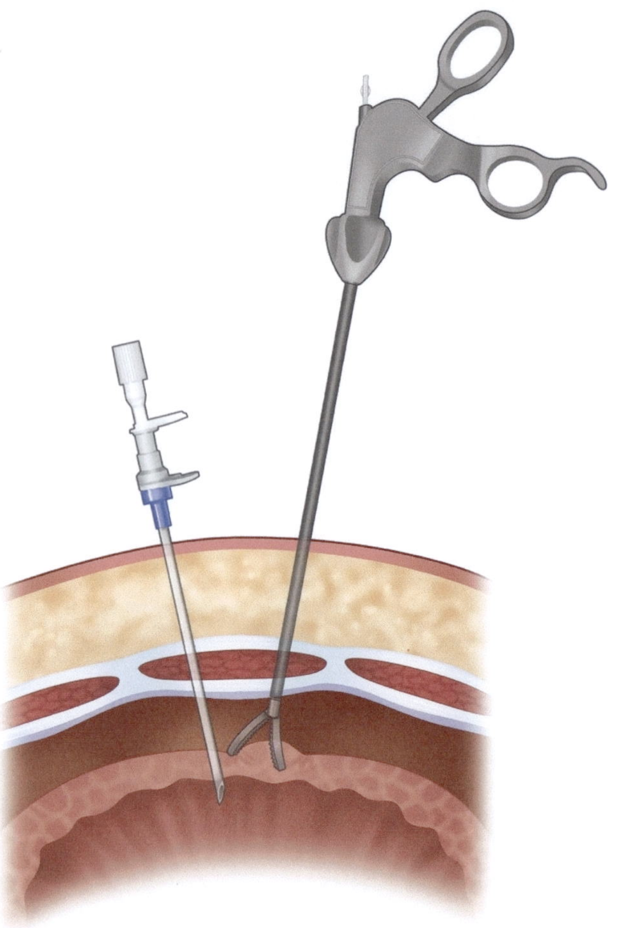

Fig. 2.11 Sagittal depiction of a laparoscopic grasper used to facilitate placement of the angiocatheter into the gastric lumen during pneumoperitoneum

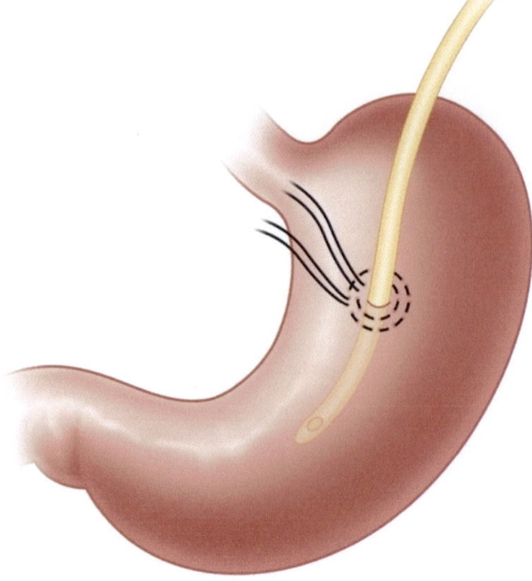

Fig. 2.12 Two concentric purse string sutures are placed around an 18 Fr Foley catheter for gastrostomy tube placement

wall can be covered with a sterile towel to minimize any contamination of the field. The laparoscopic procedure is terminated and the trocars sites closed and dressed prior to placing the outer flange and cap on the PEG tube.

Laparoscopic Gastrostomy Tube Placement

When either obstructing mass or prior surgery (e.g., Roux en Y Gastric Bypass) prevents pre-pyloric enteral access endoscopically, a fully laparoscopic gastrostomy approach can be employed. After establishment of pneumoperitoneum and survey of the abdomen, a place for tube placement is sited along the anterior aspect of the stomach, close to the greater curvature and two concentric purse string sutures are placed around this using a laparoscopic needle driver and 2-0 silk sutures. As an alternative to a laparoscopic needle driver and suture, the Endostich (Ethicon) device can be used for purse string placement. A skin incision is then made at an appropriate site in the left upper quadrant and an 18 Fr Latex Foley catheter is placed through this into the abdominal cavity.

Next a gastrotomy is made within the purse string sutures and the catheter is placed into the gastric lumen (Fig. 2.12). The balloon of the catheter is inflated and irrigation and aspiration is performed to ensure proper intragastric positioning. The purse string sutures are tied sequentially with the second/outer one ensuring the first/inner one is covered by serosa. Four sutures are then sequentially placed in the seromuscular layer of the gastric wall around the tube exit site and secured to the abdominal wall using a trans-fascial suture-passing technique (Fig. 2.13). This creates a laparoscopic modification of the Stamm gastrostomy tube and the procedure is complete after it is secured to the skin with non-absorbable suture.

Laparoscopic GJ Tube

A laparoscopic GJ tube (Fig. 2.14) can be placed in much the same way as described for the laparoscopic G-tube. Once its intragastric balloon and proximal aspect are firmly secured as previously described, endoscopy can be utilized to pass the jejunal tube distally and secure it within the jejunum in much the same way as was described in the PEG-J technique. The pediatric colonoscope is used to intubate the stomach and an endoscopic clip is passed through the instrument channel and grasps a loop on the end of the jejunal tube (loop is either premanufactured or a suture placed previously). The endoscopic clip holding this loop is then driven out into the duodenum and as far as possible, ideally into the proximal jejunum—the endoscopic clip holding the loop at the tip of the j-tube ensures that it is in tow. C-arm fluoroscopy can be used adjunctively to ensure that reasonable depth of intubation is achieved. Once the proper depth of intubation is

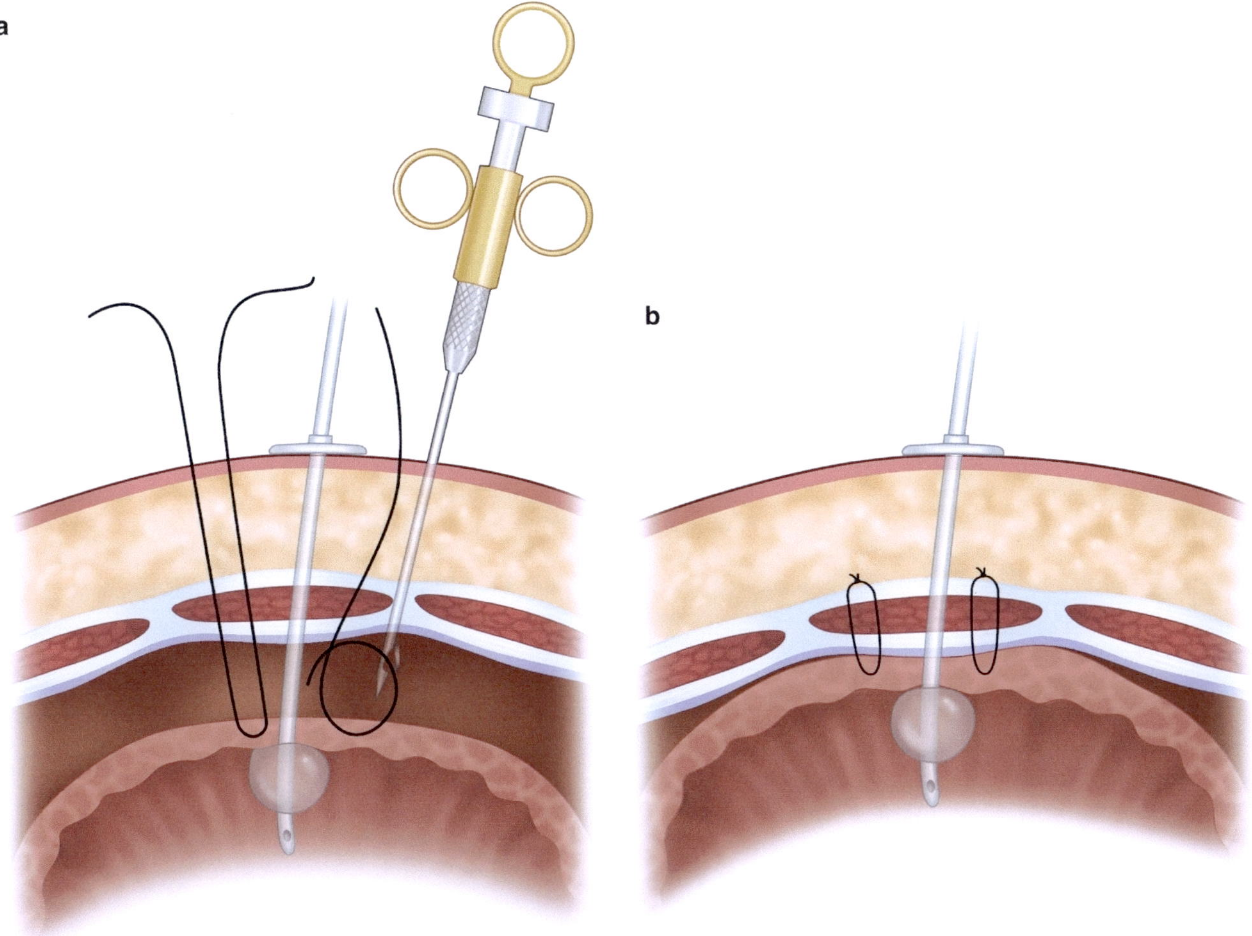

Fig. 2.13 (**a**) After the purse string sutures are tied and the gastrostomy tube is secured, four 2-0 silk suture are laparoscopically placed in the seromuscular layer before being secured via suture passer to the fascia. (**b**) Each is placed sequentially before tying all four in place

achieved, the endoscopic clip is used to secure the tube to the small bowel mucosa. The scope is then withdrawn; the endoscopic clip ensures that j-tube migration is minimized both with scope withdrawal as well as in the postoperative period.

J-Tube

A large number of laparoscopic jejunostomy techniques have been described. Once trocars are placed and the abdomen is surveyed, a segment of jejunum distal to the ligament of Treitz is carefully identified and evaluated to ensure it can reach the abdominal wall. Once this is established, a purse-string of 2-0 silk is placed on the anti-mesenteric aspect of the small intestine using a laparoscopic needle driver or an Endostitch (Ethicon). A 1 cm incision is made at an appropriate position in the abdominal wall and a 16 Fr red rubber catheter is introduced through this incision into the peritoneal cavity. An enterotomy is made within the previously placed pursestring and the j-tube is threaded through the enterotomy distally into the small bowel lumen. The purse-

string is tied and subsequently a number of imbricating seromuscular sutures are placed creating a Witzel tunnel approximately 2 cm in length (Fig. 2.15). Two sutures are then sequentially placed in the seromuscular layer of the bowel wall proximal and distal to the Witzel tunnel and secured to the abdominal wall using the previously described trans-fascial suture-passing technique (see Fig. 2.14). The tube is flushed and aspirated to ensure patency prior to securing the catheter to skin.

Postoperative Care

Perioperative antibiotics as appropriate.
 Early feeding.
 Flushing routinely to maintain patency.
 Avoidance of crushed meds, etc. depending on Tube diameter.
 Avoidance of inadvertent traction/dislodging of tube.

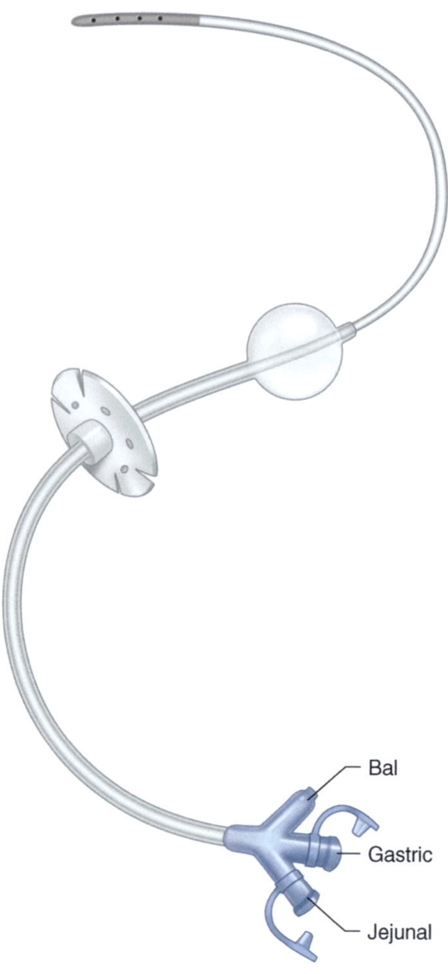

Fig. 2.14 Picture of a gastrojejunostomy (GJ) tube with dual ports for gastric decompression/aspiration and a distal port for jejunal feeding

Common Complications

Tube clogging.

Tube dislodgement or accidental removal.

Tube exit site Infection, leakage, or irritation.

Buried bumper syndrome—clinical picture resulting from partial or complete growth of gastric mucosa over the internal bolster of a PEG.

Suggested Reading

DiSario JA. Endoscopic approaches to enteral nutritional support. Best Pract Res Clin Gastroenterol. 2006;20(3):605–30.

Fan AC, Baron TH, Rumalla A, Harewood GC. Comparison of direct perctuaneous endoscopic jejuostomy and PEG with jejunal extension. Gastrointest Endosc. 2002;56(6):890–4.

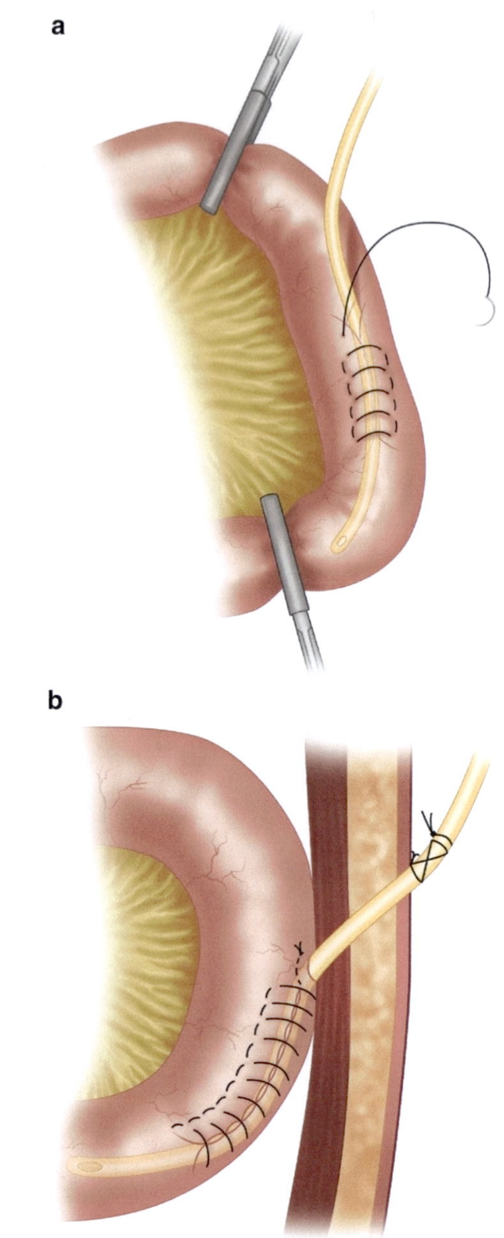

Fig. 2.15 Diagram of the Witzel tunnel created laparoscopically at time of jejunostomy tube creation

Hirdes MM, Monkelbaan JF, Haringman JJ, van Oijen MG, Siersema PD, Pullens HJ, et al. Endoscopic clip-assisted feeding tube placement reduces repeat endoscopy rate: results from a randomized cotrolled trial. Am J Gastroenterol. 2013;107(3):1220–7.

Nagle AP, Murayama KM. Laparoscopic gastrostomy and jejunostomy. J Long Term Eff Med Implants. 2004;14(1):1–11.

Paski SC, Dominitz JA. Endoscopic solutions to challenging enteral feeding problems. Curr Opin Gastroenterol. 2012;28(5):427–31.

Stewart JA, Hagan P. Failure to transilluminate the stomach is not an absolute contraindication to PEG insertion. Endoscopy. 1998;30(7):621–2.

Endomucosal Resection of Colon Polyps and Control of Postpolypectomy Bleeding

Ronald A. Gagliano Jr. and Patrick R. Kenny

Indications

Colorectal cancer (CRC) remains the fourth most common cancer and the second leading cause of cancer-related death in the USA. However, colorectal cancer screening has made a positive impact on the natural history of this cancer. Longitudinal studies have shown a decrease in CRC incidence, a decreased rate of late stage disease, and a decrease in CRC-related mortality. CRC screening modalities include tests that screen for cancer such as stool guaiac cards, tests that detect cancer and polyps (virtual CT) and those that detect cancer and polyps and are preventative (endoscopy). The decreasing incidence of CRC is in large part due to the prevention of cancer through endoscopic polypectomy. Because of the preventative nature of endoscopic polypectomy, multiple societies have endorsed colonoscopy with polypectomy as the preferred method of CRC screening and treatment of resectable colonic polyps. This chapter will review the various techniques available when performing advanced polypectomy, as well as the management of the complication of postpolypectomy bleeding.

Preoperative Preparation

Endoscopic polypectomy varies in difficulty based on the size, morphology, location of the polyp, and the experience of the endoscopist. The most common methods for performing polypectomy are by cold biopsy, cold snare polypectomy, and hot snare polypectomy. The techniques and instruments used to perform standard polypectomy can be applied to advanced polyps, with some variation and additional tools and techniques. The surgeon should be familiar with the equipment available prior to the start of the procedure. Bowel preparation is required and the preferred method is by a split-dose regimen, with a ratio of 2/3–1/3 split between the evening before and the morning of the procedure. Extended preparations are described, but are needed only in patients with history of inadequate effect from an appropriately taken prep, or known significant motility disorder.

Operative Strategy

The goal of polypectomy is to prevent a precancerous (generally adenomatous) lesion from progressing to become adenocarcinoma, and can be best achieved when a complete polyp resection is performed. Small, well-visualized polyps with well-defined borders can be entirely removed with a great deal of confidence. Polyps that are >2 cm, located in difficult locations in the right colon, are flat and broad and those that have depressed centers are often associated with increasing difficulty of polyp resection. Polyps that fail to lift with a submucosal injection typically contain tumor that has already invaded into the deeper tissue, often into the muscularis propria.

Careful assessment of the ability to remove a difficult polyp should be made prior to any attempt at polypectomy and the proper equipment, the time to perform the resection, proper anesthesia support, and trained ancillary personnel are essential. Delaying an advanced polypectomy until all resources are optimal will increase success and decrease complications.

Operative Technique

Proper endoscopic positioning of a polyp is another key factor in successful polypectomy. The working channel on the colonoscope is located in the 5–6 o'clock position. Placement of the polyp in the 5–6 o'clock position drastically improves

R.A. Gagliano Jr., M.D., F.A.S.C.R.S. (✉)
Department of Surgery, General Surgery Service,
Tripler Army Medical Center, Honolulu, HI 96859, USA
e-mail: ron.gagliano@us.army.mil

P.R. Kenny, D.O.
Division of Gastroenterology, Department of Medicine,
Tripler Army Medical Center, Honolulu, HI 96859, USA

A.L. Halverson and D.C. Borgstrom (eds.), *Advanced Surgical Techniques for Rural Surgeons*,
DOI 10.1007/978-1-4939-1495-1_3, © Springer Science+Business Media New York 2015

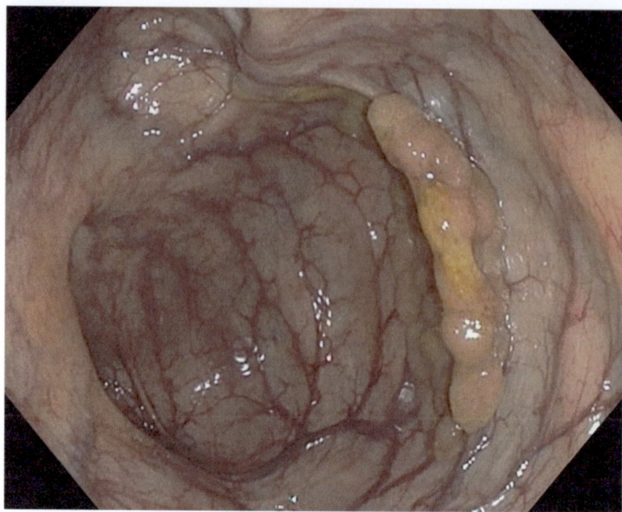

Fig. 3.1 Polyp encountered at 3 o'clock

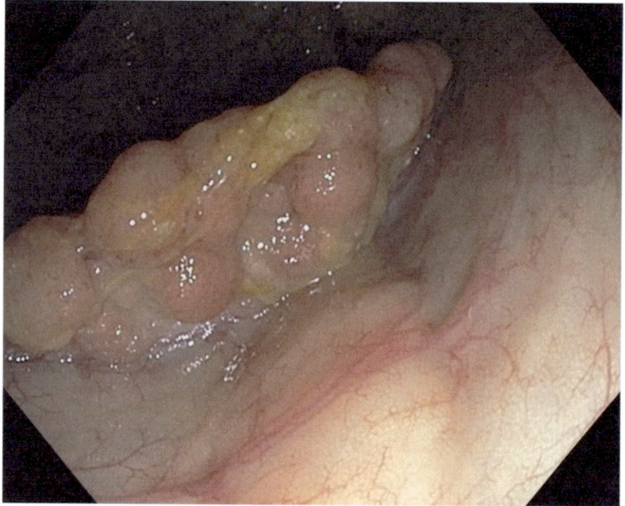

Fig. 3.2 Polyp positioned at 5 o'clock

maneuverability and visualization during polypectomy (Figs. 3.1 and 3.2). Occasionally, improved endoscopic positioning can be achieved through patient repositioning, modification of the stiffness of the endoscope, and decreasing or increasing the amount of insufflation in the colon. The use of a more flexible upper endoscope, a side-viewing scope or an endocap can be particularly beneficial in improving visualization of lesions located on the proximal aspect of a fold or on a sharp bend in the colon. The use of intravenous glucagon may increase the chance of success in cases where repeated colonic spasms make positioning challenging.

Once the lesion is determined to be resectable and is properly positioned, determination should be made about the endoscopist's ability to remove the lesion en bloc or piecemeal. The benefit of an en bloc resection is that the anatomic margins of the lesion may be preserved allowing the endoscopist and pathologist to better determine the completeness of the resection. However, there may be a slightly higher risk of perforation and bleeding, as well as an increase in difficulty retrieving larger polyps after en bloc polypectomy. Piecemeal resection allows for improved ease of polyp retrieval and decreased risk of perforation, but has also been shown to have up to a 55 % rate of early recurrence or residual polyp. In most cases the residual polyp can be completely removed with subsequent endoscopic treatment, but all polyps removed piecemeal should be re-examined in 2–6 months to ensure complete resection has been achieved.

Advanced polyps can be removed by cold scare, snare cautery, endoscopic mucosal resection (EMR), or endoscopic submucosal dissection (ESD). If a cold snare is used, it is often done in attempting a piecemeal resection, cutting through smaller sections of tissue than can be achieved with snare cautery. Due to the large size often encountered with difficult polyps, thermal energy is frequently used to assist with cutting. The use of thermal energy may increase the risk of bleeding and mural thermal injury.

EMR is generally defined as the removal of a flat or sessile polyp confined to the mucosa or submucosa, usually for lesions >2 cm in size. Injection-assisted, cap-assisted and ligation-assisted techniques have been described to perform EMR. EMR is the most widely accepted method of performing advanced polypectomy. ESD involves dissecting the polyp off the submucosal space and is a more meticulous, time-consuming and technically challenging method of performing advanced polypectomy.

EMR is currently the preferred method of performing polypectomy in large or difficult polyps. The benefit of this technique is to raise the apex of the polyp to better allow visualization and ease of capture with a snare, to predict deeper polyp invasion, and to decrease the risk of bleeding and perforation. In one study EMR led to upstaging of polyps to high grade dysplasia or adenocarcinoma in up to 44 % of cases. With the injection-assisted technique, fluid is injected into the submucosal space, thus creating a cushion between the polyp within the mucosa and the deeper muscularis propria. The cap-assisted technique is performed by placing a plastic cap over the tip of the endoscope, seating a snare into the distal tip of the cap, and then suctioning the tissue into the cap. When using this technique, the mucosa and submucosa, but not the muscularis propria are suctioned into the cap. The snare is then closed around the base of the tissue and snare cautery polypectomy is performed. The ligation-assisted technique is similar to the cap-assisted technique, but rather than a dedicated cap device, a band ligation device is used. The polyp is suctioned into the band ligation cap and a band is placed at the base of the lesion. The snare is placed either distal or proximal to the band, and snare cautery polypectomy is performed. All three techniques require

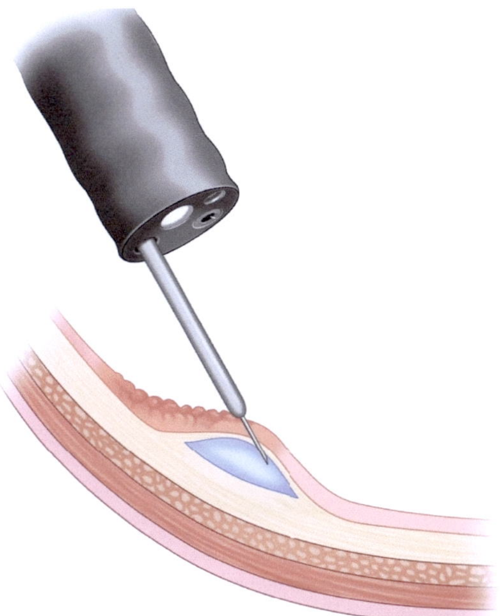

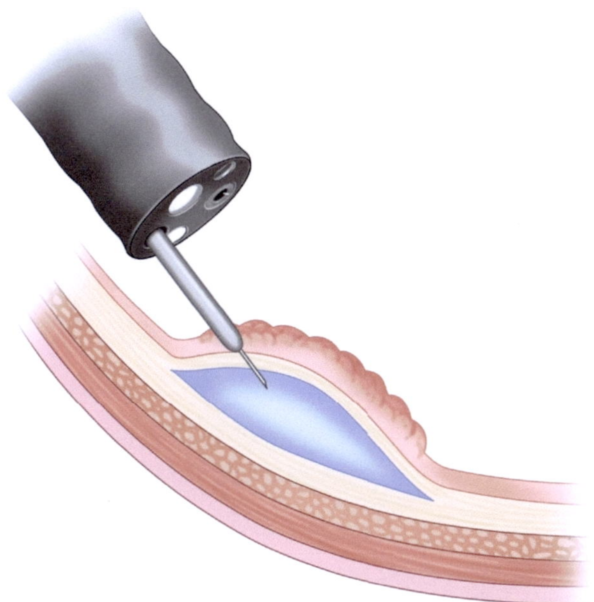

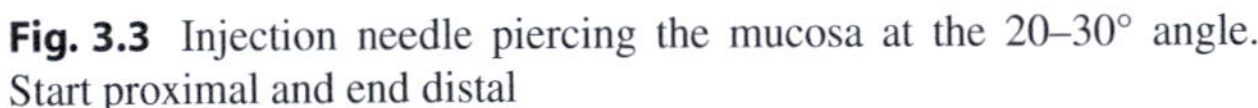

Fig. 3.3 Injection needle piercing the mucosa at the 20–30° angle. Start proximal and end distal

Fig. 3.4 Lift complete without tethered areas

similar technical skills, including performing a submucosal injection and a snare polypectomy.

The type of fluid used for submucosal injection may vary some. Osmotic agents such as hyaluronic acid, hydroxypropyl methylcellulose, glycerol, and fibrinogen solution generally remain in the submucosal space for a greater length of time, making these favorable agents to use in cases of prolonged attempts at capturing the lesion with the snare. However, these osmotic agents are expensive and not readily available in most endoscopy units, and some have also been shown to cause tissue damage. Autologous blood injections last up to seven times longer than normal saline and do not hinder visualization. In most institutions normal saline is used because of its low cost and availability. Another technique is to mix 1 mL of 1:10,000 epinephrine and 1 mL of indigo carmine or methylene blue with 8 mL of 0.9 % NS. This mixture may better aid in visualizing the resected borders of the lesion and may decrease the risk of immediate bleeding. The submucosal injection can be performed by placing the lesion at the 5–6 o'clock position and approaching the lesion with an injection needle from a 20–30° angle (Fig. 3.3). A steeper approach runs the risk of advancing the needle through the serosa and injecting fluid into the abdomen. Starting in the proximal aspect or the portion of the polyp farthest away from the scope, 3–10 mL of fluid is injected in the submucosal space, which should aid to bring the polyp into view.

Once a submucosal injection has been performed and the polyp is successfully lifted, the injection needle may be withdrawn from the scope and replaced with a snare (Fig. 3.4).

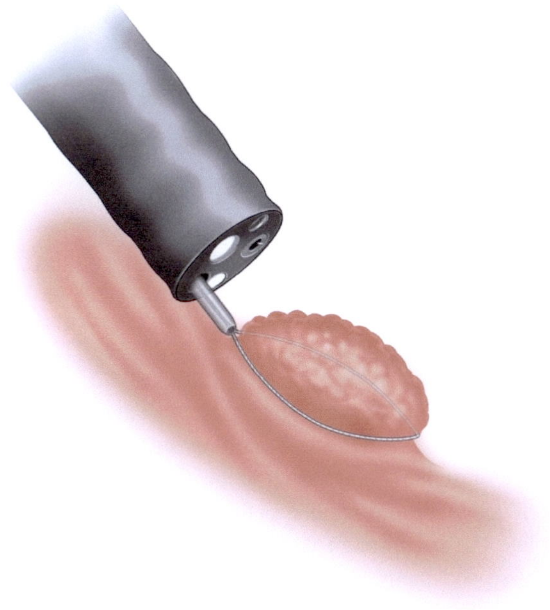

Fig. 3.5 Snare positioned around polyp while lifted

Saline will diffuse out of the submucosal space within minutes, so deliberate positioning of the snare is crucial (Fig. 3.5). If the lesion cannot be grasped with the snare prior to diffusion of the submucosal injection, repeat injection may be needed. The iSnare™ system contains both an injection needle and snare in one device, allowing for a more rapid placement of the snare after injection or repeated injections without removal of the device. Once the lesion is grasped

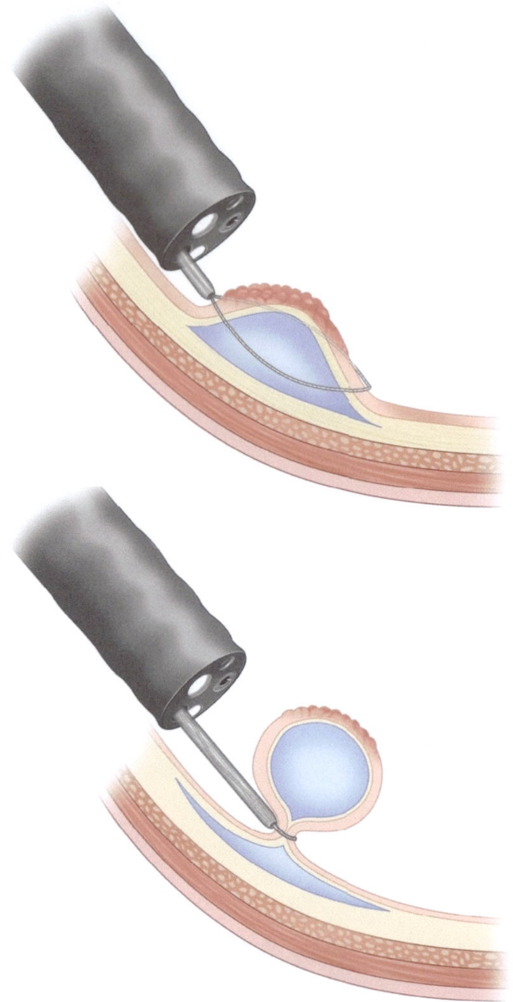

Fig. 3.6 Snare closed around polyp

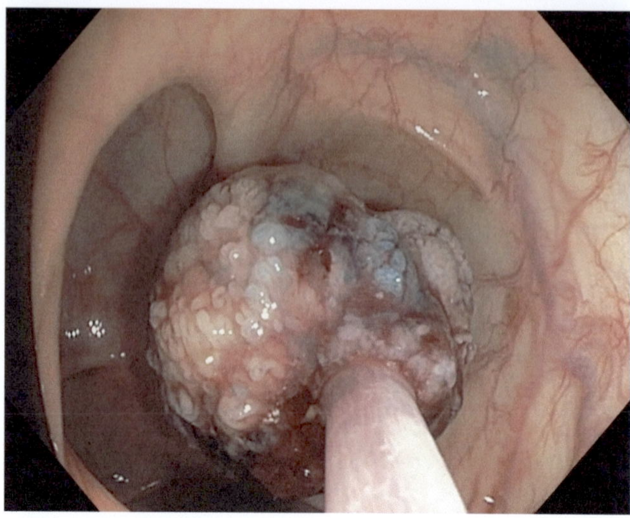

Fig. 3.7 Piecemeal excision of large right sided polyp. Snare is closed around polyp and preparing to cut through the polyp with cautery

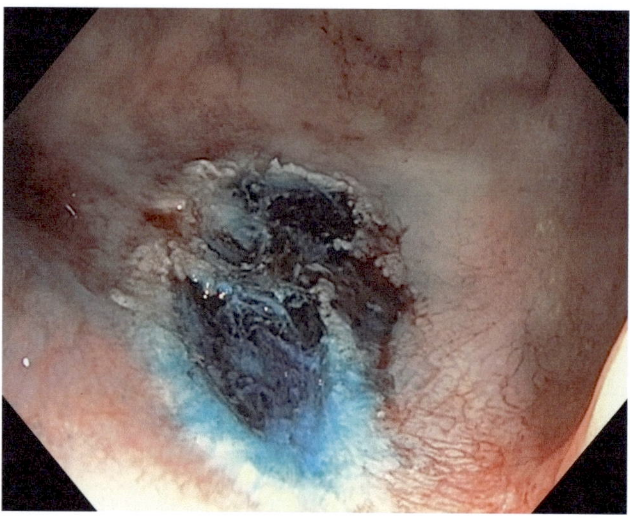

Fig. 3.8 Excised polyp after saline and methylene blue submucosal lift demonstrating good staining of submucosal tissues

firmly with the snare it should be retracted away from the wall of the colon towards the lumen, pulling the submucosa away from the muscularis and serosa (Figs. 3.6 and 3.7). A short burst of coagulation is applied as the snare is slowly closed to complete the cut through the retracted tissue. Thermal settings vary and many devices have preset levels for specific regions of the bowel, therefore the endoscopist needs to become familiar with these settings to avoid too little energy leading to a failure to cut thicker tissue, or too much energy leading to thermal injury to deeper colonic tissue. In general the coagulation mode is adequate to perform the initial resection with less of a risk for thermal injury. The cutting mode should be reserved for cases when the residual stalk is stuck to the snare (Fig. 3.8).

Appropriate snare selection depends on the size, location, and thickness of the polyp. Snares vary in size (from 1 to 3 cm), shape (from oval to hexagonal to round), and stiffness. No one snare routinely performs better than another, but having a few options to choose from may improve the ability to perform a complete polyp resection.

Once the polyp has been resected, retrieval of the entire polyp including all of the resected pieces of the polyp is critical to ruling out malignancy and assessing margins of resection. Suction ports vary in diameter from 3.2 to 3.8 mm. The polyp can then be collected in a tissue trap or by placing a gauze pad or nylon mesh between the suction nipple of the colonoscopy and the suction tubing. Tissue specimens larger than the diameter of the suction port can be compressed and pulled through the port, but typically polyps larger than 6–7 mm do not fit through suction port, and an alternate method of retrieval is needed. Although larger polyps can be cut into smaller pieces and suctioned through the scope, this further disrupts tissue, which may hinder pathologic analysis and prompt unnecessary surgery. The polyp can be held to the tip of the endoscope with suction and dragged out of the colon.

This method is often unsuccessful, especially when maneuvering the tissue through the folds in the sigmoid colon. A variety of nets and baskets have been developed to retrieve larger pieces of tissue. The Roth Net™ is one of the more common retrieval devices, but its major limitation is difficulty in capturing multiple polyps or polyp fragments at one pass. Another company has recently developed the Twister® Plus rotatable retrieval device that comes in either a 22 or 26 mm loop diameter, and can be used to scoop up polyp fragments. Once captured by a net or basket, the tissue can be pushed 1–2 cm proximal to the tip of the endoscope to allow for continued visualization of the colon as the scope and tissue capture device is withdrawn completely. Some authors suggest the use of an overtube when removing multiple tissue fragments through a challenging sigmoid colon, to facilitate repeated cecal intubations.

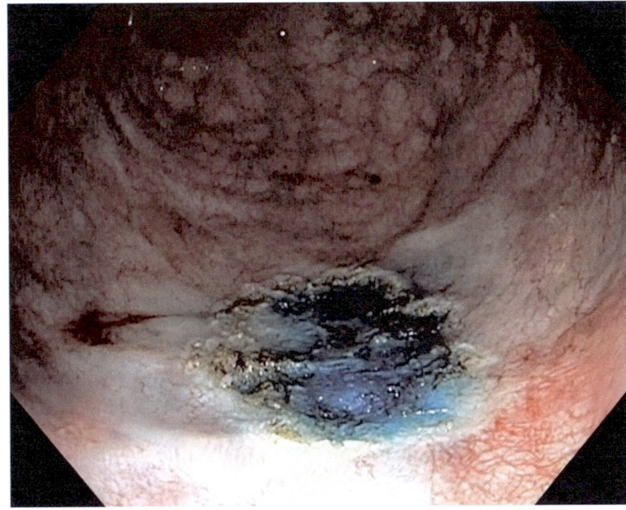

Fig. 3.9 Argon plasma coagulation after lift and hot snare excision

Potential Pitfalls

In some instances a small amount of residual polyp may be difficult to resect, or cauterized tissue may preclude determination of the completeness of resection. In these cases application of thermal destruction of tissue, often by way of argon plasma coagulation (APC), may be used. This method has been shown to reduce the risk of recurrent polyp (Fig. 3.9).

Colonic mucosa heals quite well, which can make determination of the prior site of polypectomy difficult to identify on future colonoscopy (Figs. 3.10 and 3.11). Most studies report at least a 17 % rate of residual or recurrent polyp after piecemeal resection. For this reason, a tattoo should be made at the site of the polypectomy, particularly when piecemeal resection is performed. Data from the British Bowel Cancer Screening Programme suggest that due to an increased risk of dysplasia or cancer seen in polyps that are >1 cm in size, all polyps >1 cm should be tattooed. This is done by injecting a permanent ink (such as carbon black or India ink) into the submucosal space adjacent to the site of polypectomy. Indigo carmine, methylene blue, and other solutions have been used, but due to their rapid rate of resorption they are not effective agents for tattooing. Once again, care should be taken to approach the mucosa at a shallow angle so that the needle is in the submucosal space and not the serosa. Tattoos can be placed proximal and distal or in four quadrants around the lesion.

Occasionally, resected polyps can be lost in deep pools of fluid or behind folds. Factors associated with failed polyp retrieval are small polyp size, sessile polyps, cold snare polypectomy, and proximal colon location. Adequate polyp retrieval should occur >90 % of the time per guidelines from the Bowel Cancer Screening Program. The easiest method of polyp retrieval is through the suction port of the colonoscope.

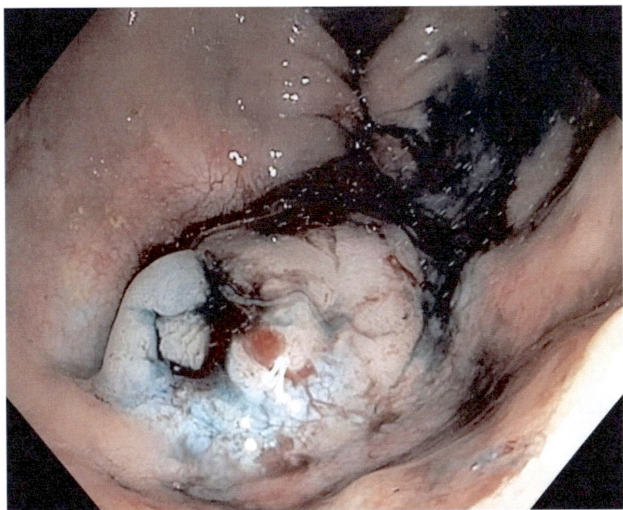

Fig. 3.10 Original polyp with saline and methylene blue submucosal lift

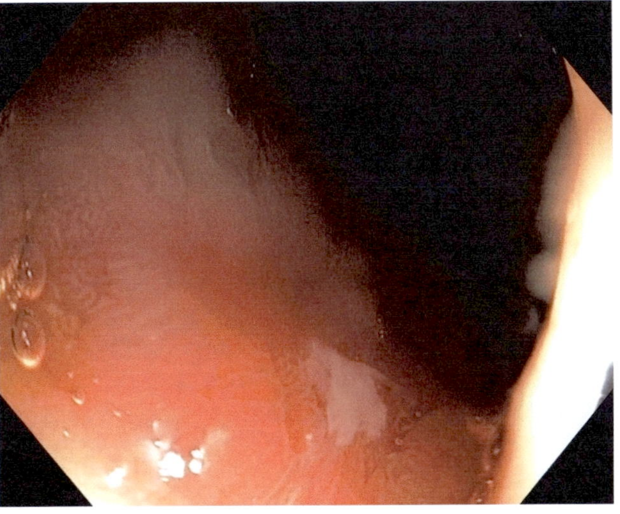

Fig. 3.11 Residual scar after only 1 month

Common Complications

Complication rates for EMR vary, with rates of bleeding in 1–45 % (10 % in larger series), delayed bleeding in 13.9 %, and perforation in 0.3–0.5 %.

Postpolypectomy bleeding (PPB) rates vary greatly depending on several factors, but occurs 1–45 % (10 % in larger series), with delayed bleeding occurring in 1–13.9 % of cases. This is the leading major complication following colonoscopic polypectomy. Therapeutic endoscopic options for treatment of PPB are divided into three categories: compression, injection, and thermal coagulation. Endovascular embolization and operative resection remain options for patients who are unstable or fail endoscopic therapies. Due to the nature of this chapter the discussion will be limited to endoscopic therapies.

Compression techniques include re-snaring the stalk of the polypectomy site in cases of pedunculated polyps, or use of one of the endoscopic clip applicators for pedunculated or sessile polypectomy sites (Fig. 3.12). Newer endoscopic clipping devices contain a grasper that can grab both sides of the cut edges of the mucosa and once approximated, a clip device is applied from an endocap. Any of these therapies can be used together as the endoscopist needs to promote hemostasis. Injection therapy with one milliliter of 1:10,000 epinephrine solution is performed as described above for submucosal therapy and is placed at and around the site(s) of bleeding. Thermal hemostasis is achieved with either contact or noncontact therapy. Contact thermal treatment can be by either bipolar coagulation or a heater probe and is applied directly to the site of bleeding, using pressure and heat to coagulate the bleeding. Noncontact therapy is done by laser or argon plasma to produce coagulation from a short distance away, and does not have to be pulled off the coagulum at the end of the procedure.

Although delayed bleeding usually occurs within 7–10 days, PPB has been reported from 0 to 29 days following therapy. Postpolypectomy bleeding is usually self-limited and over 70 % of cases resolve with only resuscitation and supportive care.

Risk factors for PPB include removal of large polyps (greater than 1 cm in diameter), age over 65 years, cardiovascular or chronic renal disease, platelet dysfunction, and coagulopathy. Multiple studies have tried to identify techniques to reduce the risk of postpolypectomy bleeding, and it

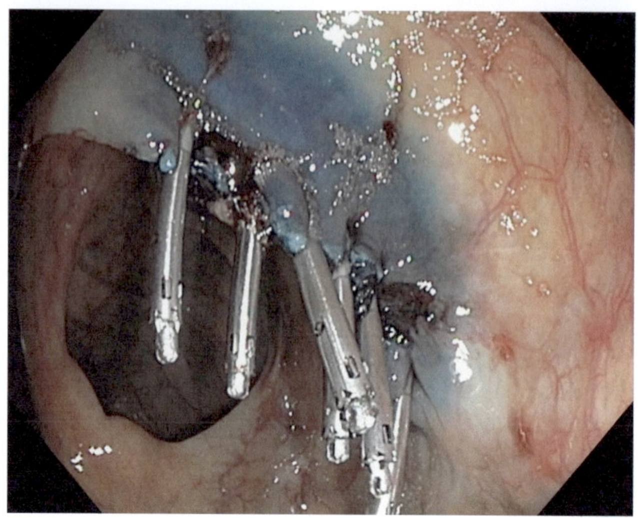

Fig. 3.12 Mucosal defect closed with endoscopic clips after PPB

is unclear whether the type of electrical current (blended vs. cutting ± APC), placement of prophylactic endoscopic clips, or use of an endoloop clearly decreases the risk of postpolypectomy bleeding, but they have all shown to be effective in the treatment of this complication. Early (within 24 h) PPB requiring therapy is often treated by immediate repeat endoscopy due to colon prep effect and rapid access to the site of bleeding. Delayed bleeding can be managed as per the algorithm below (Fig. 3.13). The techniques of colonoscopic EMR and control of PPB are manageable by the rural surgeon and can extend and improve the care delivered locally for our patients.

When to Transfer

The time to transfer the patient is prior to the polypectomy. If the polypectomy difficulty is beyond the skill of the endoscopist, simple biopsy can be done for diagnostic purposes and referral arranged to an endoscopist skilled in advanced techniques if the tissue diagnosis does not mandate operation.

Note: The views expressed in this publication/presentation are those of the author(s) and do not reflect the official policy or position of the Department of the Army, Department of Defense, or the US Government.

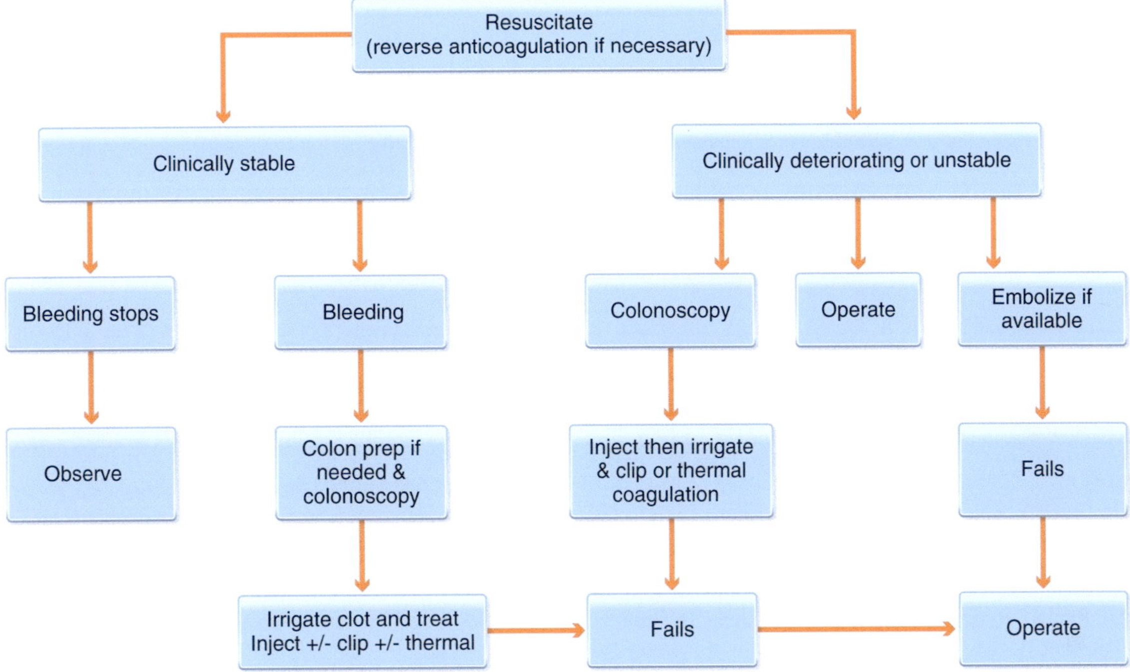

Fig. 3.13 Treatment algorithm for delayed post polypectomy bleeding (PPB). Modified from Gastrointest Endosc Clin N Am, 42(3), Church J, Complications of Colonoscopy, 639–57, Copyright 2013, with permission from Elsevier

References

1. Ahmed NA, Kochman ML, Long WB, Furth EE, Ginsberg GG. Efficacy, safety, and clinical outcomes of endoscopic mucosal resection: a study of 101 cases. Gastrointest Endosc. 2002;55(3): 390–6.
2. Baillie J. Postpolypectomy bleeding. Am J Gastroenterol. 2007;102:1151–3.
3. Benson BC, Myers JJ, Laczek JT. Postpolypectomy electrocoagulation syndrome: a mimicker of colonic perforation. Case Rep Emerg Med. 2013;2013:687931. http://dx.doi.org/10.1155/2013/687931.
4. Brooker JC, Saunders BP, Shah SG, Thapar CJ, Suzuki N, Williams CB. Treatment with argon plasma coagulation reduces recurrence after piecemeal resection of large sessile colonic polyps: a randomized trial and recommendations. Gastrointest Endosc. 2002;55(3): 371–5.
5. Carpenter S, Petersen BT, Chuttani R, Croffie J, DiSario J, Liu J, Mishkin D, Shah R, Somogyi L, Tierney W, Song LM. Polypectomy devices. Gastrointest Endosc. 2007;65:741–9.
6. Church J. Complications of Colonoscopy. Gastrointest Endosc Clin N Am. 2013;42(3):639–57.
7. Di Giorgio P, De Luca L, Calcagno G, Rivellini G, Mandato M, De Luca B. Detachable snare versus epinephrine injection in the prevention of postpolypectomy bleeding: a randomized and controlled study. Endoscopy. 2004;36(10):860–3. PMID: 15452780.
8. Fatima H, Rex DK. Minimizing endoscopic complications: colonoscopic polypectomy. Gastrointest Endosc Clin N Am. 2007;17: 145–56.
9. Feagins LA, Iqbal R, Harford WV, Halai A, Cryer BL, Dunbar KB, Davila RE, Spechler SJ. Low rate of postpolypectomy bleeding among patients who continue thienopyridine therapy during colonoscopy. Clin Gastroenterol Hepatol. 2013;11(10):1325–32. doi:10.1016/j.cgh.2013.02.003. Epub 2013 Feb 9. PMID: 23403011.
10. Frimberger E, von Delius S, Rosch T, Schmid RM. Colonoscopy and polypectomy with a side-viewing endoscope. Endoscopy. 2007;39(5):462–5.
11. Fyock CJ, Draganov PV. Colonoscopic polypectomy and associated techniques. World J Gastroenterol. 2010;16(29):3630–7.
12. Gimeno-García AZ, de Ganzo ZA, Sosa AJ, Pérez DN, Quintero E. Incidence and predictors of postpolypectomy bleeding in colorectal polyps larger than 10 mm. Eur J Gastroenterol Hepatol. 2012;24(5):520–6. doi:10.1097/MEG.0b013e328350fcdc. PMID: 22465971.
13. Ginsberg GG, Barkun AN, Bosco JJ, Burdick JS, Isenbert GA, Nakao NL, Petersen BT, Silverman WB, Slivka A, Kelsey PB. Endoscopic tattooing. Gastrointest Endosc. 2002;55(7):811–4.
14. Iishi H, Tatsuta M, Iseki K, Narahara H, Uedo N, Sakai N, Ishikawa H, Otani T, Ishiguro S. Endoscopic piecemeal resection with submucosal saline injection of large sessile colorectal polyps. Gastrointest Endosc. 2000;51:697–700.
15. Jeon JW, Shin HP, Lee JI, Joo KR, Pack KM, Cha JM, Park JJ, Lim JU, Lim K. The risk of postpolypectomy bleeding during colonoscopy in patients with early liver cirrhosis. Surg Endosc. 2012;26(11):3258–63. doi:10.1007/s00464-012-2334-0. Epub 2012 May 31. PMID: 22648106.
16. Kantsevoy SV, Adler DG, Conway JD, Diehl DL, Farraye FA, Kwon R, Mamula P, Rodriquez S, Shah RJ, Wong Kee Song LM, Tierney WM. Endoscopic mucosal resection and endoscopic submucosal dissection. Gastrointest Endosc. 2008;68(1):11–8. doi:10.1016/j.gie.2008.01.037.
17. Kapetanos D, Beltsis A, Chatzimavroudis G, Katsinelos P. Postpolypectomy bleeding: incidence, risk factors, prevention, and management. Surg Laparosc Endosc Percutan Tech. 2012;22(2):102–7. doi:10.1097/SLE.0b013e318247c02e. PMID: 22487620.
18. Kedia P, Waye JD. Colon polypectomy: a review of routine and advanced techniques. J Clin Gastroenterol. 2013;47:657–65.

19. Khashab M, Eid E, Rusche M, Rex DK. Incidence and predictors of "late" recurrences after endoscopic piecemeal resection of large sessile adenomas. Gastrointest Endosc. 2009;70:344–9.

20. Kim HS, Kim TI, Kim WH, Kim YH, Kim HJ, Yang SK, Myung SJ, Byeon JS, Lee MS, Chung IK, Jung SA, Jeen YT, Choi JH, Choi KY, Choi H, Han DS, Song JS. Risk factors for immediate postpolypectomy bleeding of the colon: a multicenter study. Am J Gastroenterol. 2006;101(6):1333–41. PMID: 16771958.

21. Komeda Y, Suzuki N, Marshall S, Thomas-Gibson S, Vance M, Fraser C, Patel K, Saunders BP. Factors associated with failed polyp retrieval at screening colonoscopy. Gastrointest Endosc. 2013;77:395–400.

22. Kouklakis G, Mpoumponaris A, Gatopoulou A, Efraimidou E, Manolas K, Lirantzopoulos N. Endoscopic resection of large pedunculated colonic polyps and risk of postpolypectomy bleeding with adrenaline injection versus endoloop and hemoclip: a prospective, randomized study. Surg Endosc. 2009;23(12):2732–7. doi:10.1007/s00464-009-0478-3. Epub 2009 May 9. PMID: 19430833.

23. Lee SH, Cho WY, Kim HJ, Kim HJ, Kim YH, Chung IK, Kim HS, Park SH, Kim SJ. A new method of EMR: submucosal injection of a fibrinogen mixture. Gastrointest Endosc. 2004;59(2):220–4.

24. Lee SH, Chung IK, Kim SJ, Kim JO, Ko BM, Kim WH, Kim HS, Park DI, Kim HJ, Byeon JS, Yang SK, Jang BI, Jung SA, Jeen YT, Choi JH, Choi H, Han DS, Song JS. Comparison of postpolypectomy bleeding between epinephrine and saline submucosal injection for large colon polyps by conventional polypectomy: a prospective randomized, multicenter study. World J Gastroenterol. 2007;13(21):2973–7. PMID: 17589949.

25. Lee TJW, Rutter MD, Blanks RG. Colonoscopy quality measures: experience from the NHS Bowel Cancer Screening Programme. Gut. 2012;61:1050–7.

26. Levin B, Lieberman DA, McFarland B, Smith RA, Brooks D, Andrews KS, Dash C, Giardiello FM, Glick S, Levin TR, Pickhardt P, Rex DK, Thorson A, Winauer SJ. Screening and surveillance for the early detection of colorectal cancer and adenomatous polyps, 2008; A joint guideline from the American Cancer Society, the US Multi-Society Task Force on Colorectal Cancer, and the American College of Radiology. CA Cancer J Clin. 2008;58:130–60.

27. Lukens FJ, Gómez V, Patel MK, Achem SR, Picco MF. Colonoscopic postpolypectomy bleeding in patients that resumed warfarin: not as frequent as we may think. J Clin Gastroenterol. 2013;47(3):290–2. doi:10.1097/MCG.0b013e31826baaec. No abstract available. PMID: 23059412.

28. Misra SP, Dwivedi M. Colonoscopy and colonoscopic polypectomy using side-viewing endoscope: a useful, effective and safe procedure. Dig Dis Sci. 2008;53:1285–8.

29. Nishihara R, Wu K, Lochhead P, Morikawa T, Liao X, Qian ZR, Inamura K, Kim SA, Kuchiba A, Yamauchi M, Imamura Y, Willett WC, Rosner BA, Fuchs CS, Giovannucci E, Ogino S, Chan AT. Long-term colorectal-cancer incidence and mortality after lower endoscopy. N Engl J Med. 2013;369(12):1095–105.

30. Park SY, Kim HS, Yoon KW, Cho SB, Lee WS, Park CH, Joo YE, Choi SK, Rew JS. Usefulness of cap-assisted colonoscopy during colonoscopic EMR:a randomized, controlled trial. Gastrointest Endosc. 2011;74:869–75.

31. Parra-Blanco A, Kaminaga N, Kojima T, Endo Y, Uragami N, Okawa N, Hattori T, Takahashi H, Fujita R. Hemoclipping for postpolypectomy and postbiopsy colonic bleeding. Gastrointest Endosc. 2000;51(1):37–41. PMID: 10625793.

32. Paspatis GA, Paraskeva K, Theodoropoulou A, Mathou N, Vardas E, Oustamanolakis P, Chlouverakis G, Karagiannis I. A prospective, randomized comparison of adrenaline injection in combination with detachable snare versus adrenaline injection alone in the prevention of postpolypectomy bleeding in large colonic polyps. Am J Gastroenterol. 2006;101(12):2805; quiz 2913. Epub 2006 Oct 6. PMID: 17026560.

33. Paspatis GA, Tribonias G, Konstantinidis K, Theodoropoulou A, Vardas E, Voudoukis E, Manolaraki MM, Chainaki I, Chlouverakis G. A prospective randomized comparison of cold vs hot snare polypectomy in the occurrence of postpolypectomy bleeding in small colonic polyps. Colorectal Dis. 2011;13(10):e345–8. doi:10.1111/j.1463-1318.2011.02696.x. PMID: 21689363.

34. Qaseem A, Denberg TD, Hopkins Jr RH, Humphrey LL, Levine J, Sweet DE, Shekelle P, Clinical Guidelines Committee of the American College of Physicians. Screening for colorectal cancer; a guidance statement from the American College of Physicians. Ann Intern Med. 2012;156(5):378–86.

35. Rabeneck L, Paszat LF, Hilsden RJ, et al. Bleeding and perforation after outpatient colonoscopy and their risk factors in usual clinical practice. Gastroenterology. 2008;135(6):1899–906. PMID 18938166.

36. Rex DK, Johnson DA, Anderson JC, Schoenfeld PS, Burke CA, Inadomi JM, American College of Gastroenterology. American College of Gastroenterology guidelines for colorectal cancer screening. Am J Gastroenterol. 2009;104(3):739–50.

37. Sawhney MS, Salfiti N, Nelson DB, Lederle FA, Bond JH. Risk factors for severe delayed postpolypectomy bleeding. Endoscopy. 2008;40(2):115–9. doi:10.1055/s-2007-966959. PMID: 18253906.

38. SEER Stat Fact Sheet; colon and rectum. National Cancer Institute. Available at: http://seer.cancer.gov/statfacts/html/colorect.html. Accessed 23 Oct 2013.

39. Shatz BA, Thavorides V. Colonic tattoo for follow-up of endoscopic sessile polypectomy. Gastrointest Endosc. 1991;37:59–60.

40. Singaram C, Torbey CF, Jacoby RF. Delayed postpolypectomy bleeding. Am J Gastroenterol. 1995;90(1):146–7. PMID: 7801918.

41. Singh M, Mehta N, Murthy UK, Kaul V, Arif A, Newman N. Postpolypectomy bleeding in patients undergoing colonoscopy on uninterrupted clopidogrel therapy. Gastrointest Endosc. 2010;71(6):998–1005. doi:10.1016/j.gie.2009.11.022. Epub 2010 Mar 11PMID: 20226452.

42. Sonnenberg A. Management of delayed postpolypectomy bleeding: a decision analysis. Am J Gastroenterol. 2012;107(3):339–42. doi:10.1038/ajg.2011.426. PMID: 22388016.

43. Strate LL. Lower GI bleeding: epidemiology and diagnosis. Gastroenterol Clin North Am. 2005;34:643–64.

44. Van Gossum A, Cozzoli A, Adler M, Taton G, Cremer M. Colonoscopic snare polypectomy: analysis of 1485 resections comparing two types of current. Gastrointest Endosc. 1992;38:472–5.

45. Waye J. It ain't over 'til it's over: retrieval of polyps after colonoscopic polypectomy. Gastrointest Endosc. 2005;62:257–9.

46. Whitlow CB. Endoscopic treatment for lower gastrointestinal bleeding. Clin Colon Rectal Surg. 2010;23:31–6.

47. Wu XR, Church JM, Jarrar A, Liang J, Kalady MF. Risk factors for delayed postpolypectomy bleeding: how to minimize your patients' risk. Int J Colorectal Dis. 2013;28(8):1127–34. doi:10.1007/s00384-013-1661-5. Epub 2013 Feb 26. PMID: 23440363.

48. Yamamoto H, Kawata H, Sunada K, Satoh K, Kaneko Y, Ido K, Sugano K. Success rate of curative endoscopic mucosal resection with circumferential mucosal incision assisted by submucosal injection of sodium hyaluronate. Gastrointest Endosc. 2002;56(4):507–12.

49. Zafar A, Mustafa M, Chapman M. Colorectal polyps: when should we tattoo? Surg Endosc. 2012;26(11):3264–6.

50. Zlatanic J, Waye JD, Kim PS, Baiocco PJ, Gleim GW. Large sessile colonic adenomas: use of argon plasma coagulator to supplement piecemeal snare polypectomy. Gastrointest Endosc. 1999;49(6):731–5.

Suggested Reading

Carpenter S, Petersen BT, Chuttani R, Croffie J, DiSario J, Liu J, Mishkin D, Shah R, Somogyi L, Tierney W, Song LM. Polypectomy devices. Gastrointest Endosc. 2007;65:741–9.

Church J. Complications of colonoscopy. Gastrointest Endosc Clin N Am. 2013;42(3):639–57.

Fatima H, Rex DK. Minimizing endoscopic complications: colonoscopic polypectomy. Gastrointest Endosc Clin N Am. 2007;17:145–56.

Fyock CJ, Draganov PV. Colonoscopic polypectomy and associated techniques. World J Gastroenterol. 2010;16(29):3630–7.

Kedia P, Waye JD. Colon polypectomy: a review of routine and advanced techniques. J Clin Gastroenterol. 2013;47:657–65.

Waye J. It ain't over 'til it's over: retrieval of polyps after colonoscopic polypectomy. Gastrointest Endosc. 2005;62:257–9.

Laparoscopic Common Bile Duct Exploration

4

Ezra N. Teitelbaum and Eric S. Hungness

Indications

Choledocholithiasis (common bile duct or common hepatic duct stones).

Preoperative Preparation

Establish the likely presence of choledocholithiasis via history and physical exam (jaundice, light-colored stools, prior episodes of pancreatitis, scleral icterus), laboratory values (elevated direct bilirubin, transaminases, and/or lipase), and transabdominal ultrasound (dilated common bile duct >6 mm, choledocholithiasis visualized). The use of preoperative magnetic resonance cholangiopancreatography (MRCP) is rarely, if ever, required.

Assemble the equipment required for intraoperative cholangiography (catheter, Olsen clamp, contrast) and laparoscopic common bile duct exploration (LCBDE) (second video tower, guide wire, balloon dilator, choledochoscope, and wire basket).

Arrange for intraoperative fluoroscopy and position the operating room table to allow for introduction of the "c-arm" (this may require reversing the head and foot of the table, depending on the model).

Operative Strategy

Begin the operation in the same manner as a standard laparoscopic cholecystectomy, with trocar insertion and dissection of the triangle of Calot to a "critical view of safety."

E.N. Teitelbaum, M.D. (✉) • E.S. Hungness, M.D., F.A.C.S.
Department of Surgery, Northwestern University Feinberg School of Medicine, Chicago, IL 60611, USA
e-mail: ezratei@gmail.com

Then perform a cholangiogram to confirm the presence of choledocholithiasis. Attempt to flush the common duct stones using saline, aided by intravenous glucagon. If flushing is unsuccessful, determine the optimal approach method for LCBDE (transcystic versus transcholedochal). If a transcystic approach is possible, introduce a guide wire through the cholangiogram catheter and then perform a balloon dilation of the cystic duct. Advance the choledochoscope through the cystic ductotomy and capture the common duct stone using an endoscopic wire basket. If a transcholedochal approach is indicated, dissect the common bile duct clear and make a longitudinal choledochotomy to allow for direct introduction of the choledochoscope. After stone removal, determine the need for t-tube insertion and then close the choledochotomy using intracorporeal suturing. Once the LCBDE is finished (either transcystic or transcholedochal), perform a completion cholangiogram to confirm ductal clearance and proceed with the cholecystectomy.

Operative Technique

Trocar Placement and Initial Dissection

Position the patient supine, with the surgeon on the patient's left side and the assistant on the right. Gain abdominal access and establish a pneumoperitoneum through a periumbical incision using either an open Hasson or closed Veress needle technique. Then place trocars in an identical configuration to that used during a standard laparoscopic cholecystectomy: a 10 mm trocar at the umbilicus, a 10 mm in the epigastrium, and two right-sided subcostal 5 mm ports, in the mid-clavicular and anterior-axillary lines. Have your assistant retract the gallbladder fundus cephalad and over the liver with their left hand and drive the laparoscope with their right hand.

Place the patient in steep reverse-Trendelenburg position with the left-side down. Use a two-handed technique to retract the gallbladder infundibulum laterally and inferiorly,

A.L. Halverson and D.C. Borgstrom (eds.), *Advanced Surgical Techniques for Rural Surgeons*,
DOI 10.1007/978-1-4939-1495-1_4, © Springer Science+Business Media New York 2015

while using a combination of blunt and electrocautery dissection to clear the triangle of Calot of fibrous and fatty tissue. It is essential to continue this dissection until a "critical view of safety" is established, in which (1) the triangle of Calot has been cleared, (2) the gallbladder has been dissected off of the liver bed, and (3) two, and only two, tubular structures are seen entering the gallbladder. Completing this dissection initially not only confirms the identity of the cystic duct, but also allows for greater mobility in retraction of the cystic duct, making the subsequent cholangiogram and LCBDE easier to perform.

Intraoperative Cholangiogram

Once a critical view has been achieved, next perform a cholangiogram. Place a 10 mm clip at the cystic duct-gallbladder junction to prevent spillage of bile and stones from the gallbladder and then make a partial cystic ductotomy using laparoscopic shears. This ductotomy should be performed as close to the gallbladder as possible, in order to preserve cystic duct length and keep subsequent manipulations and instrumentation away from the common bile duct. Insert a cholangiogram catheter through the mid-axillary port and feed it into the cystic duct. It is helpful to use an Olsen-type cholangiography clamp that can occlude the cystic duct after introducing the catheter. If choledocholithiasis is suspected, use a cholangiogram catheter that is at least 5 Fr in diameter, so that can accommodate subsequent guide wire passage.

Once the cholangiogram catheter is secured in place, flush saline through it to ensure that there is minimal resistance and no retrograde leak from the ductotomy. Then position the draped c-arm above the upper abdomen. Ensure that everyone in the operating room is appropriately shielded and take a still radiograph to check positioning of the c-arm. The cholangiography clamp should be to the left side of the image and at its approximate midpoint vertically. Check the cholangiography tubing to ensure that no air bubbles are present. Then inject a 50 %/50 % mixture of contrast and saline while visualizing with fluoroscopy. If the cholangiogram is normal, the cystic-common duct junction should be clearly seen, the common duct should fill completely and empty into the duodenum, and the common hepatic duct should fill with clear bifurcation and arborization proximally. Any discrete filling defect in the biliary tree is either a stone or an air bubble. In contrast to stones, air bubbles are perfectly round, usually small, and will move with small amounts of flow. This can be tested by oscillating the cholangiography syringe plunger back and forth while observing fluoroscopically. If a stone is impacted at the ampulla, a meniscus sign can be seen and the duodenum will not fill with contrast.

Attempt Flushing

A portion of common duct stones, especially small ones (<4 mm) can be flushed from the common duct into the duodenum, obviating the need for LCBDE. Use the cholangiogram catheter and syringe to flush several hundred milliliters of saline under pressure. Glucagon (1–2 mg) can be given intravenously in order to relax the Sphincter of Oddi prior to flushing. Next, repeat a cholangiogram in order to evaluate whether the stones have passed the ampulla.

Determination of LCBDE Approach

If the presence of stones in the biliary tree has been established via cholangiogram and flushing is unsuccessful, the optimal approach for LCBDE and stone retrieval must be decided upon. In general, a transcystic approach is preferred because it avoids a ductotomy and closure of the common bile duct. However, the following situations are contraindications to a transcystic approach: a large (>10 mm) common duct stone, more than five common duct stones, a stone in the common hepatic duct or proximal hepatic ducts, and aberrant cystic duct anatomy that would preclude passage of the choledochoscope (e.g., cystic duct entry on the left side of the common bile duct). If any of these contraindications exist, a transcholedochal LCBDE can be performed or the patient can be referred for postoperative ERCP. The main contraindication to a transcholedochal approach is a nondilated (<8 mm) common bile duct.

Transcystic LCBDE

Guide Wire Access

After intraoperative cholangiogram confirms the presence of choledocholithiasis that is amenable to transcystic LCBDE, obtain guide wire access through the cholangiogram catheter. A 0.035″ hydrophilic flexible-tip guide wire is used and should be advanced under fluoroscopic visualization. Lubricate the guide wire with saline, and then pass it through the cholangiogram catheter into the distal common bile duct, and ideally past the ampulla and into the duodenum. Once the guide wire is in position, unclamp and remove the cholangiogram catheter. As the catheter is being removed, hold onto the guide wire with a laparoscopic grasper to avoid losing access. A "spot check" with fluoroscopy can be used between operative steps to check wire position.

Cystic Duct Dilation

If the cystic duct is already dilated from the biliary obstruction, it may not be necessary to perform additional mechanical dilation. However, the tortuosity of the cystic duct itself often

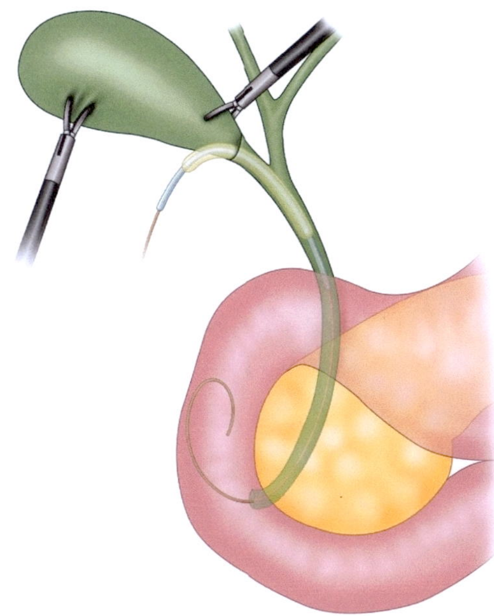

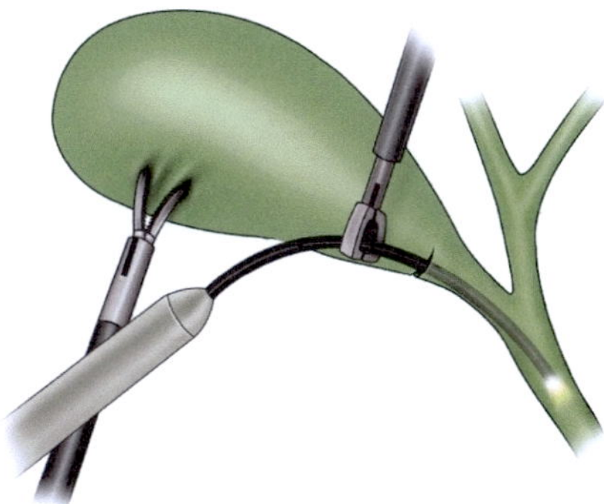

Fig. 4.2 A padded grasper is used to gently advance the choledochoscope distally under direct visualization. It is important to guide the scope in parallel with the cystic and common bile ducts to avoid ductal injury. The scope should not be advanced unless the lumen of the duct is clearly visualized endoscopically

Fig. 4.1 A dilating balloon is passed over the guide wire and through the cystic ductotomy. The position of the balloon is checked fluoroscopically to ensure that it is traversing the entire length of the cystic duct. The balloon is then held inflated for at least 3 min to maximally dilate the duct and obliterate any values and tortuosity

impedes choledochoscope insertion and performing routine dilation will likely save time in the long run. A balloon dilator with an 8 mm diameter and 4 cm length is used. Pass the balloon over the guide wire and position it across the entirety of the cystic duct using fluoroscopy. Using a pressure injector, inflate the balloon to its recommended dilation pressure (between 3 and 12 atm) and hold it in place inflated for at least 3 min (Fig. 4.1). Next, deflate and remove the balloon, again holding the guide wire in place with a grasper.

Choledochoscope Setup and Insertion

Connect the choledochoscope to a pressurized saline bag. Check to ensure adequate flow through the working channel, and then clamp the irrigation during insertion. Use a picture-in-picture setup on the main monitor, so that the laparoscopic and choledochoscopic images can be viewed simultaneously. Feed the guide wire through the scope's working channel and then pass the scope along the wire and through the cystic ductotomy. Use one hand to advance the scope and control torque, while the other operates the scope flexion dial. Once the scope is within the cystic duct, turn on the irrigation and scope light source. Usually an illumination intensity of only 30 % is required. Slowly advance the choledochoscope, while using torque and flexion to keep the ductal lumen centered. Usually the scope can be advanced by manipulating it external to the trocar; however, if this is not possible, a padded laparoscopic grasper can be used to gently pass it internally (Fig. 4.2). Once the scope is within the common duct,

remove the guide wire from the working channel. Advance the scope until the first common duct stone is encountered.

Stone Capture and Extraction

Pass a three- or four-wire stone extraction basket through the working channel of the choledochoscope. Advance the closed basket beyond the stone and then have your assistant open it. Slowly trawl the open basket back toward the scope until the stone falls within it (Fig. 4.3). Often a back-and-forth jiggling motion is required to make the stone drop within the wires of the basket. Once the stone is centered within the wires, slowly close the basket around it. Withdraw the scope from ducts, while keeping the stone pinned against the face of the scope. Often there will be some resistance at the cystic-common duct junction, which can be overcome with steady, gentle pressure. Once the stone is delivered out of the cystic ductotomy, it can be deposited in the peritoneal cavity and removed using a stone-grasper or with the gallbladder in an endoscopic bag after completion of the cholecystectomy. If multiple stones were present on cholangiogram, reintroduce the scope through the cystic ductotomy and repeat the process of capture and extraction. Usually once the cystic duct has been dilated, the scope can be reintroduced manually without the need to regain guide wire access.

Completion Cholangiogram and Cystic Duct Ligation

Even if all common duct stones were thought to have been removed, it is important to perform a repeat cholangiogram after LCBDE to confirm and document ductal clearance and antegrade flow of contrast into the duodenum. As the cystic duct was dilated to at least 8 mm, use two suture loops to ligate it (rather than clips). Then proceed with the cholecystectomy as usual. It is not necessary to leave a drain after transcystic LCBDE.

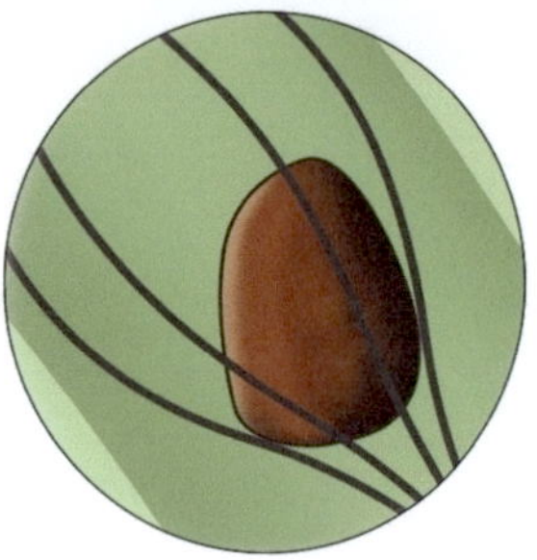

Fig. 4.3 The wire basket is advanced distal to the stone and opened. It is then slowly pulled back, and in this figure we can see the stone has fallen within the wires of the basket. The basket is then closed to capture the stone against the face of the choledochoscope

Transcholedochal LCBDE

If a transyctic approach is not feasible based on stone size or patient anatomy, a transcholedochal approach can be utilized. However, this should not be attempted unless the surgeon has adequate experience with advanced intracorporeal suturing, as well as the ability to perform an open repair of the common bile duct. Alternatively, the patient can always be referred first for ERCP without "burning any bridges," with transcholedochal LCBDE reserved in case the duct cannot be cleared endoscopically.

Common Duct Dissection and Choledochotomy

First, dissect along the cystic duct to identify the cystic-common duct junction. As the common duct is approached, the use of electrocautery should be avoided completely to prevent injury via thermal spread. Bluntly clear any fatty tissue overlying the anterior surface of the common duct and identify the course of the proper hepatic artery in relation to the common duct. Once the common duct has been cleared, perform a longitudinal choledochotomy. Specialized microshears or Potts-type laparoscopic scissors can be used in order to help ensure a linear and precise ductotomy. The ductotomy should be made inferior to the cystic-common duct junction and should be just long enough to allow for passage of the largest stone seen on cholangiography.

Choledochoscope Insertion and Stone Capture and Extraction

When performing LCBDE via a transcholedochal approach, it is usually possible to pass the choledochoscope directly through the ductotomy without first gaining guide wire access. The choice of which trocar to use for scope passage (either epigastric or mid-clavicular) will depend on the angle and course of the common duct. Once the scope is within the common duct, stones are captured and extracted as described above for transcystic LCBDE.

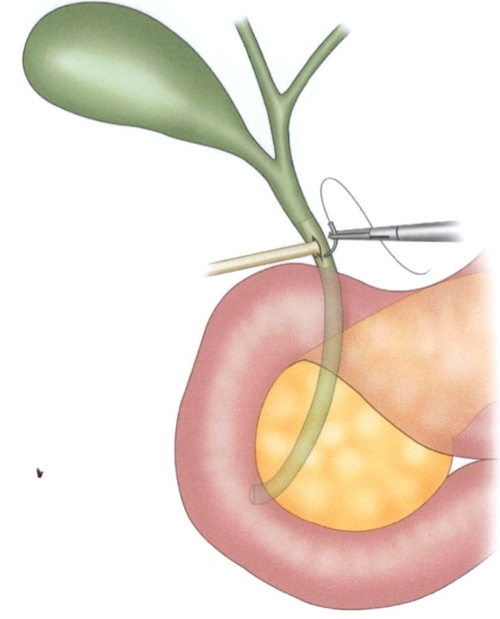

Fig. 4.4 Once the t-tube has been inserted, the choledochotomy is closed using interrupted sutures. The first stitch is placed just distal to the t-tube to hold it in place during the remainder of the closure. Care is taken to avoid incorporating the tube into this initial closure stitch

Choledochotomy Closure (With or Without T-Tube Insertion)

Recent studies have shown that it is not necessary to routinely place a t-tube during choledochotomy closure, and that placement may lead to unnecessarily longer hospitalizations and increased costs. Indications for t-tube drainage include residual sludge or debride within the common bile duct or a lack of duodenal filling on completion cholangiogram.

If a t-tube is required, fashion a 10–14 Fr tube with a long and short end. Internalize the tube completely and then use graspers to place it into the ductotomy with the long end pointed distally, toward the ampulla. Close the ductotomy using interrupted stitches with 4-0 monofilament absorbable suture. Placing an additional port in the right mid-abdomen may create a better angle for performing the closure. If a t-tube has been placed, push the tube to the cephalad edge of the ductotomy and place the first stitch immediately distal to the tube so that it holds the tube securely in position during subsequent suturing (Fig. 4.4). Take care to avoid catching the tube in the suture closure. Use an intracorporeal knot tying technique to secure each stitch and work distally until the ductotomy is closed completely. The t-tube can then be left in position and externalized through one of the subcostal trocars after the cholecystectomy is completed.

Completion Cholangiogram and Cystic Duct Ligation

As with a transcystic approach, a completion cholangiogram must be performed after stone clearance. If a t-tube was placed during ductotomy closure, either perform the cholangiogram through the t-tube or occlude the t-tube and pass the catheter through the cystic ductotomy. If a primary closure was performed without t-tube placement, perform the cholangiogram in the standard fashion through the cystic ductotomy. Although the cystic duct was not mechanically dilated during a transcholedochal approach, it is probably still best to use suture loops to ligate it. After duct ligation, proceed with the cholecystectomy as usual.

Potential Pitfalls

Not having the required equipment assembled prior to beginning the operation.

Failure to achieve a "critical view of safety" during initial dissection, resulting in a misidentification of anatomy.

Misinterpretation of the cholangiogram images.

Failure to gain guide wire access or perform cystic duct dilation during transcystic LCBDE, resulting in difficulty passing the choledochoscope.

Incorporating the t-tube into the choledochotomy closure after transcholedochal LCBDE.

Failure to perform a completion cholangiogram after stone extraction.

Using clips, rather than suture loops, to ligate the cystic duct after a dilation was performed.

Postoperative Care

Patients are provided with pain control and antiemetics as needed, similar to after a standard laparoscopic cholecystectomy. If the completion cholangiogram demonstrated a clear common duct without evidence of biliary obstruction, patients can be started on a clear liquid diet postoperatively. Patients should remain in the hospital and a bilirubin level should be checked the following day to ensure a downward trend. As long as there is no evidence of ongoing biliary obstruction and patients are tolerating a diet with adequate pain control, they can be discharged as early as postoperative day one.

Common Complications

Retained common bile duct stones.
Biliary leak.

When to Transfer

Patient with cholangitis and ERCP is not available.

Suspected or observed common bile duct injury.

Transcystic LCBDE fails to remove a common duct stone and surgeon is not experienced in performing transcholedochal LCBDE.

Suggested Reading

Bingener J, Schwesinger WH. Management of common bile duct stones in a rural area of the United States: results of a survey. Surg Endosc. 2006;20(4):577–9.

Crawford DL, Phillips EH. Laparoscopic common bile duct exploration. World J Surg. 1999;23(4):343–9.

Grubnik VV, et al. Laparoscopic common bile duct exploration versus open surgery: comparative prospective randomized trial. Surg Endosc. 2012;26(8):2165–71.

Lezoche E, Paganini AM. Technical considerations and laparoscopic bile duct exploration: transcystic and choledochotomy. Semin Laparosc Surg. 2000;7(4):262–78.

Poulose BK, et al. National analysis of in-hospital resource utilization in choledocholithiasis management using propensity scores. Surg Endosc. 2006;20(2):186–90.

Rogers SJ, et al. Prospective randomized trial of LC+LCBDE vs ERCP/S+LC for common bile duct stone disease. Arch Surg. 2010;145(1): 28–33.

Partial Cholecystectomy

5

Christine E. Van Cott and Randall S. Zuckerman

Indications

Partial cholecystectomy (PC) is an operative technique that may be necessary if significant inflammation/bleeding is encountered between the gallbladder and liver parenchyma or if anatomy cannot be fully dissected risking damage to portal structures and other visceral organs.

Preoperative Preparation

PC can be used as a safe alternative procedure when the anatomy within the triangle of Calot, otherwise known as the critical view of safety, cannot be obtained (Fig. 5.1).

There is no additional preparation needed than that done for a laparoscopic or open cholecystectomy.

Consent for a laparoscopic cholecystectomy should always include possible conversion to an open procedure, bile duct/vascular injury, and need for a drain.

Operative Strategy

Partial cholecystectomy can be performed using either an open or laparoscopic technique. We will address the open technique but the general principles can be applied to a laparoscopic approach. PC allows for amputation of either just the anterior wall of the gallbladder or removal of the gallbladder at the level of the infindibulum. Once resected the contents of the gallbladder and cystic duct are cleared, the mucosa obliterated and the stump closed.

Operative Technique

Make a Kocher incision two finger breaths below the right costal margin, incising fascia and rectus abdominis and lateral muscles. Maintain hemostasis of abdominal wall vasculature as the peritoneal cavity is entered.

One may need to locate and divide the falciform ligament to aid exposure and assist with retraction.

A self-retaining retractor should be used to facilitate visualization and allow the surgeon and assistant use of both hands. The authors prefer a Thompson or Omni retractor; however, a Bookwalter may be used.

Any adhesions not already incised should be taken down allowing clearance of the infindubulum as low as safely possible (Fig. 5.2).

Gallbladder distension may be relieved with either needle or suction decompression. Bile leakage should be minimized by occluding the opening with a stitch or hemostat.

If dissection is difficult between the gallbladder and liver bed, it is possible to leave the posterior wall of the gallbladder intact. The gallbladder is first entered approximately 1 cm from liver edge and the full thickness of the gallbladder is transected parallel to the liver to a safe level (Figs. 5.3 and 5.4).

The transection is then brought around the anterior surface of the gallbladder exposing both the posterior wall and infindibulum mucosa (Fig. 5.5).

Any remaining contents including stones are then removed. The cystic duct orifice should be appreciated and using either a right angle or small catheter/fogarty intubated to assure that there are no stones within. Using half strength contrast with either intraoperative fluoroscopy or X-ray a cholangiogram should be preformed to assure that the biliary system has not been damaged. A complete cholangiogram

C.E. Van Cott, M.D., F.A.C.S.
Frank H. Netter MD School of Medicine, Quinnipiac University, North Haven Campus, 370 Bassett Road, North Haven, CT 06473, USA

St. Vincent's Medical Center, 2800 Main Street, Bridgeport, CT 06606, USA

R.S. Zuckerman, M.D., F.A.C.S. (✉)
St. Vincent's Medical Center, 2800 Main Street, Bridgeport, CT 06606, USA
e-mail: randall.zuckerman@stvincents.org

A.L. Halverson and D.C. Borgstrom (eds.), *Advanced Surgical Techniques for Rural Surgeons*,
DOI 10.1007/978-1-4939-1495-1_5, © Springer Science+Business Media New York 2015

should visualize left and right hepatic ducts, common bile duct, and contrast flowing freely into the duodenum.

Mucosa within the remnant is then cauterized to help in preventing future mucocele formation (Figs. 5.6 and 5.7).

The gallbladder neck is then sutured closed with an absorbable suture in either an interrupted or continuous fashion. Closure will be difficult if not impossible at times with a high risk of bile leakage. A closed suction abdominal drain should be placed in the area of the neck of gallbladder, brought out through the abdominal wall and secured (Figs. 5.8 and 5.9).

If the reason for necessitating a partial cholecystectomy is because of inability to discern portal structures it is possible to amputate just the fundus of the gallbladder. The visceral peritoneum of the gallbladder is incised approximately 1 cm from the liver edge extending along the gallbladder parallel

to the liver. This is continued until the gallbladder is fully mobilized from the liver bed as low as is safely possible. The now free portion of the gallbladder is amputated. Again the remaining gallbladder and cystic duct should be cleared, cholangiogram preformed, and mucosa cauterized. The gallbladder neck is then sutured closed with an absorbable suture; alternatively it may also be stapled closed after fundal amputation. A closed suction drain should be placed (Figs. 5.10 and 5.11).

The abdomen should be irrigated copiously to avoid bile irritation to the abdominal cavity.

Potential Pitfalls

One should not consider partial cholecystectomy as an operative failure but rather an alternative approach that may help to avoid the most devastating of bile duct injuries.

Bleeding from the cut surface of the gallbladder can be significant at times especially in the setting of sever inflammation. Maintaining continual hemostasis will allow the surgeon improved visualization.

Closure of the gallbladder remnant can be difficult and bile leak from the remnant would be common; the importance of operative placement of a closed suction drain cannot be stressed more.

Postoperative Care

As per standard open cholecystectomy plus monitoring the abdominal drain for evidence of bile.

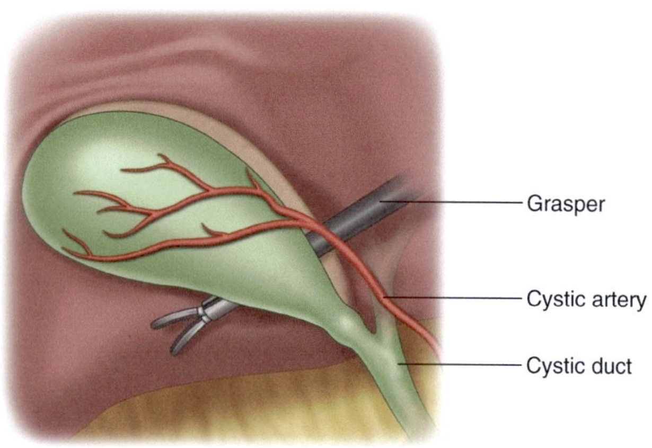

Fig. 5.1 Critical view of safety as defined by strassberg

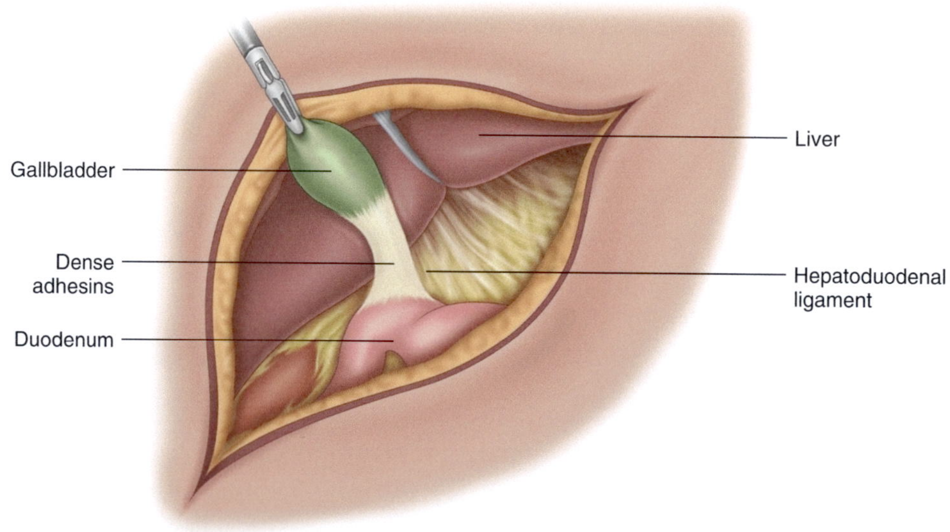

Fig. 5.2 Dense adhesions making a traditional cholecystectomy high risk for biliary injuries

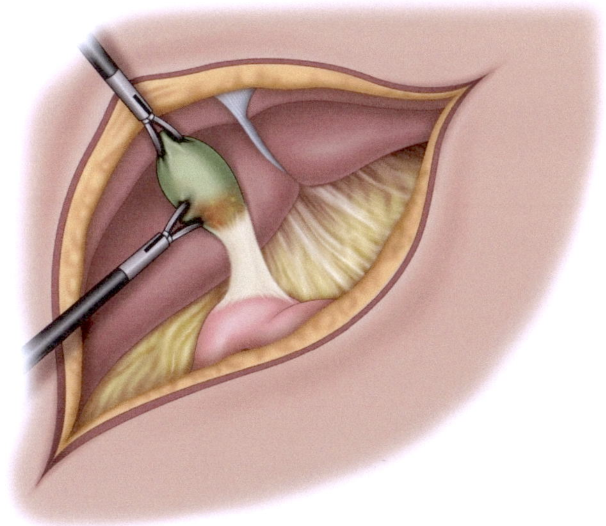

Fig. 5.3 Entering the gallbladder at the fundus. One can appreciate the lack of a dissection plane between the liver and the gallbladder

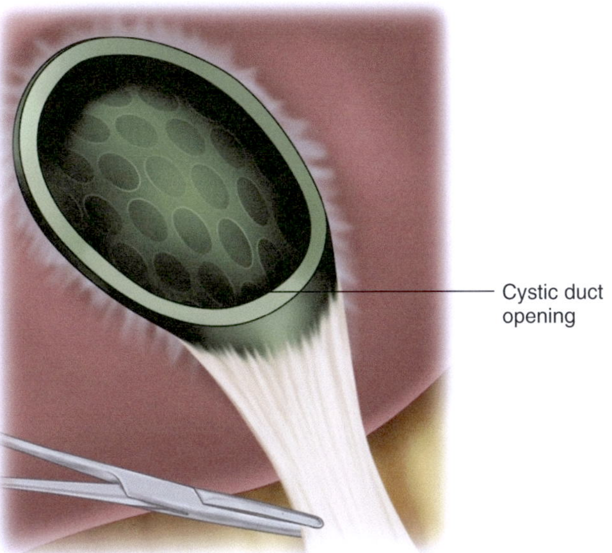

Fig. 5.5 Transection has now exposed the mucosal surface of the gall-bladder and the cystic duct orifice

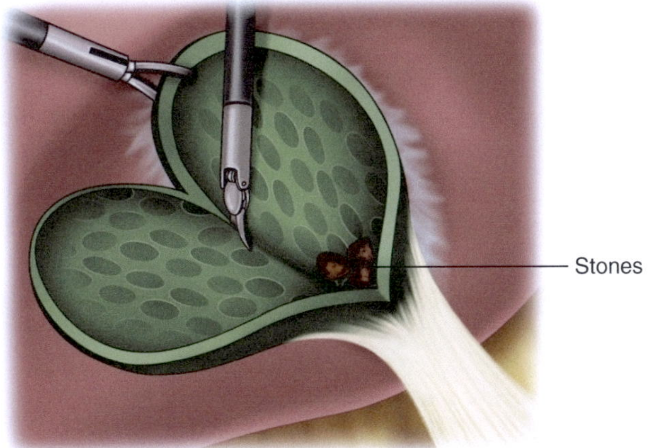

Fig. 5.4 Transection is continued through the full thickness of the gall-bladder wall parallel to the liver surface. Stones can sometimes be appreciated

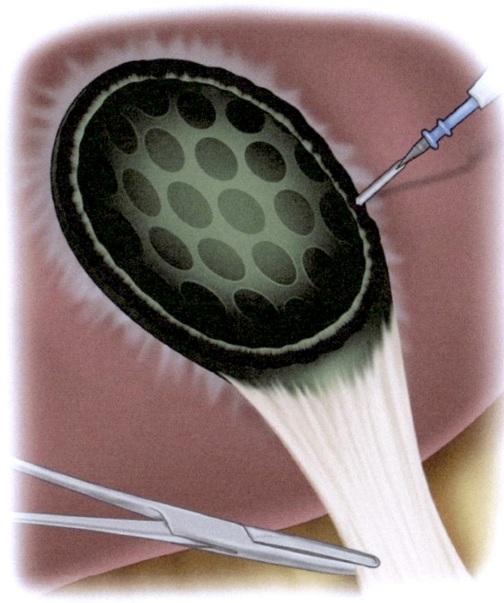

Fig. 5.6 Cauterization of transected edge of gallbladder

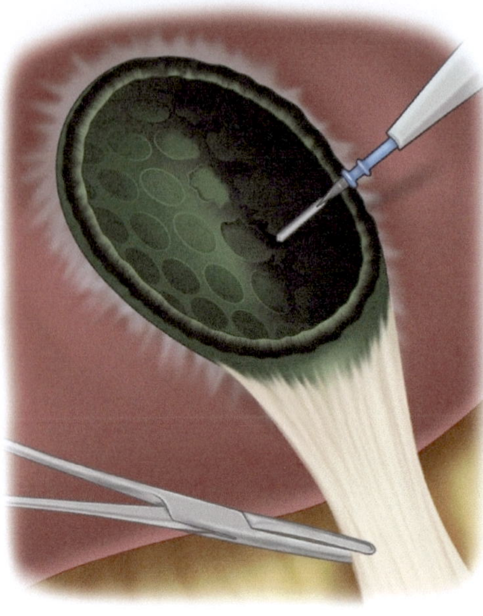

Fig. 5.7 Cauterization of remnant posterior wall mucosa

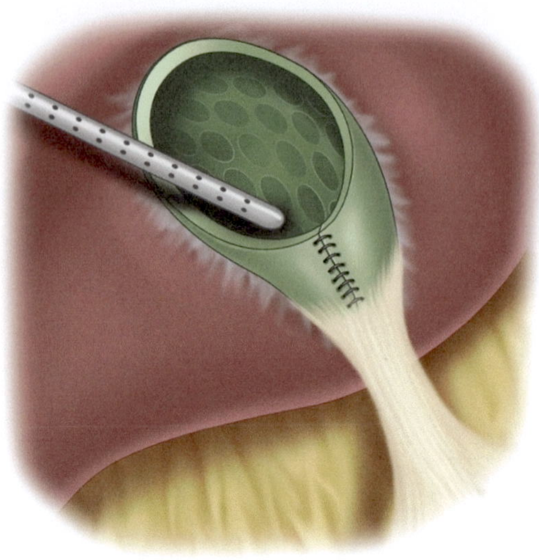

Fig. 5.9 A closed suction drainage catheter is placed to allow for formation of a controlled bile fistula

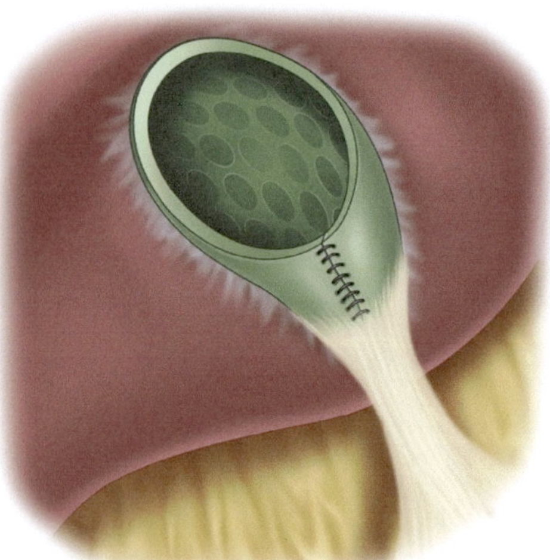

Fig. 5.8 Infundibulum of the gallbladder is closed in an interrupted fashion with absorbable sutures

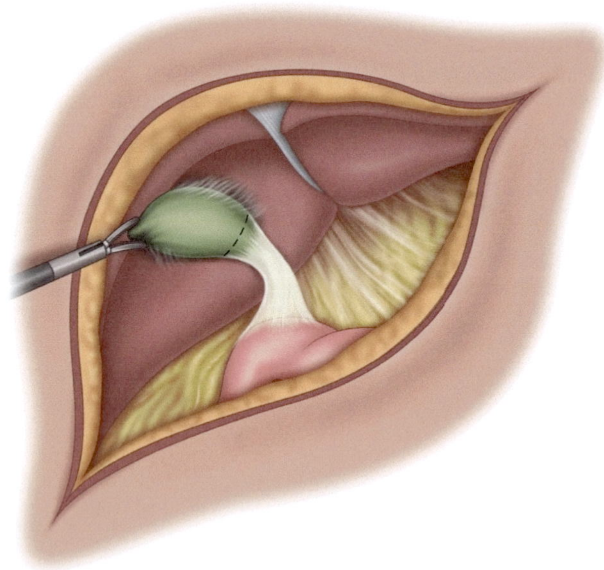

Fig. 5.10 Full mobilization of the fundus of the gallbladder from the liver bed

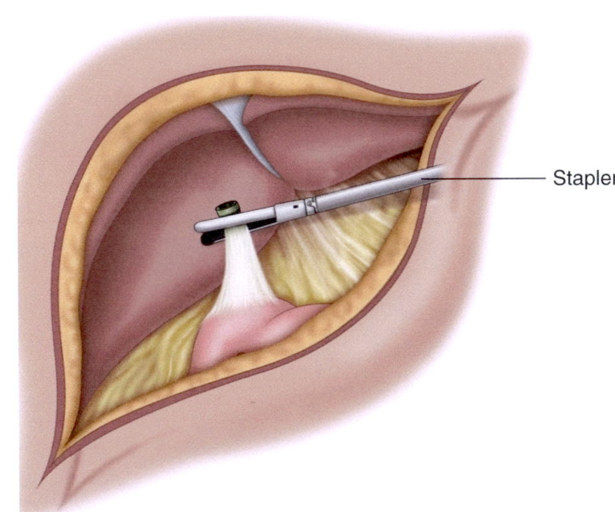

Fig. 5.11 Amputation of the gallbladder being closed with a stapling device

Common Complications

Hemorrhage
Infection
Wound infection

Hernia
Retained stones
Visceral injury
Vascular injury
Bile duct injury
Bile duct leak

When to Transfer

With a persistent bile leak transfer to a facility with ERCP capabilities may be necessary to facilitate closure with common bile duct stent placement.

Transfer to a tertiary care facility is of paramount importance in the setting of a bile duct injury.

Suggested Reading

McAneny D. Open cholecystectomy. Surg Clin North Am. 2008; 88(6):1273–94.
Strausberg SM. The "hidden cystic duct" syndrome and the infundibular technique of laparoscopic cholecystectomy—the danger of the false infundibulum. J Am Coll Surg. 2000;191:661–7.
Strausberg SM, Brunt LM. Rational and use of the critical view of safety in laparoscopic cholecystectomy. J Am Coll Surg. 2010; 211(1):132–8.

Percutaneous Cholecystostomy

6

Christine E. Van Cott and Randall S. Zuckerman

Indications

Percutaneous cholecystostomy (PC) is an image-guided method for placement of a drainage catheter into the gallbladder lumen for decompressing the gallbladder either definitively or as a temporizing method. Indications include management of cholecystitis and/or gallbladder access for dissolution/removal of stones.

Preoperative Preparation

PC can be used as an alternative to cholecystectomy in those patients that are high risk for an operation or general anesthesia, such as those with sepsis, organ system failure, acalculous cholecystitis due to critical illness, or those with complications of cholecystitis, such as perforation empyema or abscess. In view of the compromised health of most patients undergoing this procedure, it is imperative that coagulopathies be evaluated for and corrected or improved prior to this procedure. For the majority of patients, the procedure can be done at the bedside; however, it may be preferential to be performed in either radiological suite or operating room depending on the clinical scenario.

For best outcomes, it would be recommended that the practitioner has some training in ultrasound technologies such as the American College of Surgeons Ultrasound for Surgeons: A Basic Course.

C.E. Van Cott, M.D., F.A.C.S.
Frank H. Netter MD School of Medicine, Quinnipiac University,
North Haven Campus, 370 Bassett Road, North Haven,
CT 06473, USA

St. Vincent's Medical Center, 2800 Main Street,
Bridgeport, CT 06606, USA

R.S. Zuckerman, M.D., F.A.C.S. (⊠)
St. Vincent's Medical Center, 2800 Main Street,
Bridgeport, CT 06606, USA
e-mail: randall.zuckerman@stvincents.org

Operative Strategy

Using portable ultrasound equipment and the Seldinger technique, a drainage catheter can be placed in a transhepatic fashion into the gallbladder to achieve immediate drainage and decompression. A curved probe starting at a frequency of 3.5 MZh and adjusting per body habitus is recommended. The transhepatic approach is favored over the transperitoneal route to reduce the risk of bile leakage into the peritoneal cavity and to better anchor the catheter. However, with the transhepatic approach there is an increased risk of hemorrhage and future catheter manipulations are more difficult. While the transperitoneal route does in fact have a lower risk of hemorrhage, it is associated with an increased risk of bile leakage and damage to the adjacent hollow viscus.

Operative Technique

Equipment Needed

Ultrasound machine.
Portable fluoroscopy machine if available.
Sterile ultrasound cover and sterile ultrasound gel.
Local anesthesia.
7–10 Fr general use locking pigtail catheter.
21-Gauge needle (long) on an empty syringe.
0.018 Guidewire with soft tip.
0.035 (or smaller) guidewire with a soft tip.
6–9 Fr dilator.
Gravity drainage bag.

For most patients, this procedure can be performed in the supine position. However prior to skin preparation, the practitioner should determine there route of access because it may be necessary to place some patients in a slight decubitus position.

The patient should be prepped and draped in the usual sterile fashion.

A.L. Halverson and D.C. Borgstrom (eds.), *Advanced Surgical Techniques for Rural Surgeons*,
DOI 10.1007/978-1-4939-1495-1_6, © Springer Science+Business Media New York 2015

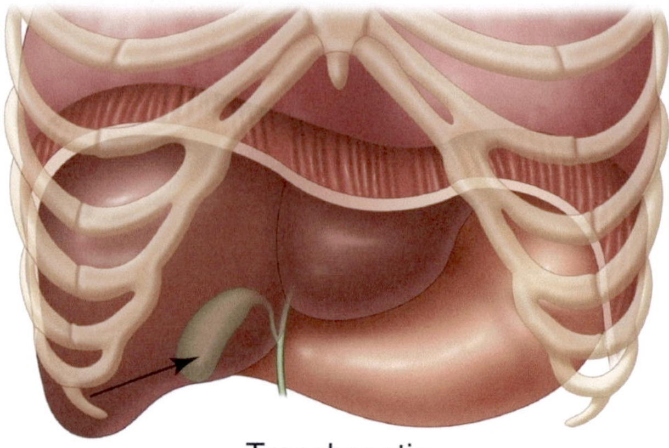

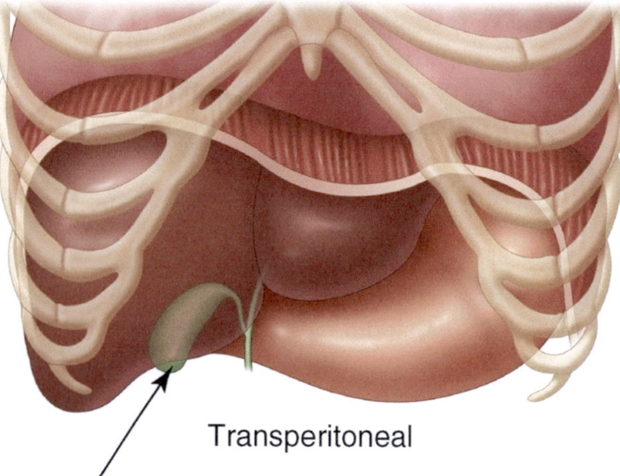

Fig. 6.1 Difference in approach for transhepatic versus transperitoneal approaches

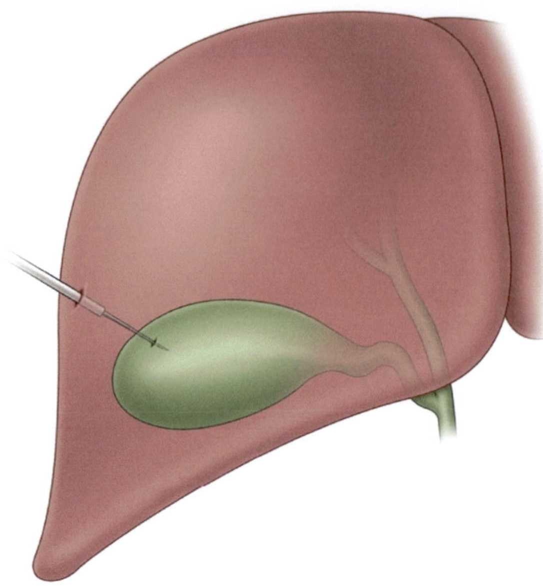

Fig. 6.2 Needle entering gallbladder lumen as seen under fluoroscopy. Contrast can be appreciated in the dependent portion of the gallbladder

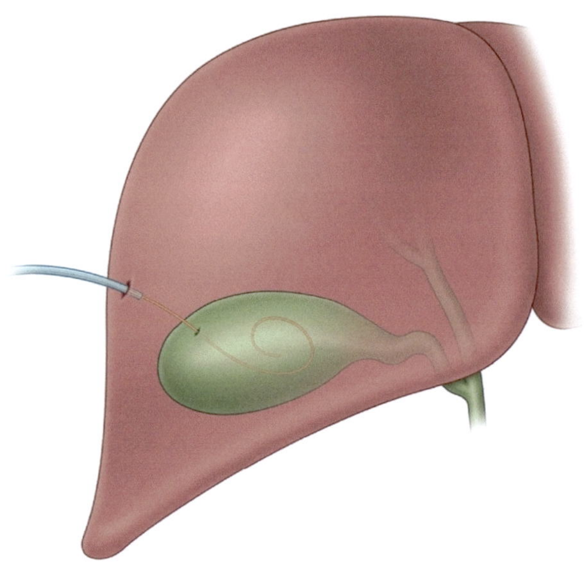

Fig. 6.3 Guidewire in gallbladder lumen as seen under fluoroscopy

Pre-procedural antibiotics according to your hospital guidelines should be administered.

Using ultrasound guidance, the transhepatic route should be determined. The transhepatic route should begin in a subcostal position in the right mid-axillary line aiming to the bare area of the gallbladder where the gallbladder is attached to the liver capsule. Care should be taken to avoid the neurovascular bundle that lies on the inferior surface of each rib. Local anesthetic should be used to not only anesthetize this ultimate catheter tract but also the liver capsule itself. If using the transperitoneal route, access should start in the subcostal position below the liver edge where the gallbladder is best visualized against the anterior abdominal wall (Fig. 6.1).

Under real-time ultrasound guidance, the 21-gauge needle is advanced through the hepatic parenchyma into the gallbladder. Aspiration of either bile or purulent aspirate confirms proper position (Fig. 6.2).

The syringe is then removed from the access needle and soft J-tipped guidewire inserted into the gallbladder. Insertion of the 0.018 guidewire into the gallbladder cavity should be confirmed with ultrasound guidance (Fig. 6.3). Access needle is removed and a 6 Fr sheath advanced over the wire. With the six sheath in place, the 0.018 is replaced with a 0.035 guidewire.

The sheath is removed and an appropriately sized dilator (dependent on ultimate size of final catheter) is placed over the guidewire. The dilator is then removed; pigtail catheter inserted over the guidewire; the guidewire is removed leaving the catheter in position (Fig. 6.4).

Again aspiration of bile or purulent material confirms position. The catheter is also able to be identified in proper

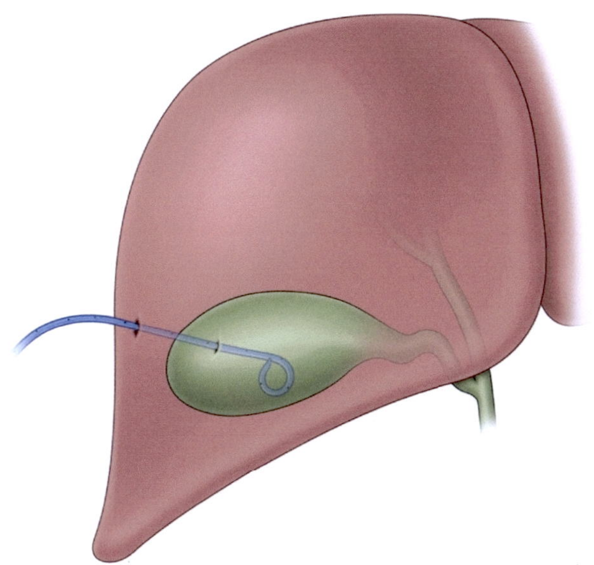

Fig. 6.4 Pigtail catheter in final position within gallbladder lumen. Contrast can be appreciated filling the gallbladder

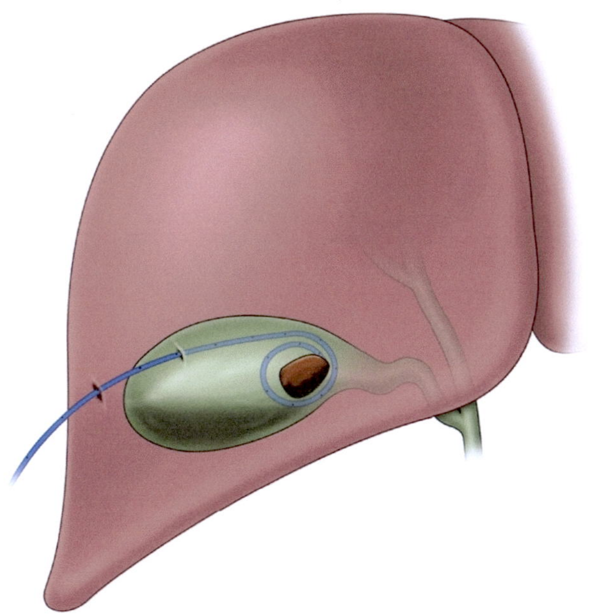

Fig. 6.5 Gallbladder lumen filling with contrast. One can appreciate a single large gallstone occupying the entirety of the gallbladder lumen

position within the gallbladder lumen with ultrasound. If portable fluoroscopy is available, then injection of one half strength contrast into the catheter under real-time fluoroscopy will allow visualization of not only the catheter but the gallbladder lumen itself (Fig. 6.5). If one is experienced with cholangiography, it may be possible at this time to appreciate patency of the cystic duct. If fluoroscopy is not available, then a single X-ray can be taken after administration of contrast.

Once proper position is confirmed the pigtail catheter needs to be securely attached to the skin using either simple locking sutures and an adhesive cover or a commercial fixation device.

If clinically indicated, the catheter can be aspirated and bile/purulent material can be sent for analysis.

The catheter should then be attached to gravity drainage bag.

Potential Pitfalls

Gallbladder manipulation is associated with hypotension and bradycardia in the most critically ill. Atropine should be readily available during the procedure.

Repeat punctures with the access needle should be avoided to decrease the chance of leakage of gallbladder contents into the peritoneal cavity and inadvertent gallbladder decompression making subsequent access more difficult.

Securing the catheter after placement will ensure unnecessary manipulation and avoid the most common complication of dislodgment.

Catheter should be flushed every 6–8 h with 10 cm³ of sterile flush to prevent blockages.

Postoperative Care

PC is technically successful in 90–93 % of cases with an intent to treat success ranging from 65 to 90 % depending on the clinical indication.

Definitive treatment for calculus cholecystitis is a cholecystectomy. PC may be all that is needed for acalculous cholecystitis.

Time to tract maturation is not established and recommendations varies anywhere from 7 days to 6 weeks. Prior to removal of the tube it should be clamped for 24–48 h and patient evaluated for patency of cystic duct (Figs. 6.6 and 6.7) or increasing pain, fevers or elevated WBC. The tube should be removed over a wire after injection of contrast checking for tract maturation. If extravasation is noted, the catheter should be replaced and attempt at removal made again in 2 weeks.

Common Complications

Overall complication rate	5 %
Catheter dislodgement	<1–2 %
Sepsis	2.5–5 %
Hemorrhage	2.2–5 %
Inflammation/Infection (including peritonitis)	2.9–6 %
Damage to other organs	1.6–2 %
Death	2.5–3 %
30 day post-procedural mortality rate	8–36 %

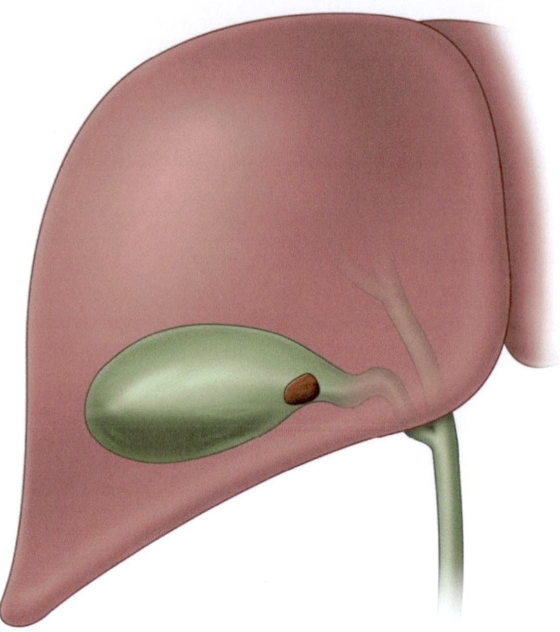

Fig. 6.6 Contrast outlining a large solitary stone in the gallbladder lumen. The common bile duct can now be seen confirming patency of the cystic duct

When to Transfer

Transfer should be considered when either the equipment is not available or when the practitioner does not have proper ultrasound training.

Persistent hemobilia that does not respond to correction of coagulopathy.

Suggested Reading

Abi-Haidar Y, Sanchez V, Williams SA, Itani KMF. Revisiting percutaneous cholecystostomy for acute cholecystitis based on a 10-year experience. Arch Surg. 2012;147(5):416–22.

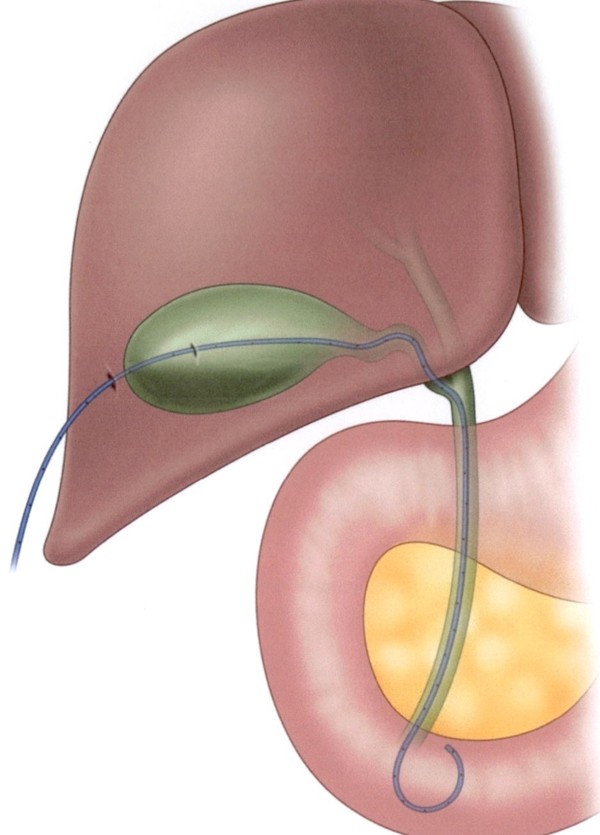

Fig. 6.7 Contrast entering small bowel, confirming patency of the cystic duct. This patient had their tube immediately removed

Jarnagin WR. Blumgart's surgery of the liver, biliary tract, and pancreas. 5th ed. Philadelphia: Elsevier Saunders; 2012. Chapter 32, Percutaneous approaches to the treatment of gallbladder disease; p. 494–496.

Saad WEA, Wallace MJ, Wojak JC, Kundu S, Cardella JF. Quality improvement guidelines for percutaneous transhepatic cholangiography, biliary drainage, and percutaneous cholecystostomy. J Vasc Interv Radiol. 2010;21:789–95.

Part II

Abdominal Wall

Mark Thomas Savarise and Daniel J. Vargo

Introduction

Laparoscopic technique can be used to repair many types of ventral hernias, as an alternative to traditional open hernia repair. It is a procedure that can be performed by surgeons in small hospitals and ambulatory surgery centers, making it appealing as a tool to be employed by rural surgeons, all of whom take care of patients with abdominal wall hernias.

Laparoscopic ventral hernia repair (LVHR), compared to open ventral hernia repair (OVHR), offers potential advantages and disadvantages. These need to be considered in the individual patient to determine the optimal surgical approach. The skill and experience of the surgeon in laparoscopic techniques will influence the choice of technique.

Advantages of LVHR include:

- Avoidance of an incision directly over the prosthesis: this is particularly important in patients with skin problems or wound healing problems that would increase the chance of exposure and infection of the mesh prosthesis in OVHR (Fig. 7.1).
- The ability to repair multiple defects with a single prosthetic through small laparoscopy incisions.
- Cosmetic advantage of laparoscopic surgery.
- Less pain and faster recovery: many studies have documented the decreased need for pain medication in the postoperative period and earlier return to normal activities with LVHR compared to OVHR.

Disadvantages of LVHR include:

- Increased cost of operative supplies.
- Need for general anesthesia in all cases.
- Typically, increased time of operation, especially early in the surgeon's experience.

- Need for specialized coated mesh: intraperitoneal placement of mesh means that it is likely to come in contact with the bowel.
- Higher risk for missed intestinal injury, with possibility of fistula, sepsis, and death.

Indications

Nearly all ventral hernias can be approached laparoscopically. As the complexity of the hernia increases and/or the number of patient comorbidities increase, the skill level required to repair the hernia will also increase. Thus the true indication for a laparoscopic ventral hernia repair is dependent on the comfort level of the surgeon. Primary ventral hernias (umbilical or epigastric) and first time incisional hernias are the most straightforward, and the vast majority of these are candidates for laparoscopic repair. Multiply recurrent hernias, incarcerated hernias, and parastomal hernias are more complicated but still may be approached with LVHR. Often these patients see the most benefit from LVHR, compared to OVHR. Complex abdominal wall reconstruction for hernia with loss of domain remains an open procedure.

Preoperative Preparation

Patient preparation is identical to that for OVHR. Patients with comorbid conditions need these optimized prior to elective repair. Smoking cessation, weight loss, and control of diabetes and metabolic deficits have the same advantages in decreased complications and increased chance for successful repair in LVHR as in OVHR. Consider a CT scan to image the hernia anatomy, but it is not absolutely necessary. Consider a bowel prep only if the patient has large intestine in the hernia. All patients should receive a dose of prophylactic preoperative antibiotics and DVT prophylaxis.

M.T. Savarise, M.D., F.A.C.S. (✉) • D.J. Vargo, F.A.C.S.
Department of Surgery, University of Utah, 30 North Medical Drive, #3B-113, Salt Lake City, UT 84132, USA
e-mail: mark.savarise@utah.edu

A.L. Halverson and D.C. Borgstrom (eds.), *Advanced Surgical Techniques for Rural Surgeons*,
DOI 10.1007/978-1-4939-1495-1_7, © Springer Science+Business Media New York 2015

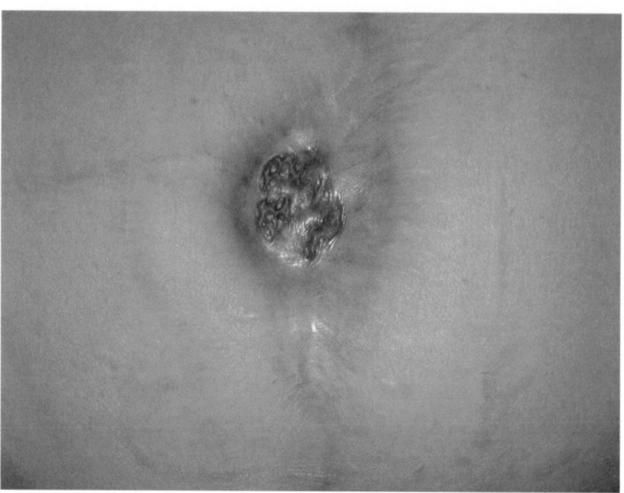

Fig. 7.1 Wound over hernia defect

Most importantly, ensure that you have the proper supplies for your operation. In addition to an angled 5 mm laparoscope and standard laparoscopy supplies, you will need a mechanical fixation device, a suture passing device, and an assortment of sizes of specialty mesh that include an adhesion barrier bonded to one side. Mesh is either polypropylene or polyester, and there are several proprietary adhesion barrier systems that are applied to one side of the mesh. It is also helpful to have access to energy sources that will help with the dissection of the hernia, such as bipolar cautery shears or ultrasonic dissection.

Operative Strategy

The hernia is approached from within the peritoneum, reduced, and repaired with an intraperitoneal onlay of permanent mesh. This mesh is then secured to the abdominal wall with transfascial fixation sutures placed through the entire abdominal wall. The mesh overlaps the healthy fascia by at least 5 cm in every direction.

Proper initial placement of the trocars is essential to facilitate completion of the procedure. Trocars should be placed away from the defect, far enough to allow the surgeon to work at a reasonable angle to fix the defect, but close enough to allow the instruments to reach the furthest part of the mesh. Surgeon and assistant typically work from one side of the defect, but must be able to alter their positions and placement of the scope and instruments through their ports to work around all sides of the hernia. Primary and slave video monitors are needed if the surgeon will be working from more than one angle, which is often the case (Fig. 7.2).

Operative Technique

The patient is placed under general anesthesia with complete muscle relaxation. The arm on the side where the surgeon plans to work should be tucked to allow the surgeon and assistant to operate without restriction. Foley catheter placement may be necessary for lower abdominal hernias and cases that are expected to take a long time. The abdomen should be prepped and draped as widely as possible. Initial planning for trocar placement is critical.

If the hernia is in the midline, the first choice for Veress needle placement is at the costal margin in the left upper quadrant. The abdominal wall is fixed at this point, the liver is not near the entry point, and most patients have not had surgery in this region. The right upper quadrant would be an alternative if prior left upper quadrant surgery has been performed. A laparoscopic port can then be placed at any desired location. If a Hasson approach is going to be utilized, then placement can be in either the right or left abdomen, depending on lowest expected adhesions. The angled 5 mm laparoscope is then inserted, and the additional 2 or 3 ports can be placed under direct vision. A 4-port technique is useful to allow the surgeon to operate with both hands, the assistant to hold the scope and provide additional retraction with a grasper. The ports are best arrayed in a semicircle around about half the circumference of the hernia. When placing the ports, consider that mesh will overlap normal fascia 5 cm away from the hernia defect; ports placed too close to the defect will not be of use to secure the mesh. One port must be at least 10 mm to accommodate introduction of the mesh (Fig. 7.3).

Once all ports are placed, the first step is reduction of the hernia and lysis of adhesions to the anterior abdominal wall. The surgeon should identify any bowel adherent or incarcerated and take special care to use only atraumatic graspers there. Omentum can be grasped with traumatic instruments. Scissor dissection, monopolar cautery, bipolar cautery, and ultrasonic dissection are all appropriate options, but care must be taken when using cautery around the bowel. Clearing away all adhesions widely around the hernia defect is important to allow placement of the mesh (Fig. 7.4).

For incisional hernias, it is not uncommon to identify additional occult defects beneath the incision. A single piece of mesh can cover the entire area. It is unnecessary to remove the hernia sac from the subcutaneous space. If there has been a previous repair, the old mesh may be apparent. Generally this can be left in situ. Rotation of the bed and use of Trendelenberg and reverse-Trendelenberg positions may aid the dissection. Moving the scope to different ports and rotating the scope's angle of view allow visualization of the hernia contents from different perspectives, which reduces the chance of bowel injury.

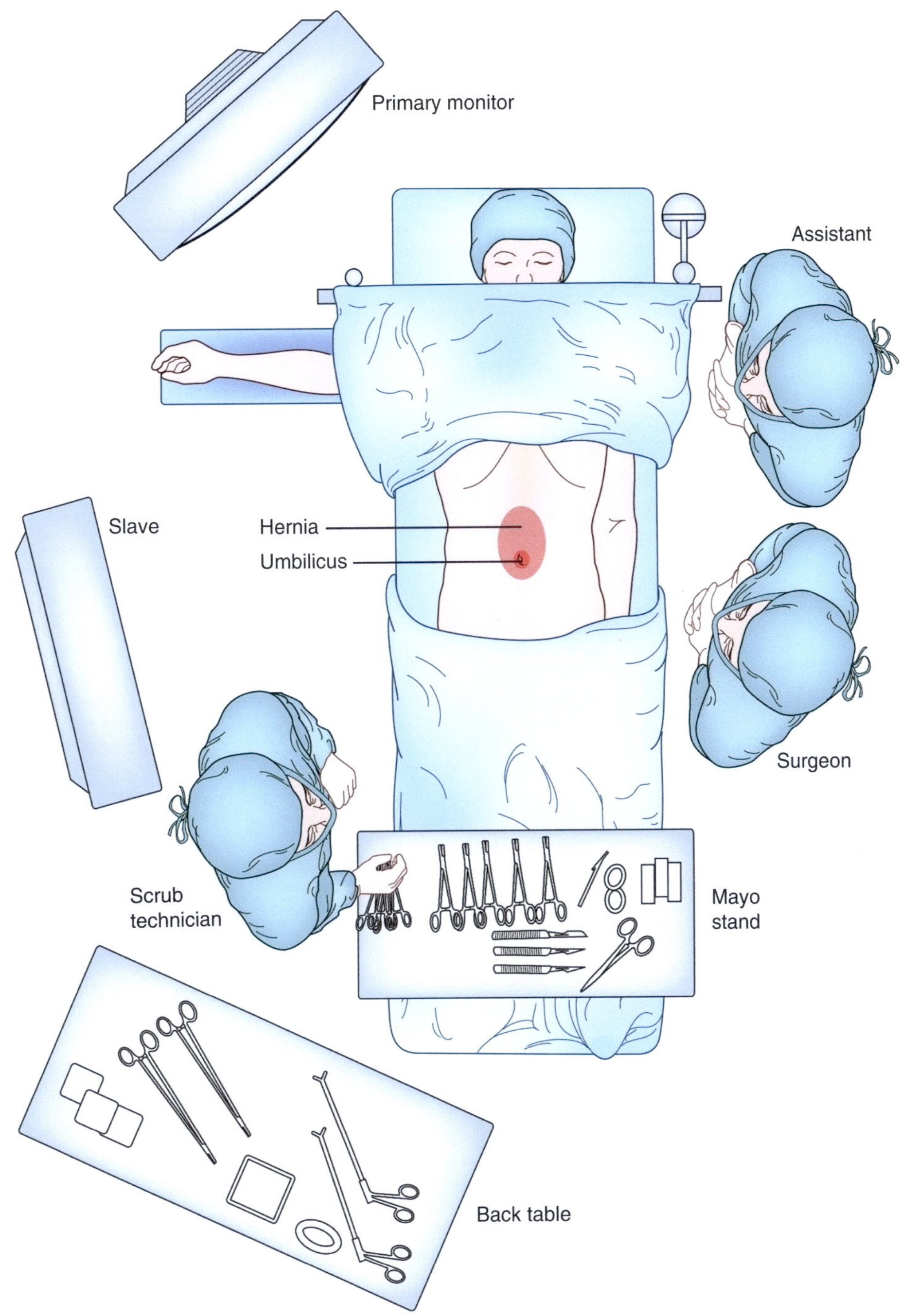

Fig. 7.2 Illustration of typical patient setup

Once the dissection has been completed, the surgeon should look down at the abdominal contents for any ongoing bleeding or any sign of bowel injury or leak. Sponges or suction and irrigation can be helpful.

The next step is measurement of the defect and appropriate mesh onlay. A ruler can be introduced into the abdomen. Alternatively, the defect size can be measured on the abdominal skin. To do this, the surgeon uses a hypodermic needle to puncture through the skin to the edges of the defect, and marks these points externally. Because the abdomen is insufflated, this will overestimate the size of the defect. The abdomen can be desufflated prior to measuring on the skin.

A mesh is then cut to the appropriate size, designed to overlap normal fascia by at least 5 cm in all directions. Four to six permanent sutures, about 10 cm long, are placed around the edges of the mesh. Mesh orientation can be assured by

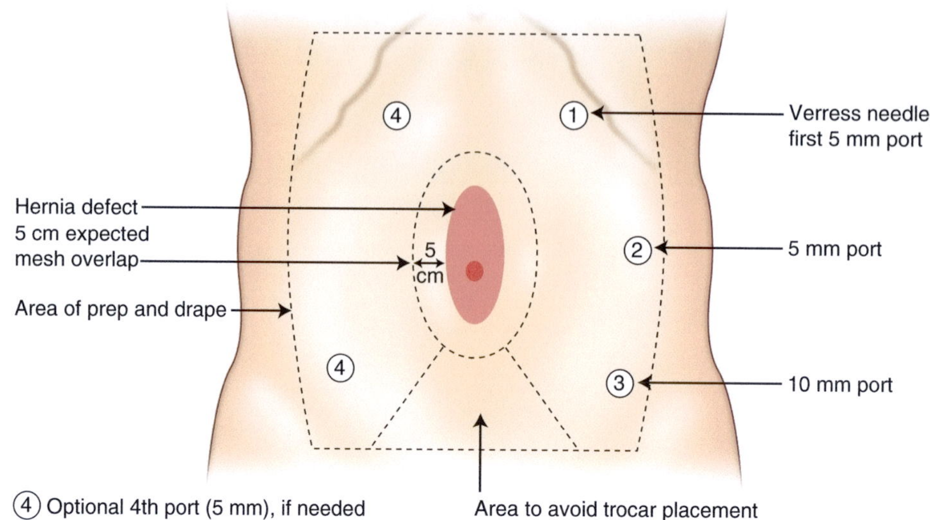

Fig. 7.3 Port placement for periumbilical midline hernia

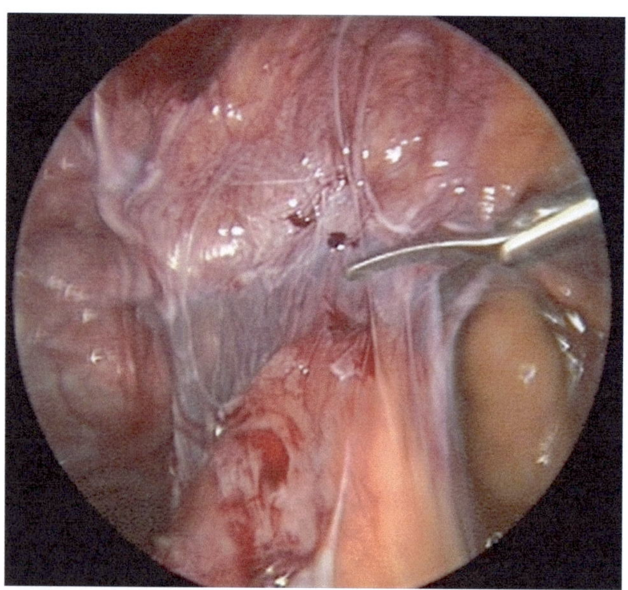

Fig. 7.4 Intraoperative view of dissection

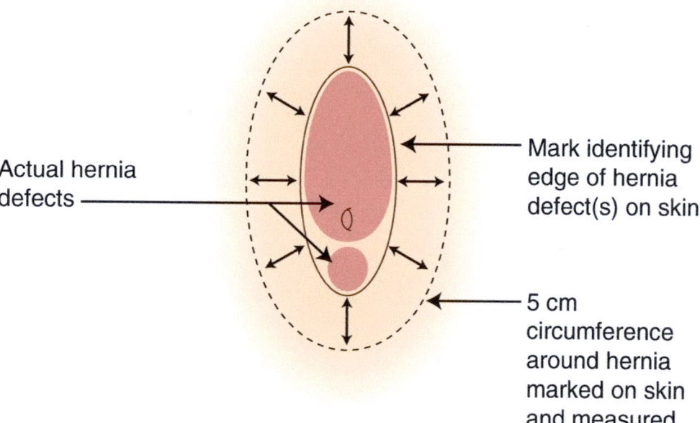

Fig. 7.5 Marking and measuring mesh size on anterior abdominal wall

marking the superior or inferior aspect of the mesh prior to insertion into the abdomen. The mesh is then rolled and placed through the larger port into the abdomen (Fig. 7.5).

At this point, it is essential that the unrolled mesh is oriented correctly in the patient. The coated side of the mesh must be down. If the mesh is not circular, the long axis must align with the long axis of the defect.

The pre-tied sutures in the mesh are used to secure the mesh to the abdominal wall. The surgeon makes small skin incisions with an 11-blade, 5 cm away from the marked edges of the hernia defect, and a suture passer grasps each suture to bring it up through the abdominal wall. The surgeon or assistant "hands" the suture end to the passer with a grasper placed through one of the trocars. Each pair of sutures is held with a hemostat and all are tied after all of the sutures have been retrieved. The mesh should be flat against the abdominal wall at this point.

Additional permanent sutures can now be placed at intervals around the circumference of the mesh. The number of sutures depends on the size of mesh. Each suture is placed through a skin stab incision, through the fascia and through the edge of the mesh. A grasper holds the suture. The passer is removed and replaced, the suture end grasped and pulled to the skin, and the suture is tied.

In addition, a mechanical fixation device can be used to place anchors to hold the mesh to the fascia. It should be noted that these anchors do not permanently secure the mesh and should not replace the transfixing suture. Absorbable

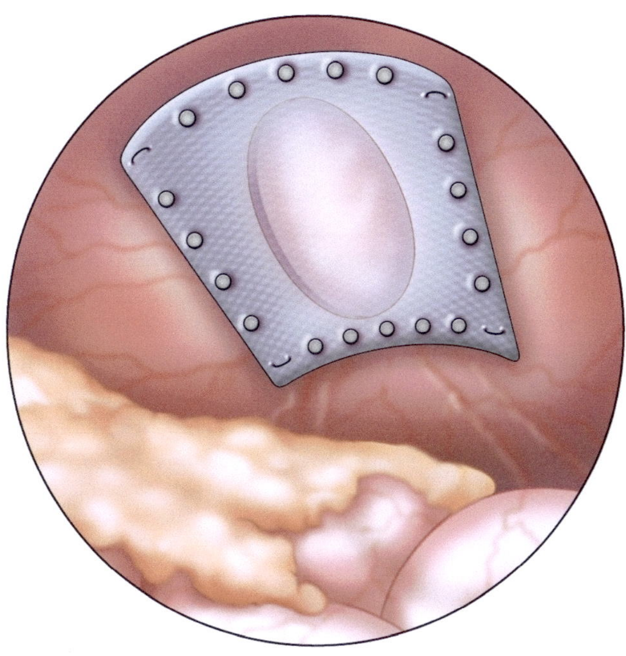

Fig. 7.6 Completed mesh repair

anchors are recommended, as permanent anchors may be associated with chronic pain (Fig. 7.6).

Once the mesh is secure and prior to desufflating the abdomen, a suture placed with the passer should be used to secure the fascia at the 10 mm port incision. Finally, the port site skin incisions are closed with absorbable sutures. The stab incisions require only steri strips.

Potential Pitfalls

A common technical problem during LVHR is limitation in the ability to use instruments placed through trocars in the lower abdomen, where the working handle of the instrument is impeded by contact with the patient's thighs. To avoid this, first resist the urge to place a comfortable pillow under the patient's knees. Second, try to avoid placing working ports below the level of the umbilicus and medial to the mid-clavicular line. Low ports should be placed under laparoscopic visualization as far lateral as possible while avoiding the colon (Fig. 7.7).

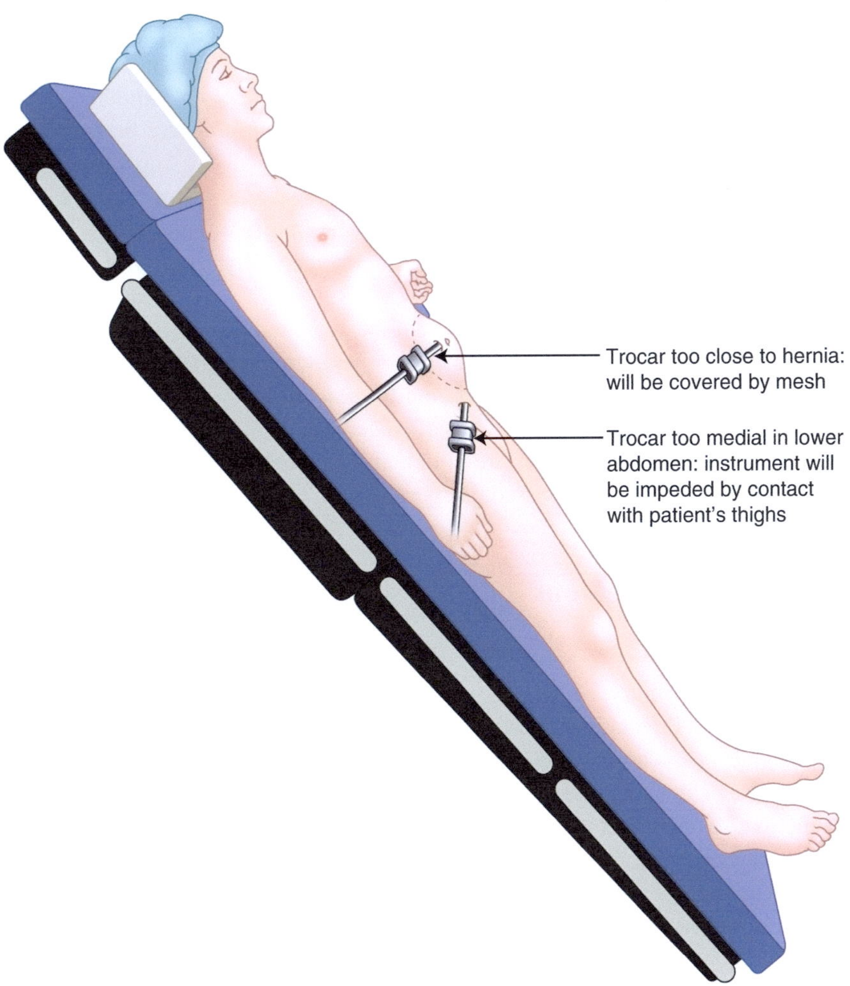

Fig. 7.7 Illustration of poor trocar placement

When placing the mesh, if the surgeon has overestimated the defect size, the mesh will not lie flat against the abdominal wall. In this case, one or more of the transfixing sutures can be released. A second skin incision is made and the sutures are re-grasped further from the fascial edges.

With larger defects, placement and fixation of the mesh at full insufflation can lead to the mesh ballooning into the defect when the abdomen is desufflated. One can avoid this by passing the sutures and placing the anchors at a lower insufflation pressure (8–10 mmHg).

The epigastric vessels and subcutaneous vessels can be injured with suture placement, so care must be taken to avoid this. If bleeding from abdominal wall vessels is encountered due to injury by either the suture passer or trocar, the vessel can be ligated with one or two transfixing abdominal wall sutures placed around the vessel with the suture passer.

Hernias that are very superior or inferior in the abdomen can also present special difficulties if one border of the hernia is the costal margin or the pubis.

In this case, adequate overlap of the mesh will require it be secured to or around a bony structure.

Postoperative Care

The size and complexity of the hernia determines to a large extent the length of recovery. Patients who undergo repair of small hernias are managed as outpatients with oral pain medications and immediate resumption of diet. All patients should be counseled to avoid heavy lifting for the first few weeks, but should also be encouraged to resume other daily activities as soon as possible.

Patients with large hernias or significant incarceration of viscera will often develop some degree of postoperative ileus. These patients may require hospitalization for several days, and intravenous narcotic pain control is often necessary.

Atelectasis and constipation are common postoperative problems that should be addressed prospectively.

Common Complications

The most serious early complication of this procedure is a missed intestinal injury, which will result in subsequent leak, possible fistula, infection of the mesh, and possible sepsis. It is absolutely essential to identify any intestinal injury. Serosal tears can be repaired, and the operation can be completed. A safe technique to avoid serious complications if a bowel injury is encountered is to complete the lysis of adhesions, reduction of the hernia and repair of the bowel at the time of initial operation. The operation is completed without repair of the hernia, and then staged with a second operation for mesh placement. In this case, the first operation is coded

44180, laparoscopy with lysis of adhesions. The second operation is coded 49652-49657, laparoscopic repair of ventral, umbilical, epigastric, spegelian, or incisional hernia, and should be appended with modifiers -52, reduced services and -58, staged procedure.

Delayed recognition of a visceral injury can result in life-threatening complications; these patients may be best managed by stabilization and transfer to a higher level of care.

Recurrent hernia is recognized as a complication in approximately 5–10 % of patients.

A common postoperative occurrence is development of a seroma at the hernia site. Because the sac is not removed, the space above the mesh fills with fluid. The patient should be counseled of this preoperatively. Generally, no action is required and the seroma is left to reabsorb.

When to Transfer

The decision to perform LVHR should be based on the surgeon's familiarity with the procedure and the patient's characteristics. A referral should be made when the patient is best served with LVHR (rather than open VHR) but the surgeon is not comfortable with the complexity of the hernia (very large hernias, or incarcerated hernias).

Another situation in which referral to a larger hospital may be appropriate arises when the surgeon must plan on using a biologic mesh, due to contamination or wound problems that increase the risk of mesh infection. Large biologic mesh prostheses can cost $20,000. Small hospitals often cannot afford to stock these products. Prior to the planned procedure, the surgeon should work with his hospital and the patient's insurance carrier to be sure the hospital will be reimbursed for the cost of the mesh.

A patient who has loss of abdominal domain, who will require complex abdominal wall reconstruction should be referred, unless the surgeon is experienced in these procedures, which are long and difficult.

Finally, a patient who develops a complication from a missed bowel injury during LVHR should be stabilized and referred to a tertiary care center. These patients will require management of their sepsis, their injured bowel, and their abdominal wall defect. These are complex patients who are at risk for many secondary complications.

Suggested Reading

Colavita PD, Walters AL, Tsirline VB, Belyansky I, Lincourt AE, Kercher KW, Sing RF, Heniford BT. The regionalization of ventral hernia repair: occurrence and outcomes over a decade. Am Surg. 2013;79(7):693–701.

Jenkins ED, Yom VH, Melman L, Pierce RA, Schuessler RB, Frisella MM, Christopher Eagon J, Michael Brunt L, Matthews BD. Clinical predictors of operative complexity in laparoscopic ventral hernia repair: a prospective study. Surg Endosc. 2010;24(8):1872–7.

Melvin WS, Renton D. Laparoscopic ventral hernia repair. World J Surg. 2011;35(7):1496–9.

Rogmark P, Petersson U, Bringman S, Eklund A, Ezra E, Sevonius D, Smedberg S, Osterberg J, Montgomery A. Short-term outcomes for open and laparoscopic midline incisional hernia repair: a randomized multicenter controlled trial: the ProLOVE (prospective randomized trial on open versus laparoscopic operation of ventral eventrations) trial. Ann Surg. 2013;258(1):37–45.

Sauerland S, Walgenbach M, Habermalz B, Seiler CM, Miserez M. Laparoscopic versus open surgical techniques for ventral or incisional hernia repair. Cochrane Database Syst Rev. 2011;3, CD007781.

Tintinu AJ, Asonganyi W, Turner PL. Staged laparoscopic ventral and incisional hernia repair when faced with enterotomy or suspicion of an enterotomy. J Natl Med Assoc. 2012;104(3–4):202–10.

Closure Repair of Complex Ventral Hernias: Open with Separation of Parts

W. Thomas Huntsman

Indications

A symptomatic ventral hernia defect that is a result of a significant loss of structural integrity or tissue: this would include delayed closures from abdominal catastrophe, multiple recurrent hernias, or loss of abdominal wall from infection, trauma, or tumor.

Preoperative Preparation

Repairs of these large defects carry unique problems with loss of abdominal domain, altered abdominal physiology, and prolonged ileus. It is very important that the risks are clearly defined as they may be greater than the benefits.

Generally, the larger the hernia, the less likely the risk of incarceration. Very careful analysis of the patient's preoperative state is critical to avoid problems. These operations should be considered elective and every attempt should be made to anticipate potential postoperative problems.

The work-up of these patients should obviously include a detailed history and physical appropriate for any major surgical procedure. Preexisting conditions that would increase the risk of recurrence, such as ascites, diabetes, smoking, prostate disease, multiple recurrences, or nutritional depletion, must be addressed. A preoperative CT scan is very important to identify the location of primary and secondary defects that may not be apparent. Reviews of previous operative notes will give clues to potential problems that are best not repeated. Use of mesh, conditions of the tissue, and previous techniques are very important for preoperative planning. In addition, pulmonary function tests are strongly indicated for large defects with possible domain loss.

The ventral hernia working group analysis helps to define the postoperative risk of a surgical site occurrence (see Table 8.1).

Anatomy

In order to plan a successful abdominal wall reconstruction (AWR), understanding the anatomy is critical. Failure rates of 30 % or more are routine. The better the surgeon understands the anatomy, the easier it is to plan an effective reconstruction.

Effective abdominal integrity requires an intact and compliant musculofascial layer. These muscles are the paired rectus abdominis, external oblique, internal oblique, and the transverse abdominis. Together with the fascial aponeuroses, these tissues create a supportive frame-up that maintains abdominal function. A disruption of the fascial support creates weakness that persistent abdominal pressure exploits (Fig. 8.1).

Understanding the orientation of the muscles is critical. The rectus abdominis is a paired, vertically oriented muscle covered by a strong fascial sheath. Two thirds down the muscle is the arcuate line. Above the arcuate line the anterior sheath consists of the entire external oblique fascia, and half of the internal oblique fascia. The posterior sheath is the other half of the internal oblique, the transversus abdominis fascia, and the transversalis fascia. However, below the arcuate line the posterior sheath consists of only transversalis fascia. This creates a potential weakness (Fig. 8.2).

The linea alba is the fusion between the two rectus fascias. This structure is important in maintaining the structural integrity of the anterior abdominal wall.

The rectus muscle has a vigorous blood supply by the superior and inferior epigastric arteries. In addition supply is from the terminal branches of the intercostals. This blood supply allows the muscle to be used in many ways. Importantly, the skin above the muscle is supplied by these epigastric perforators (Fig. 8.3).

W.T. Huntsman, M.D. (✉)
Division of Plastic Surgery, Bassett Medical Center,
1 Atwell Road, Cooperstown, NY 13326, USA
e-mail: thomas.huntman@bassett.org

A.L. Halverson and D.C. Borgstrom (eds.), *Advanced Surgical Techniques for Rural Surgeons*,
DOI 10.1007/978-1-4939-1495-1_8, © Springer Science+Business Media New York 2015

Table 8.1 As the grade increases, the potential for postoperative complications increases

Grade 1	Grade 2	Grade 3	Grade 4
Low risk	*Comorbid*	*Potentially contaminated*	*Infected*
• Low risk of complications	• Smoker	• Previous wound infection	• Infected mesh
• No history of wound infection	• Obese	• Stoma present	• Septic dehiscence
	• Diabetic	• Violation of the gastrointestinal tract	
	• Immunosuppressed		
	• COPD		

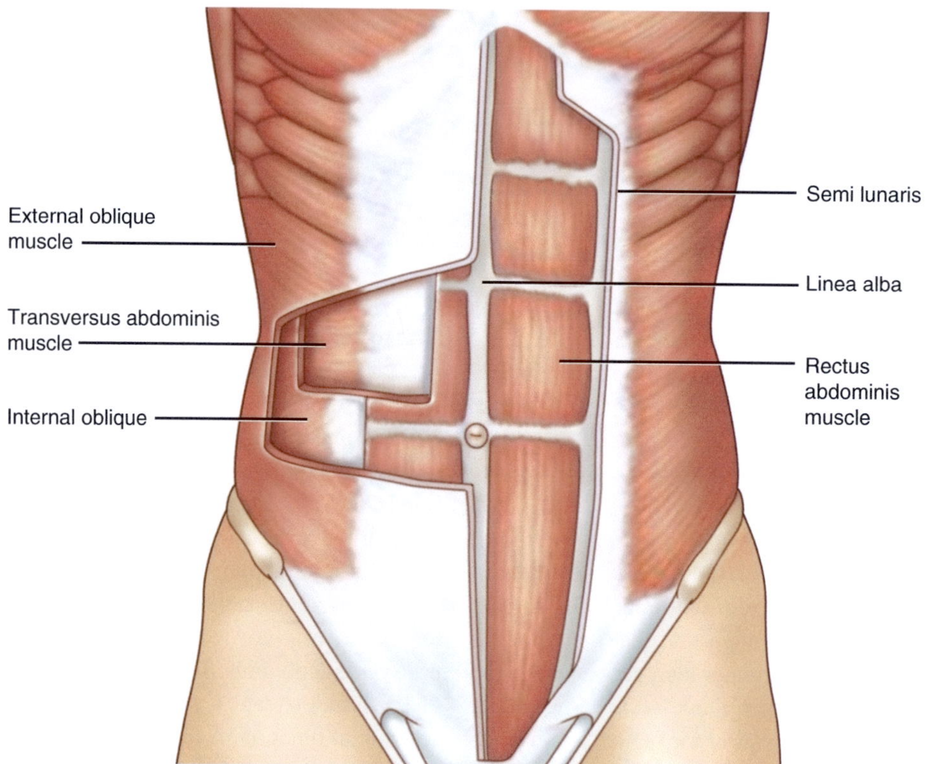

Fig. 8.1 Rectus abdominis, external, internal, and transverse abdominis anatomy

Lateral to the rectus muscle is the linea semilunaris. This is the fascial attachment of the obliques to the rectus sheath. It too is an important landmark.

The obliques can be identified by the direction of the muscles. The external oblique is the largest of the muscles. Its fibers travel from lateral to inferior medial—like hands in pockets. The internal oblique travels from lateral to superior medial. While the transversus abdominis inserts directly transversely into the rectus sheath. The blood supply and nerves to these muscles travel between the internal oblique and the transversus (Fig. 8.4).

Operative Strategy

Rather than consider hernias as simple repairs, the term AWR gives greater understanding to the complexity of the process.

The goals are to prevent strangulation/incarceration, reestablish the linea alba, and create a functional myofascial abdominal wall.

The planning of repair of ventral hernias depends on a number of considerations. If the patient has been medically stabilized, a determination should be made of the timing of repairs. If the patient has a stable hernia, then planning the repair is significantly different than if there is contamination, bowel problems, or the loss of a functional protective abdominal wall. In this situation the initial goal is to use standard surgical processes to obtain a clean wound. Once this has been achieved then temporary coverage of the wound will allow stabilization of the patient and allow a definitive reconstruction at a later time. The urge to repair an unstable patient or unstable wound is bound to fail catastrophically. The idea should be to consider every repair as a staged elective process and maximize the preoperative preparation.

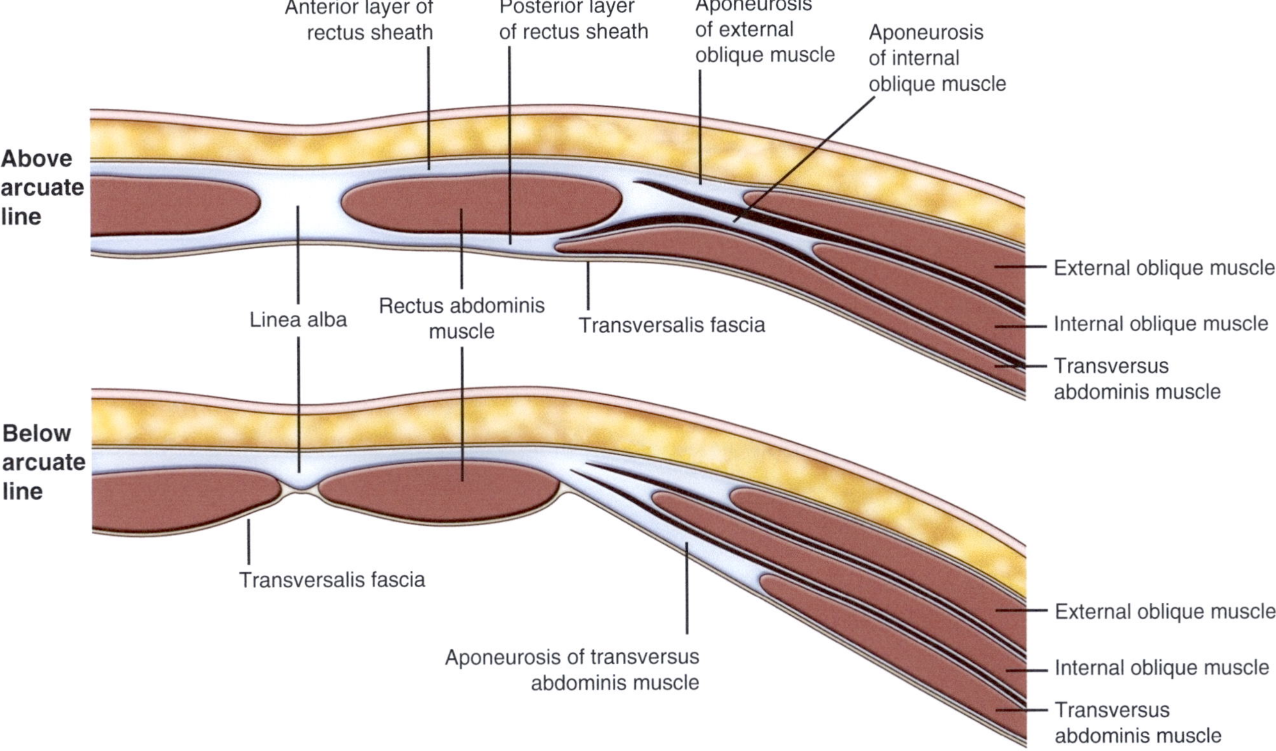

Fig. 8.2 The rectus sheath

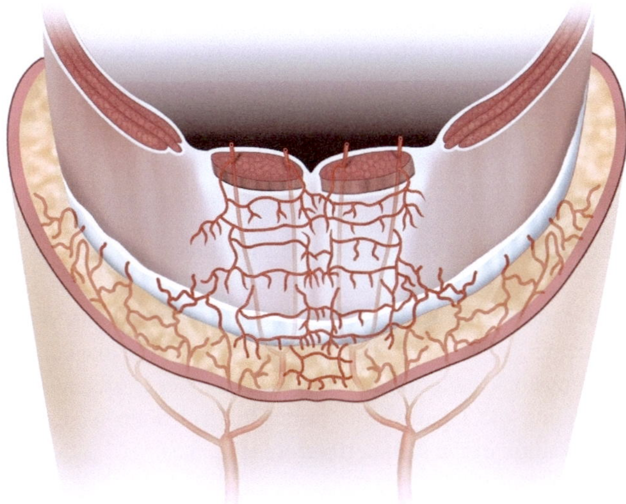

Fig. 8.3 Epigastric perforators. Note that they arise from the inferior and superior epigastric vessels close to the midline

Operative Technique

Before undergoing surgical repair, it is important to understand mesh, its different types, and its indications.

Mesh

The technique of hernia repair has changed dramatically with the introduction of mesh. The improvement in repairs with these materials has changed the management of hernias.

However, there has been an explosion of devices and products. They can be conveniently divided into two categories: prosthetic meshes and bio-prosthetics. To understand hernia repair, it is important to get an understanding of the advantages and disadvantages of both.

There are multiple studies comparing these products; unfortunately, none thus far have provided much clarity as to any clear benefit of one product over another. Therefore, the surgeon is left to practice by trial and error.

Since 1950 polypropylene has probably been the most common synthetic material. It is inexpensive, lightweight, and has a monofilament structure that aids in incorporation and decreases the risk for infection. It is used to greatest advantage in the clean wound with good soft tissue coverage. It is incorporated into the tissue wall. This process has been improved with lighter weight mesh with a macroscopic pore structure. These changes improve compliance and incorporation. However, polypropylene is frowned upon in contaminated wounds. There also is a major concern about the possibility of bowel erosion and fistula formation.

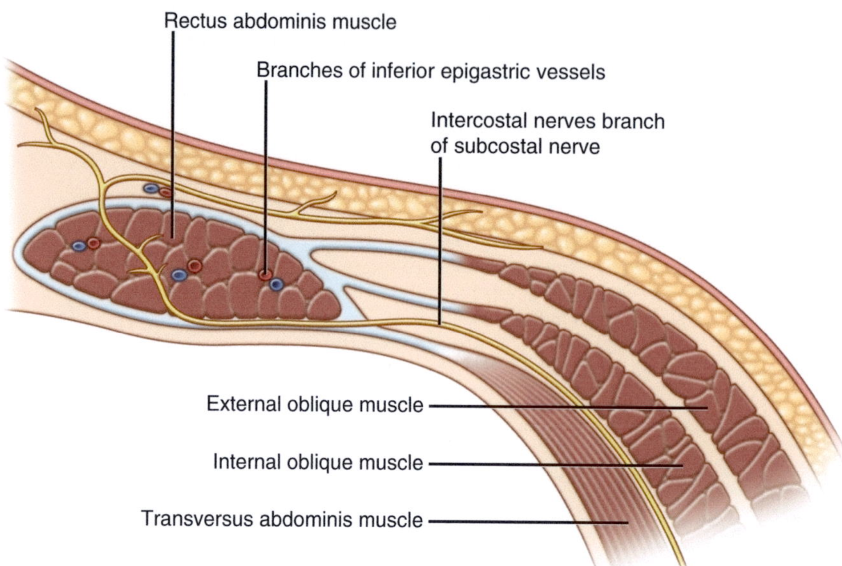

Fig. 8.4 Association of the nerves and vessels to the muscles

In contrast (PTFE) (Gore-Tex) mesh was designed to prevent tissue adherence. However, this quality is also its largest problem. The absence of tissue adherence leads to poor incorporation of the material with high rates of failure which includes infection. In contrast to tissue incorporation, encapsulation prevents the mesh from providing adequate support with poor compliance matching and high rate of failure. For this reason, it is rarely used in typical situations.

Further developments and inventions have concentrated on the use of composite materials. These are a synthetic prosthetic covered with an absorbable membrane. These products have the theoretical advantage of nonabsorbable materials, and avoid the problems of adhesion to bowel, etc. However, there are no studies that demonstrate a significant advantage of one product over the other.

Polyglactin 910 mesh (vicryl) is a completely absorbable product that was another approach to solving the infectious potential of mesh. It is inert and 95 % absorbed by one month. It is mainly used in contaminated fields to provide temporary support until a definitive repair can be set up. Its use as a permanent solution is lacking because it is completely absorbed with a recurrence of the hernia defect.

In spite of the improvement in preventing hernia recurrences, the prosthetic meshes are still troubled by recurrences and a high rate of infection. The goal was to reproduce tissue that would mimic normal wall function and as well be incorporated into the native tissue. This is the field of bio-prosthetics. These compounds are designed to be re-vascularized and integrated like native tissue. These materials come from a variety of animal or human sources. They can be cross-linked for strength or not for better tissue ingrowth. There are three major types in practice: acellular porcine dermis, acellular human dermis, and porcine small intestinal submucosa. The theoretical advantage of these products is better tissue compliance and reduced risk of infection. However, the literature suggests that there is still a higher rate of recurrence with these bio-prosthetics. They are very costly, and depending on the degree of cross-linkage have a tendency to stretch. It is hard to justify their use in the straightforward case.

Technical Repair: Positioning and Marking

The patient is positioned in a supine position with arms abducted. A Foley catheter and a gastric tube are placed. All old incisions including excess skin and scars are marked (including old laparoscopic port sites and drain locations) and location of the skin perforators (Fig. 8.5).

Initial Operative Hernia Management

Incision

A full midline laparotomy incision is made, with an elliptical skin component to remove the old scar. The incision is stopped at the level of the pubis; generally do not extend the incision onto or below the pannus where skin care issues may compromise the incision*. Safe access to the abdominal cavity is critical to avoid bowel injury and is best achieved by

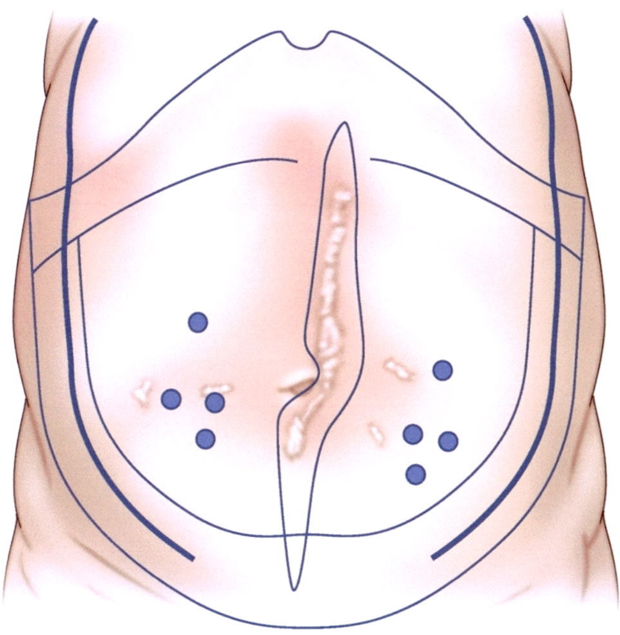

Fig. 8.5 Marking extra skin, scars, and location of the perforators

opening the fascia in an area remote from the hernia (above or below the old incision). Avoid aggressive subcutaneous dissection around the periumbilical area in order to protect the skin perforators.

*However, since many of these patients have a large abdominal pannus, this can complicate the incisional approach. The weight of this skin and its poor quality will interfere with wound healing. A transverse incision above the groin crease can allow a conservative panniculectomy. Removing the skin below the umbilicus gives excellent exposure, protects the skin perforators, removes troublesome old incisions, and places the skin closure perpendicular to the hernia closure. This can minimize wound healing problems in some patients.

Addressing Foreign Bodies and Adhesions

Visceral adhesions to the anterior abdominal wall and pelvis are fully lysed. This is critical to allow full medial mobility of the posterior abdominal wall components. Avoid unnecessary injury to the posterior layers of the abdominal wall (peritoneum and transversalis fascia) during this portion of the procedure. Take down adhesions that interfere with the fascial edges. Remove all foreign bodies (old sutures, mesh, etc.).

Retrorectus Dissection

An incision is made in the posterior rectus sheath within 0.5 cm of its medial border. This incision is extended superiorly and inferiorly, spanning the entire length of the rectus

muscle (Fig. 8.6a). Working from medial to lateral, the plane is continued using blunt and atraumatic dissection. Care must be taken to avoid injury to the epigastric vessels, which should remain with the muscle, not the posterior sheath, during the dissection (Fig. 8.6b). The lateral limit of this dissection is the linea semilunaris at the lateral boarder of the rectus muscle, where the anterior and posterior rectus sheaths fuse (Fig. 8.6c). Identification and preservation of the intercostal neurovascular structures as they enter the posterior aspect of the rectus muscle is crucial. Superiorly, this plane is extended into the retroxyphoid space. Inferiorly, the plane extends into the space of Retzius. Blunt dissection in this avascular plane permits exposure to the midline, symphysis pubis, and Cooper's ligaments bilaterally. Care must be exercised here to avoid injury to the inferior epigastric vessels at their origin on the iliac vessels.

Reconstruction of Posterior Layer

The posterior rectus sheath is reapproximated in the midline (Fig. 8.7). Any holes created in the posterior layer during dissection must be closed. Defects in the posterior layer are common in areas where the abdominal wall has been traversed (laparoscopic port sites, drain sites, old incisions) and below the arcuate line (where there is no transversus abdominis muscle within the posterior layer). Small holes that cannot be repaired primarily with suture can be closed with native tissue such as omentum or the hernia sac. Larger holes are best closed by patching the defect with absorbable mesh such as (vicryl).

Mesh Placement

For patients with clean wounds, a large light-weight, macroporous, polypropylene mesh is used. In potentially contaminated wounds the use of biological mesh may be considered. The mesh is trimmed as appropriate and is anchored inferiorly using a single transfascial stitch just above the pubic ramus or bilateral sutures placed into Cooper's ligaments using absorbable suture (0 PDS or equivalent) to secure the mesh. The mesh should be positioned with at least 4 cm overlap. If other concurrent hernias exist, the mesh can be positioned to cover those as well. Working on one side and then the other, full thickness transfascial sutures are placed to secure the mesh (Fig. 8.8). The sutures can be brought out through the skin through small stab wounds to avoid aggressive subcutaneous undermining. Tension on the medial rectus muscle toward midline is needed as the transfascial sutures are placed. This allows the mesh to absorb much of the force needed to move the rectus muscles toward the midline. This not only permits primary fascial closure over the

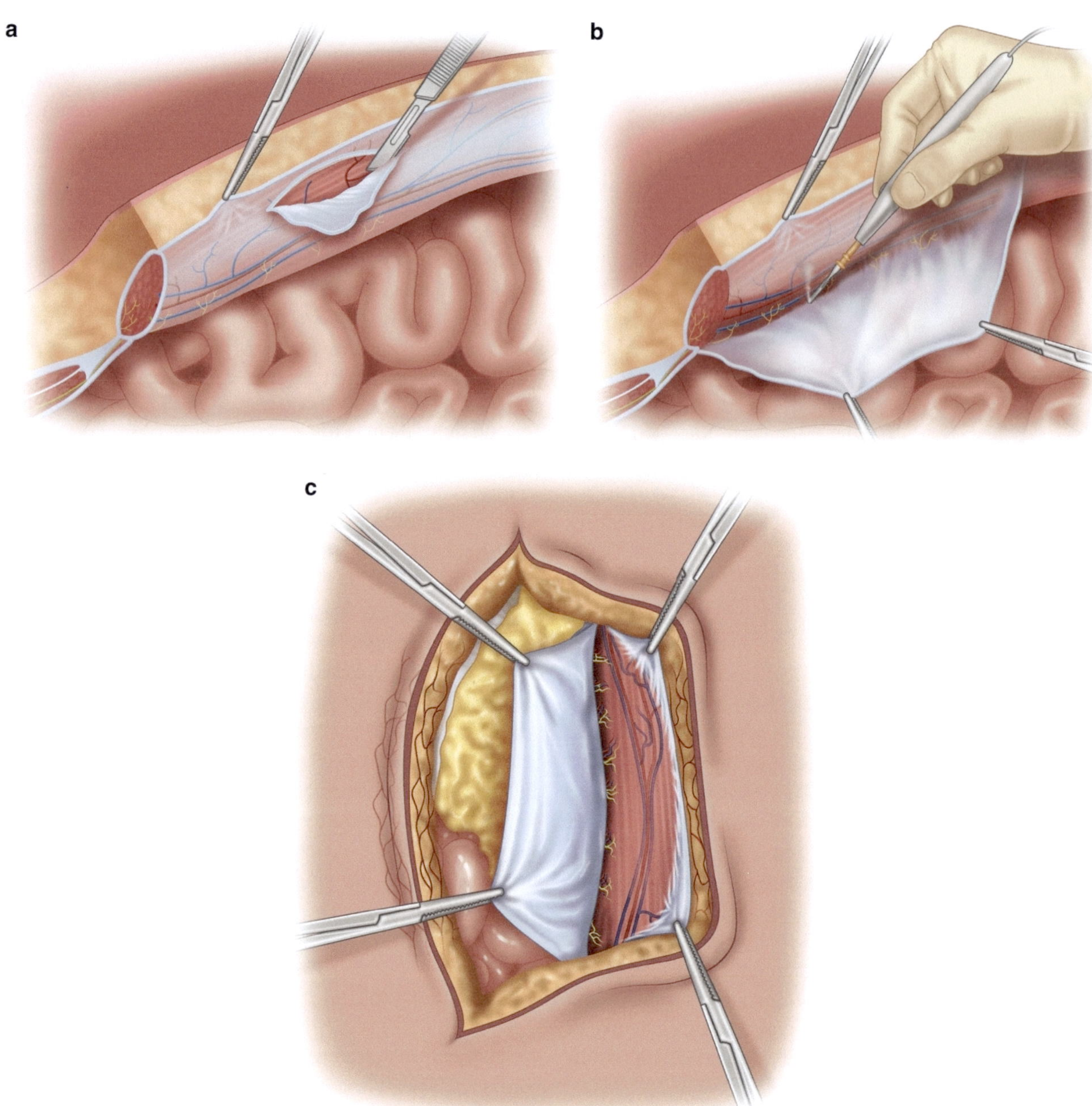

Fig. 8.6 (**a**) Incising the posterior sheath figure. (**b**) Releasing to the semilunar line, protecting the neurovascular structures. (**c**) Showing the extent of the dissection, retrorectus above posterior sheath, limit of lateral dissection

mesh, but also reduces the tension on the midline closure. The mesh will not buckle or wrinkle when the *linea alba* is recreated, reducing the space for seroma to accumulate (Fig. 8.9).

In many circumstances, dissection in the retrorectus space just to the *linea semilunaris* is insufficient to permit adequate AWR due to the following considerations. There may be insufficient medial advance of both the posterior rectus sheath (to exclude the mesh from the peritoneal cavity) and of rectus muscles (to permit reconstruction of the *linea alba*

anterior to the mesh). In this situation either an anterior component separation or a posterior component separation is necessary.

Anterior Component Separation

Anterior exposure of the linea semilunaris is the next step. It is important to preserve the periumbilical blood supply to the skin (Fig. 8.10). Note how they are transposed laterally by

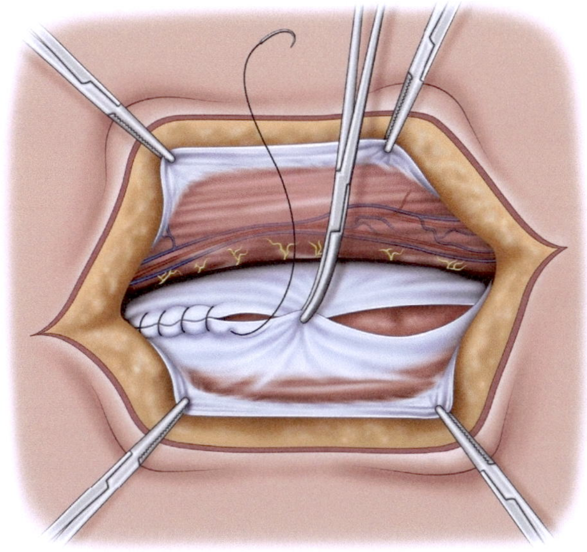

Fig. 8.7   Closing the posterior sheath

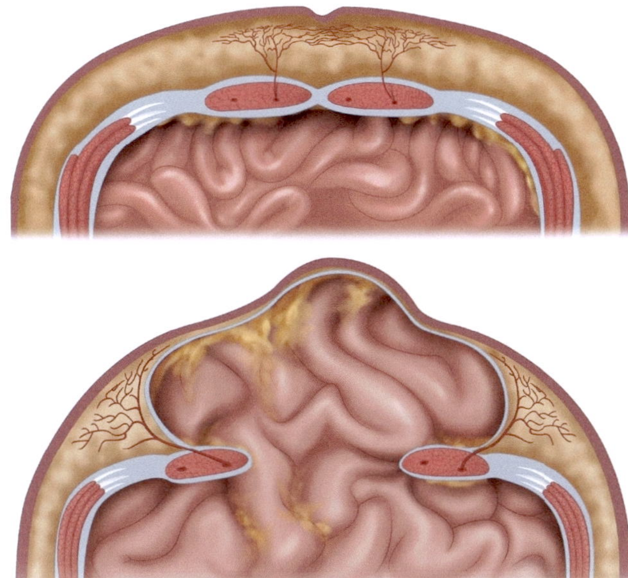

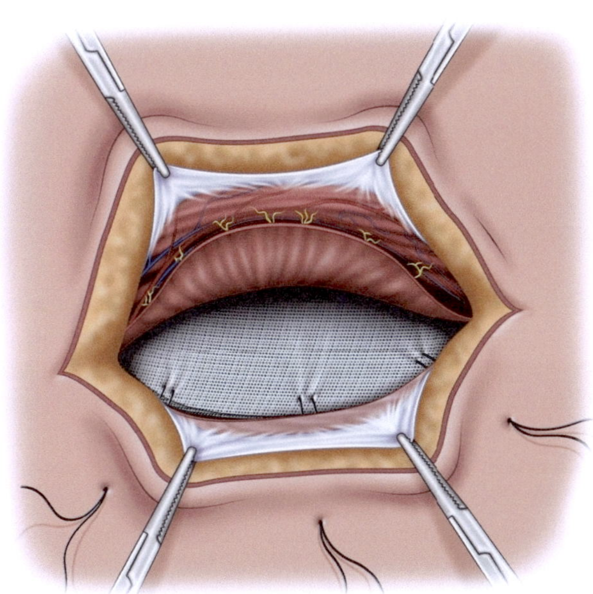

Fig. 8.8   Placement of the mesh and full thickness transfascial sutures

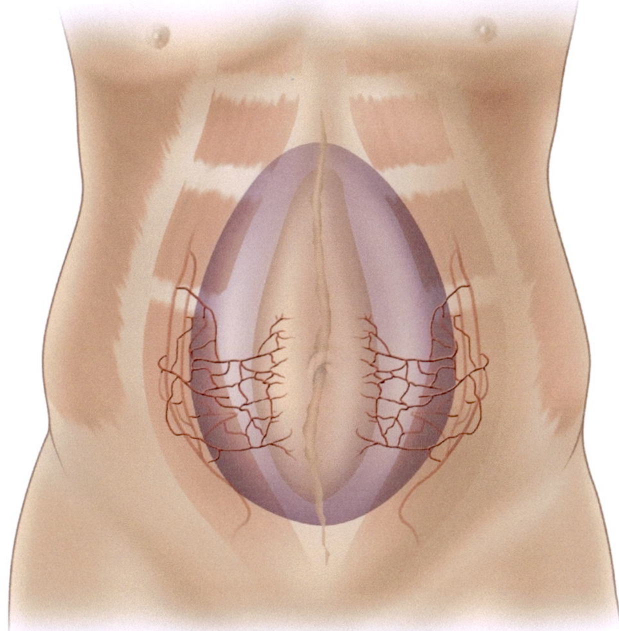

Fig. 8.10   Location of the periumbilical perforators

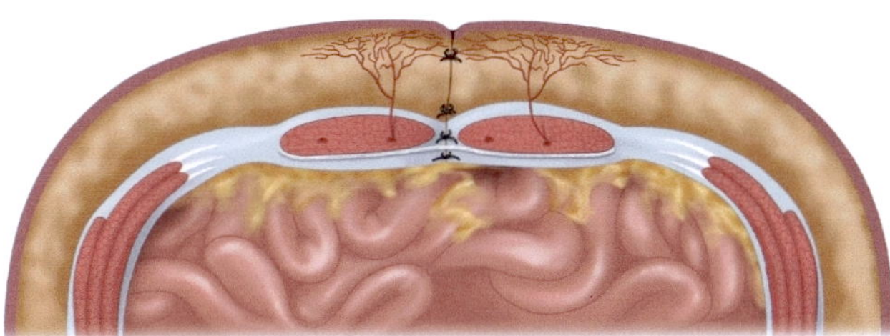

Fig. 8.9   Retrorectus mesh placement

the hernia. There are a number of ways to do this. One is to make a small counter incision over the lower lateral ribs and expose the linea semilunaris this way. Also, windows can be made around the perforators to get exposure laterally (Fig. 8.11). Laparoscopes have also been used to create the exposure. In each of the methods, a 1–2 cm incision is made lateral to the linea semilunaris through the myofascial portion of the external oblique (Fig. 8.12). The dissection should start on the lower ribs and extend to the groin. It is important

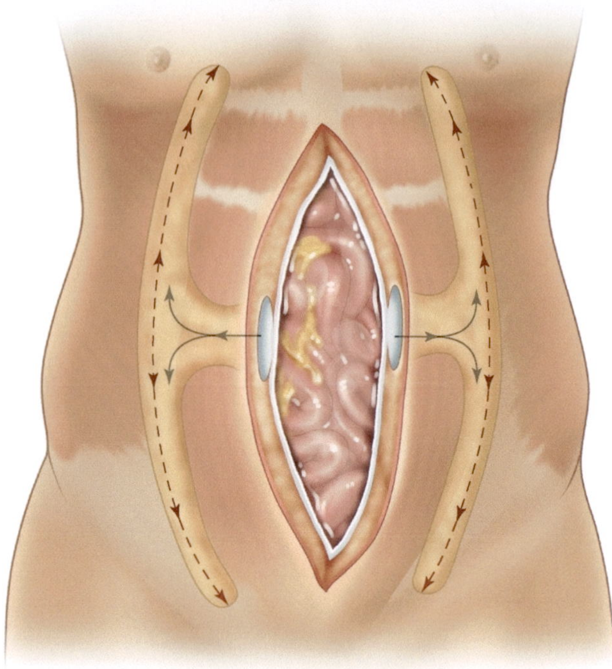

Fig. 8.11 Subcutaneous windows to preserve the perforators

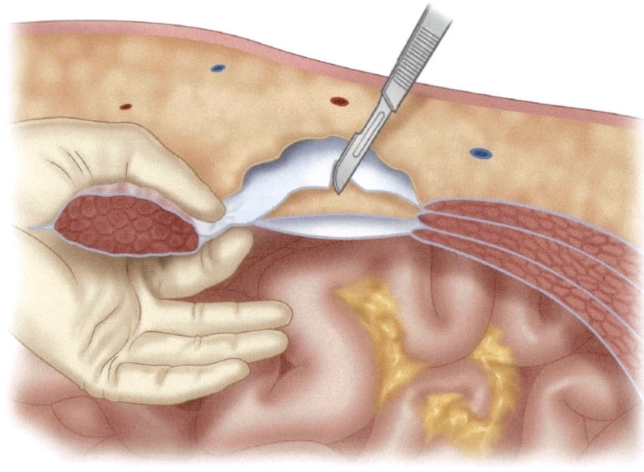

Fig. 8.12 Incision through the myofascial portion of the external oblique, lateral to the linea semilunaris

to remember that the rectus may be curved since it is not attached at the linea alba. The plane is avascular and easy to dissect inferiorly and then laterally to the anterior axillary line. Dissection can be done bluntly with a suction catheter (Fig. 8.13). This will release the rectus and allow it to move 10 cm or more to the midline (Fig. 8.14). If the tissue has

been sufficiently released, the anterior fascia should be able to be brought together with minimal tension (Fig. 8.15). Alternatively, if the anterior skin and fascia is of poor quality, then a transversus abdominis release (TAR) may be a better choice. This has the advantage of less dissection of the abdominal skin and preserves the neurovascular support of the rectus and the skin.

Posterior Component Separation: TAR

From the retrorectus position approximately one-half cm medial to the linea semilunaris, the posterior sheath is released exposing the transversus muscle (Fig. 8.16). This is most easily accomplished in the upper half of the abdomen where the muscle belly is well defined. The transversus abdominis muscle is transected (Fig. 8.17). Care must be taken to avoid injury to the transversalis fascia/peritoneal layer that lays deep to this. Once divided, the muscle can be retracted anteriorly and the avascular retromuscular plane developed bluntly. Superiorly, this plane extends beyond the costal margin to the diaphragm, inferiorly to the myopectineal orifice and laterally to the psoas muscle. The TAR is then completed on the contralateral side (Fig. 8.18). The posterior rectus sheath is now reapproximated with monofilament suture. Mesh is placed as mentioned above (Fig. 8.19)

Reconstruction of the Anterior Layers

The linea alba is recreated by suturing the anterior rectus sheaths to each other in the midline. Before these stitches are tied, closed suction drains (typically 2) are positioned anterior to the mesh and in the dependent portions of the repair. The skin and subcutaneous tissues are then closed.

Generally this approach will manage most of the uncomplicated abdominal wounds. However, in the situation of the frozen abdomen or contaminated wounds the process should be to obtain tissue control. Here a VAC dressing can be invaluable in stabilizing the wound. After the wound and the patient are stabilized, usually skin grafts can then be used to control the wound. This will allow time for a definitive repair at a more optimal date.

Potential Pitfalls

Mesh should be used as a supporting matrix and not as the primary repair. The type of mesh is not so important as its application. Generally the synthetic meshes provide excellent support at a reasonable cost. The restoration of a

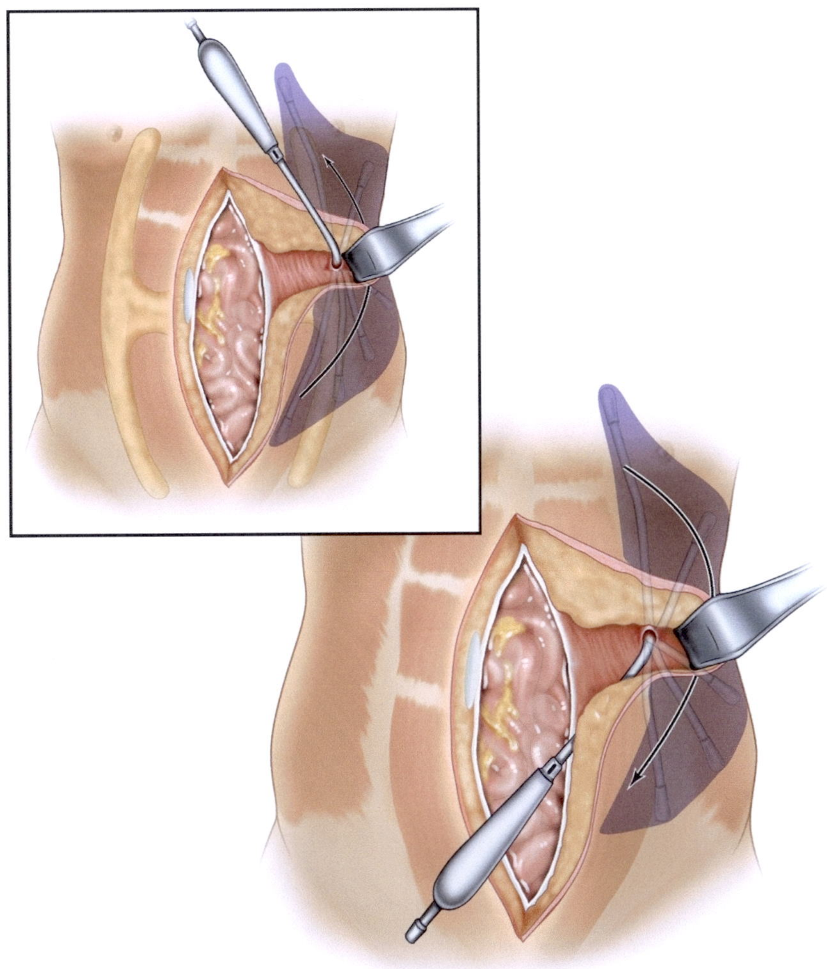

Fig. 8.13 Blunt dissection releasing the avascular plane between the internal and external obliques

compliant, strong functioning myofascial unit is critical to decrease the risks of recurrence. Trying to obtain normal positional anatomy and function of rectus is key to this. Mesh should be placed always as a retrorectus layer supported by muscle and fascia. In case there is no posterior sheath, then an inlay biologic mesh is the next option. Only as a last resort should mesh of either type be used as a bridging material or as an onlay.

Study of hernia failures reveals that they fail at the tissue interface between the fascia and the mesh: This is usually from pullout of the sutures. The sutures damage the fascial tissue and literally pull through. More sutures placed atraumatically with wide tissue bites creates less tissue stress.

It is important to consider how the abdominal muscles work together. The pull of the obliques balances and supports the functions of the abdominal wall. If there is a defect or injury to the abdominal wall, the pull of these muscles can increase the defect. This vector force effectively pulls against the midline and may be a substantial cause of the creation of the hernia defect. By decreasing this pull, less tension is placed on the midline fascial closures.

Preservation of the skin perforators is very important. Dissection around the periumbilical area will protect these and improve skin healing.

Postoperative Care

Seromas are a major complication. Drains should be left in until the fluid changes to serous and is less than 20 cc per day for approximately 2 days. At times drains need to remain in place for 4 weeks or longer. Minimizing subcutaneous dis-

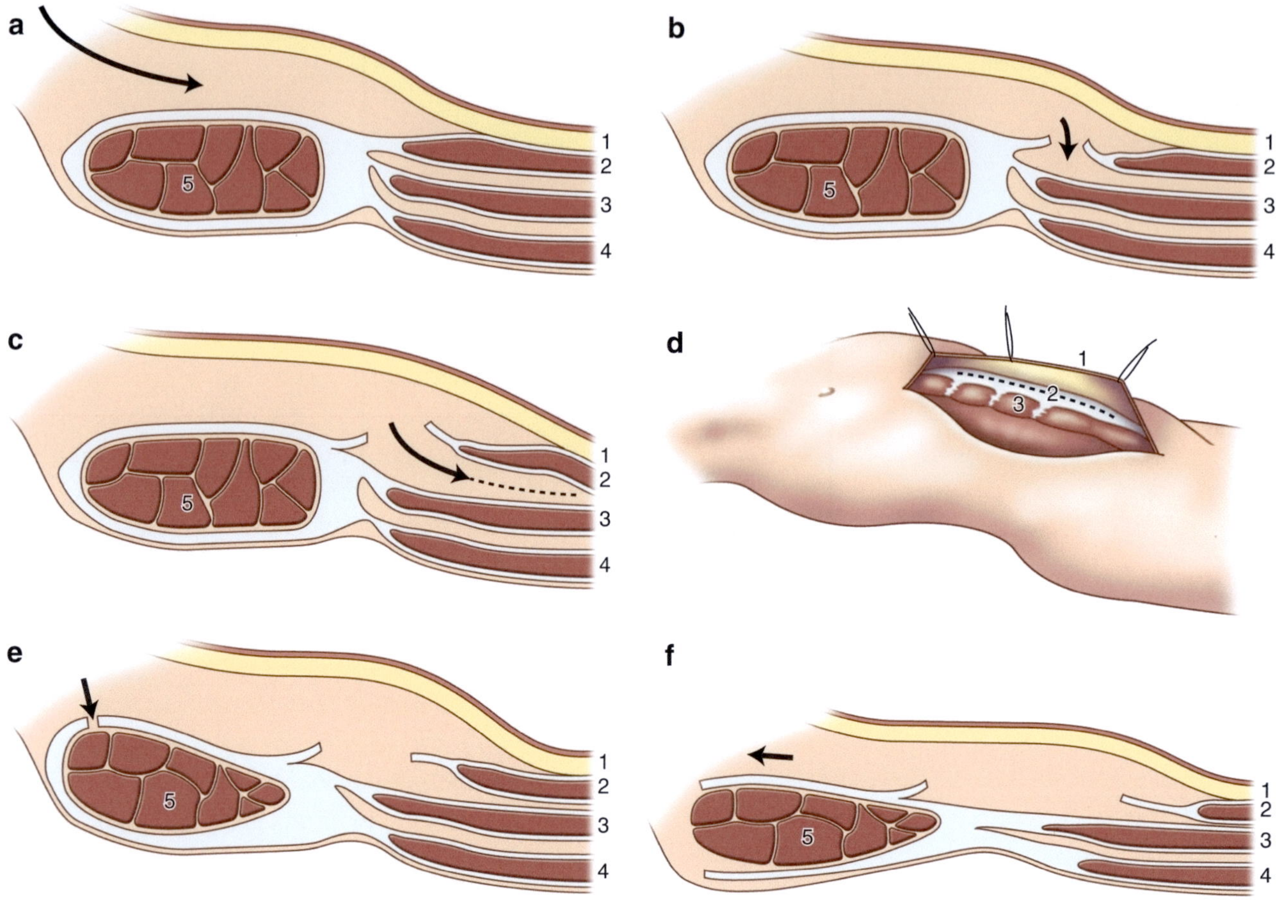

Fig. 8.14 Release of the anterior sheath

section and placing mesh retrorectus also decreases the potential for seroma.

It is also helpful to keep in mind that the fascia of the abdominal wall is essentially a tendon. Tendon repairs take a minimum of 6 weeks to begin healing, and up to 6 months to reach maximal strength. Understanding tendon management shows that some tissue tension may actually improve healing. Therefore activities that gently and gradually increase core strength are very important for healthy muscle function. The inactivity associated with large hernias, coupled with surgical trauma to these structures, weakens these muscles. Physical therapy to improve core strength is very useful to restore myofascial health.

Common Complications

In addition to the usual surgical complications, those of AWR are extensive and unique. The loss of domain for a period of time can decrease the effective abdominal cavity space. Also chronic low grade bowel obstruction or inflammation can create chronic dysmotility of the bowel, making it more susceptible to injury from increase in abdominal pressure. This can lead to ischemia and bowel injury. The most concerning is the creation of intra-abdominal hypertension. This is the result of compression of the inferior vena cava. In its extreme form this creates the abdominal compartment syndrome. If abdominal pressures exceed 25 mmHg this leads rapidly to multi-organ failure. Lesser increases in thoracic pressure lead to ventilation difficulties, raise intracranial pressure, and can lead to hepatorenal failure.

Since these patients often have many comorbidities, the risk of surgical site infection is increased. This presents increased problems with potential infection of the mesh.

When to Transfer

AWR are generally elective procedures. For this reason, if one is not equipped for a prolonged operation, then consider transfer to a center that is comfortable treating these complex

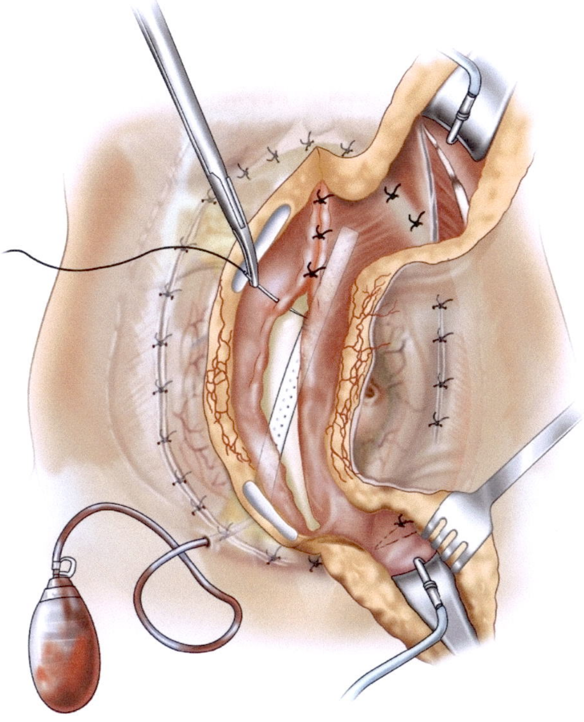

Fig. 8.15 Closure of midline

Fig. 8.16 Posterior sheath dissection past the semilunar line

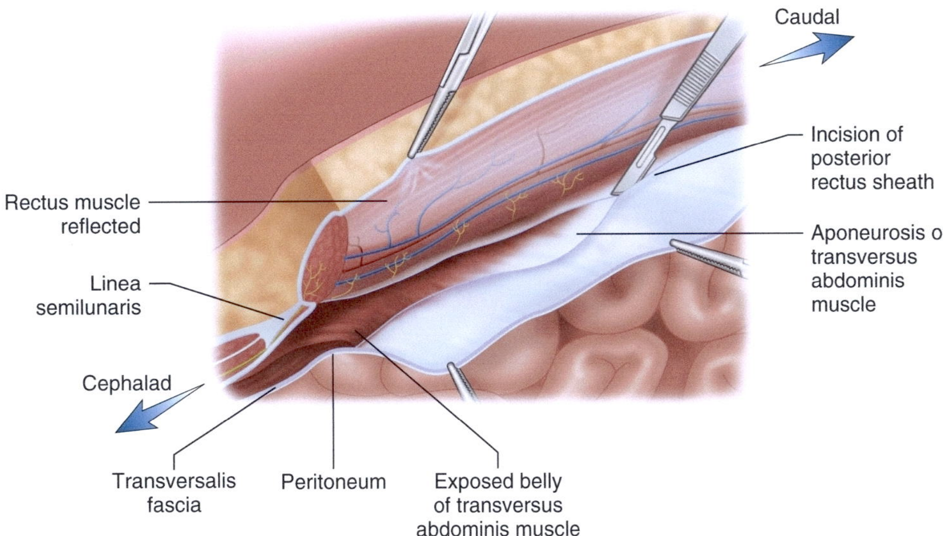

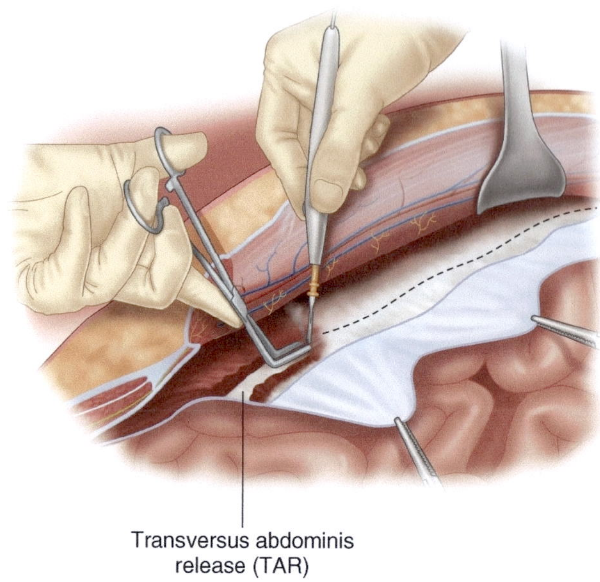

Fig. 8.17 Release of the transversus abdominis muscle

Fig. 8.18 Closure of the posterior sheath

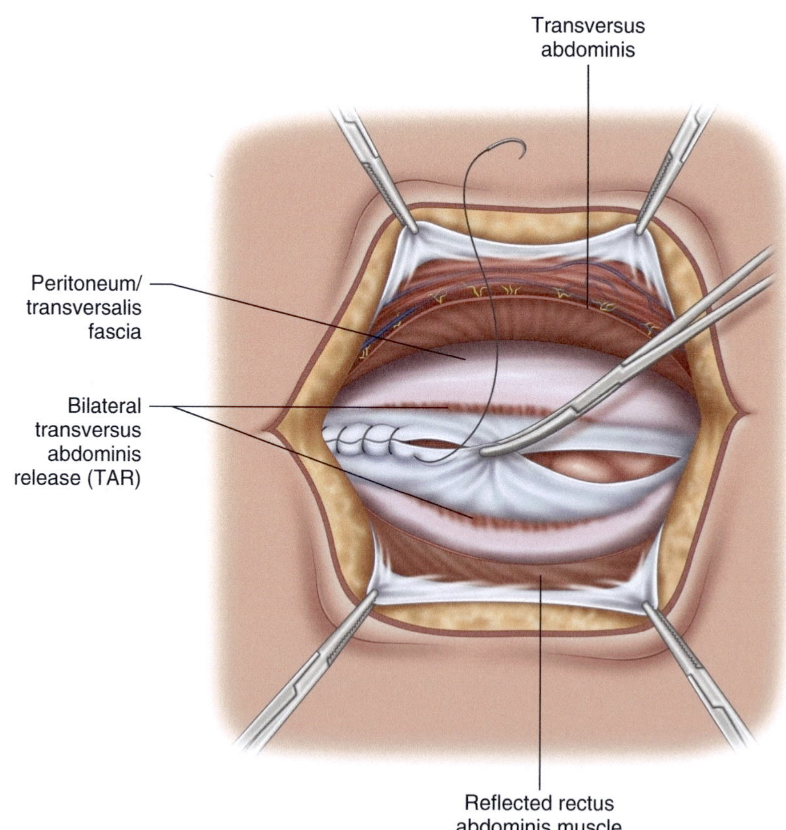

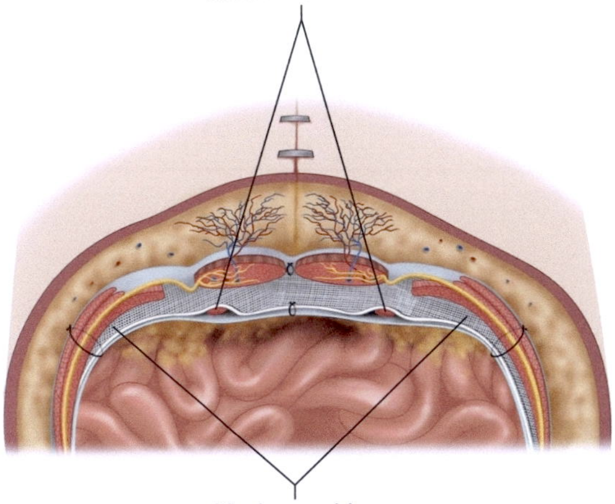

Bilateral released
edges of transversus
abdominis muscle

Mesh as sublay
in retromuscular
space

Fig. 8.19 Closure of the anterior sheath in the midline

problems. Often a team of general and plastic surgeons and medicine physicians are needed to safely address these problems. With recurrence rates of 15–20 % even in good series, careful planning is critical to the successful management of these cases.

Suggested Reading

Ceydeli A, Rucinski J, Wise L. Finding the best abdominal closure: an evidence based review of the literature. Curr Surg. 2005;62:220–5.

Finan KR, Vick CC, Kiefe CL, Neumayer L, Hawn MT. Predictors of wound infection in ventral hernia repair. Am J Surg. 2005;190:676–81.

Ramirez OM, Ruas E, Dellon L. Component separation method for closure of abdominal wall defects: an anatomic and clinical study. Plast Reconstr Surg. 1990;86:519–26.

Reid RR, Dumanian GA. Panniculectomy and the separation-of-parts hernia repair: a solution for the large infraumbilical hernia in the obese patient. Plast Reconstr Surg. 2005;116:1006–12.

Rosen MJ, Williams C, Jin J, McGee MF, Schomisch S, Marks J, Ponsky J. Laparoscopic versus open-component separation: a comparative analysis in a porcine model. Am J Surg. 2007;194(3):385–9.

Saulis AS, Dumanian GA. Periumbilical rectus abdominis perforator preservation significantly reduces superficial wound complications in 'separation of parts' hernia repairs. Plast Reconstr Surg. 2002;109:2275–80.

Shestak KC, Edington HJ, Johnson RR. The separation of anatomic components technique for the reconstruction of massive midline abdominal wall defects: anatomy, surgical technique, applications, and limitations revisited. Plast Reconstr Surg. 2000;105:731–8.

The Ventral Hernia Working Group, Breuing K, Bulter CE, Ferzoco S, Franz M, Hultman CS, Kilbridge JF, Rosen M, Silverman RP, Vargo D. Incisional ventral hernias: review of the literature and recommendations regarding the grading and technique of repair. Surgery. 2010;148(3):544–58.

Rosen MJ, editor. Atlas of abdominal wall reconstruction. Philadelphia: Saunders; 2011

Eric K. Mooney

Introduction

Squamous cell and basal cell cancers of the face are a common problem in rural practice. Despite the growing popularity of specialty techniques, such as Mohs surgery, the rural practitioner can confidently manage most of these lesions.

General Principles

The general principles of cancer management apply to the management of facial carcinomas. That is to say that the rural surgeon must: (1) establish the diagnosis; (2) provide adequate resection; and (3) close the defect adequately. Diagnosis can be established by simple punch biopsy, shave biopsy, or excisional biopsy. Occasionally it is useful to do several punch biopsies in poorly defined area of generalized or subtle skin changes ("field cancerization," for instance on the scalp or the retroauricular region) to help delineate the area of cancer. Shave biopsy sometimes can provide definitive resection but may also obscure the region of involvement because normal healing changes may mimic cancerous changes, requiring a larger area of resection. This is not so much of a problem in areas of skin excess but can be a problem in areas of little excess such as the ala. Lastly, in areas of skin excess (such as the cheek, temple, and forehead), primary excision may serve as clearance as well as diagnosis (Fig. 9.1). The excision may be planned as an ellipse with the long axis parallel to the Relaxed Skin Tension Lines (RSTL). The patient is marked in the sitting position, animating the face (smiling, feownig, puzsing etc.) to delineate the RSTL (Fig. 9.2).

E.K. Mooney, M.D. (✉)
Department of Surgery, Bassett Healthcare,
One Atwell Road, Cooperstown, NY 13326, USA
e-mail: eric.mooney@bassett.org

The surgeon must decide how he will manage margins. In most cases, particularly in areas of excess skin, a well-defined lesion can be primarily excised with comfortable margins. The specimen should, of course be tagged with a stitch and oriented for the pathologist in permanent margins are positive. If a lesion is poorly defined or a complex flap closure is planned, frozen sections can be used to ensure clearance. If these are unavailable, the wound can be safely left open and closed secondarily a week later when permanent section results are available. In the interim, the wound should not be allowed to desiccate.

Once the diagnosis is made and the resection accomplished, adequate closure is then accomplished. Closure may be achieved by direct primary closure, skin grafting, or local flaps. Direct closure is applied in areas of relative skin excess (e.g., cheek, forehead, temple, lip) so as to limit anatomic distortion. Closure should be tensionless particularly near the lower lid and craniad cheek to avoid ectropion. If there is any question, a full thickness graft or flap should be used. Generous undermining (of the scalp or forehead) and even scoring the galea (scalp) can facilitate the process.

Direct closure is accomplished in areas of skin excess (cheek) or specialized areas such as the lip, the helix of the ear, and the eyelid.

In repairing defects, the general principle of "like replaces like" should be applied. For instance, the ideal donor site for a skin graft of the eyelid is the contralateral eyelid (or ipsilateral other lid). Other donor sites are relative areas of skin excess such as pre- or postauricular skin, the temple, and the neck (Fig. 9.3). When skin grafts are used, they should be full thickness grafts. Grafts should be generous, at least the same size as the defect to prevent contracture distortions, particularly around the eyelids (Fig. 9.3). Small grafts on the nose can be taken from the preauricular skin or the lateral forehead, although thick sebaceous nose skin is hard to match. One may consider excision of the whole aesthetic subunit to avoid a noticeable unnatural geographic appearance of small flaps. This should be considered in the nose (Fig. 9.4). A disadvantage of skin grafting, particularly on

A.L. Halverson and D.C. Borgstrom (eds.), *Advanced Surgical Techniques for Rural Surgeons*,
DOI 10.1007/978-1-4939-1495-1_9, © Springer Science+Business Media New York 2015

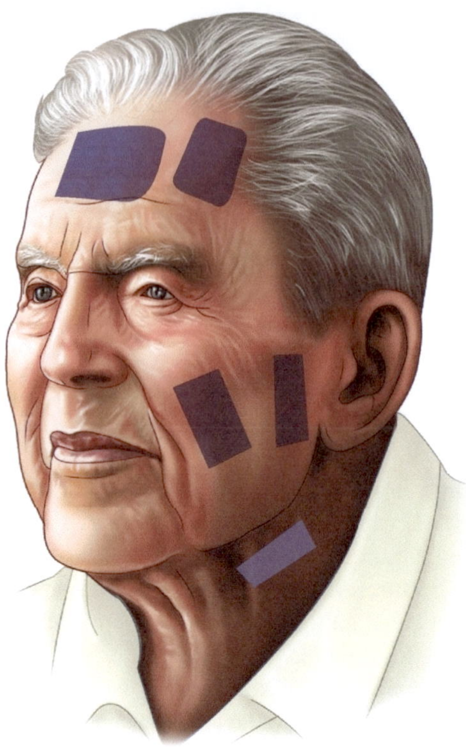

Fig. 9.1 Relative areas of skin excess

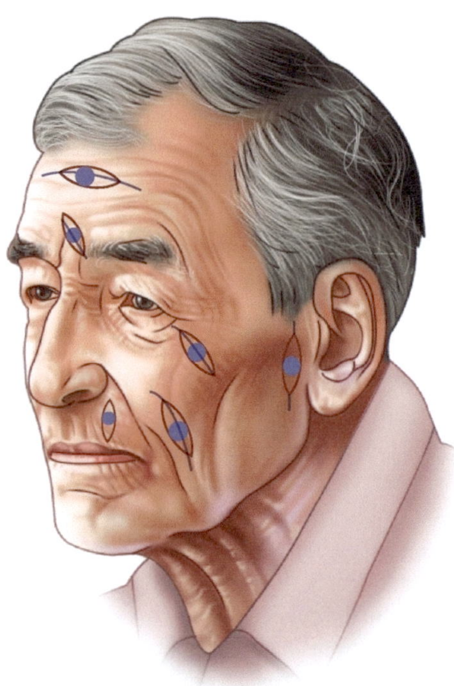

Fig. 9.2 Relaxed skin tension lines can be used to plan excision and primary closure

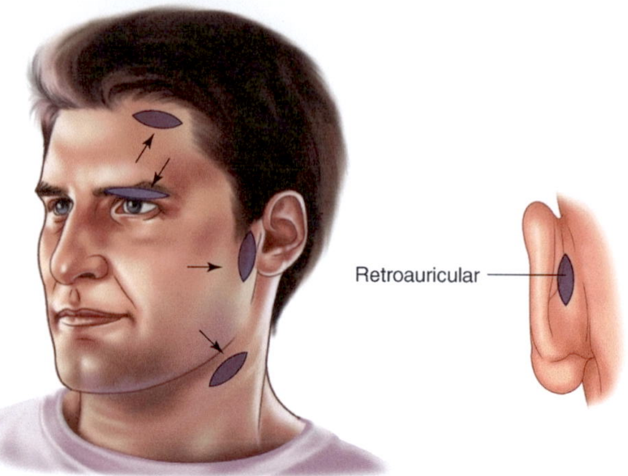

Fig. 9.3 Potential Graft donor sites. An additional site lies behind the ear (retroauricular scalp)

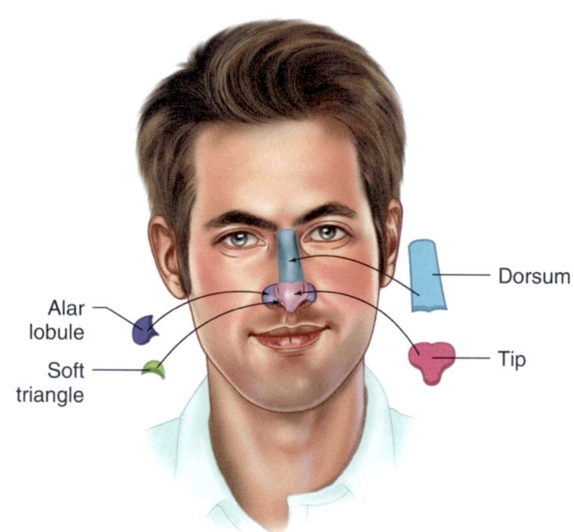

Fig. 9.4 Aesthetic units of the nose

the nose, is that grafts often do not match the color or texture of the original or surrounding skin.

Local flaps have the advantages of color and texture match. This is particularly useful for the nose. They are vascularized so that they can cover full thickness defects straight down to cartilage or bone, allowing for aggressive cancer resection. They are planned to take advantage of relative areas of skin excess. In planning flap closure, one must anticipate the line of maximum tension and make sure that the donor area will close using a "pinch test" (Fig. 9.5). The arc of transposition should be tested or measured to make sure the flap is long enough to close the defect. Because of the generous blood supply of the face and the viscoelastic properties of skin, closure can be performed even under moderate tension as skin creep will allow for eventual capillary refill.

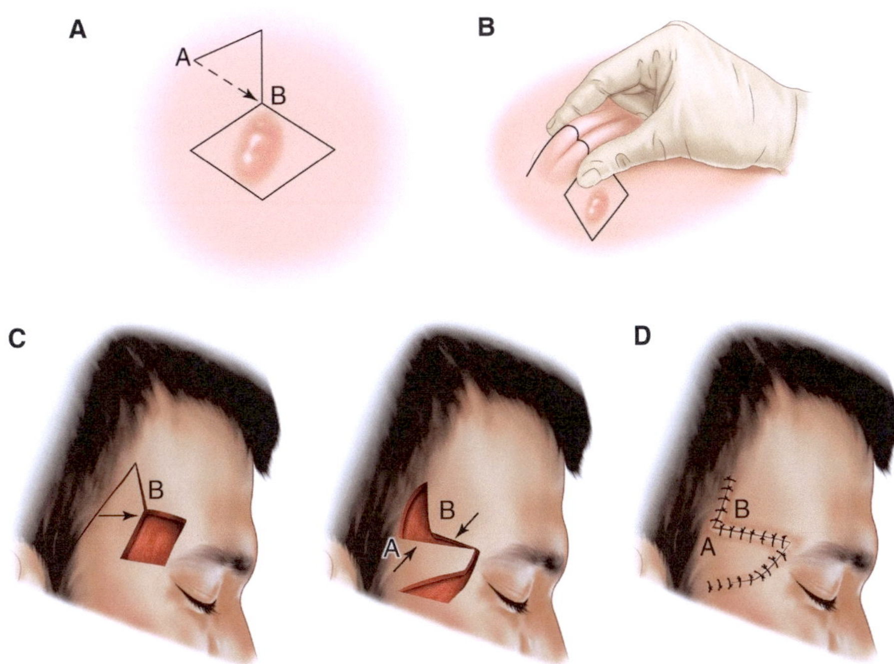

Fig. 9.5 Using a "pinch test" test for adequate closure. *A*: A rhomboid flap is planned to close an excision of the forehead. Line *A-B* represents the line of maximum tension. *B*: The closure is tested with a "pinch test." *C*: The flap is rotated to close the defect, while points *A* and *B* come together at the point of most tension. *D*: Final closure

Preoperative Preparation

The patient should be counseled as to the inevitability of facial scars and the possibility of positive margins necessitating further surgery should be discussed.

The patient should be off aspirin for 10 days, if possible, particularly if a graft is anticipated. A sedative may be considered if the patient has anxiety problems or high blood pressure.

The lesion is marked with the patient in the sitting position, taking the RSTL and esthetic subunits into consideration. Loupe magnification is helpful. Having the patient animate the face will accentuate the RSTL and help orient the resection. A pinch test is used when primary closure or flap closure is anticipated (across the maximum line of tension). Mark all anatomic lines to be approximated before injection (e.g., the vermillion, the alar rim, the helix of the ear, etc). Donor sites for grafts are marked.

Operative Strategy

Surgical management of facial neoplasia must focus on complete excision of the carcinoma. That is to say that excision must be perpendicular through all layers of the skin, and deeper to perichondrium or bone if necessary. Once resection is adequate, then closure is planned. One should not allow the anticipated method of closure to dictate the limits of resection, as it is the resection that must be complete. There are no magic numbers for margins. Margins can be planned so as to allow for direct closure. If adequate margins cannot afford direct closure, grafts or flaps should be used. Occasionally, excision of an entire aesthetic unit may give a better result after subsequent grafting than small, patchwork grafts. This is particularly true of the nose. All specimens are tagged with a stitch, the specimen for the pathologist. Make sure all margins are clear before closing with a flap, so as not to bury and obscure a recurrence.

Operative Technique

The eyes should be protected by moistened gauze, corneal protectors, etc. Working on the face is a fire hazard, particularly with nasal cannula oxygen. Measures should be taken to reduce that risk.

The operation is begun by setting up a "regional nerve block" supplemented by local infiltration (Fig. 9.6). For instance, the forehead is blocked by infiltrating the supraorbital rim (Fig. 9.7). The lip and medial cheek are blocked with an infraorbital nerve block by inserting the needle at the base of the ala and injecting the palpable infraorbital foramen below the inferior orbital rim. Alternately, with one hand palpating the inferior orbital rim, the needle directly injects the palpable foramen (Fig. 9.8). The lower lip is blocked by injecting the mental nerve in the labiobuccal sulcus, just under the mucosa near the first bicuspid (Fig. 9.9).

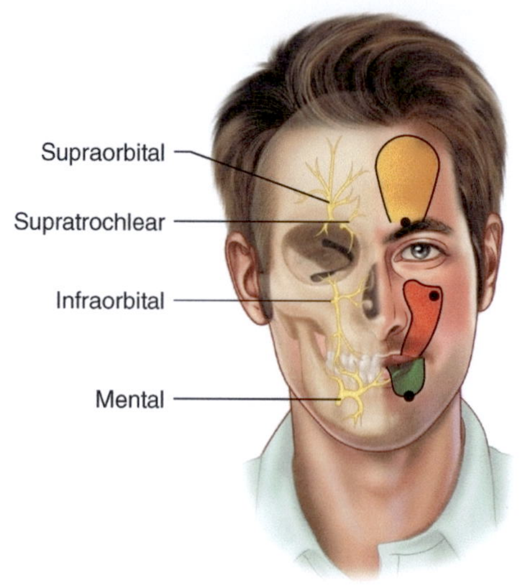

Fig. 9.6 Sensory innervations of the face

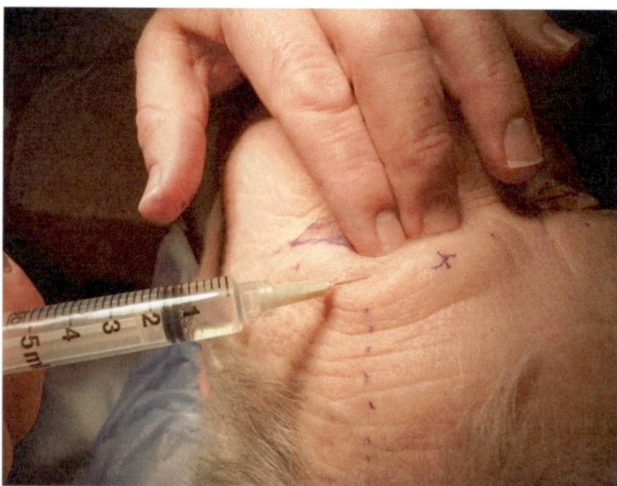

Fig. 9.7 Blocking the supraorbital and supratrochlear nerves

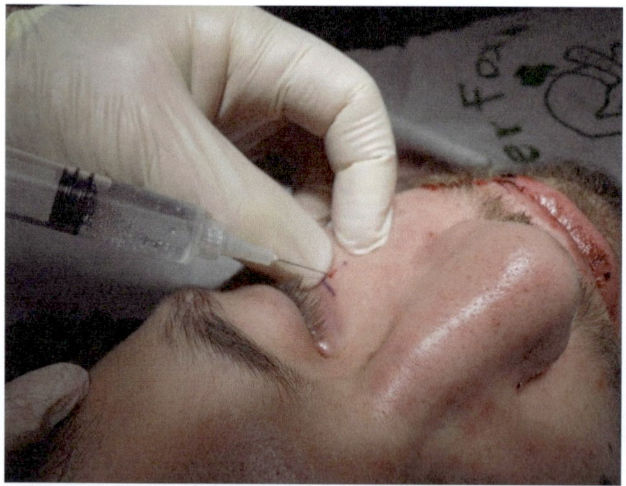

Fig. 9.8 Infraorbital nerve block

Resection is carried perpendicular through the dermis and through the subcutaneous fat layer. Deeper resections are performed for nodular or fixed lesions, right to perichondrium, periosteum, or bone. The later will require flap closure. Margins may be controlled by (1) wide excision; (2) frozen section; (3) leaving the wound open and waiting permanent section.

Grafts are taken full thickness and defatted with scissors. After insetting with rapidly dissolving 5-0 gut, a bolster of petrolatum gauze and moistened cotton is tied over it.

Flap coverage necessitates careful planning. Once the flap is marked, the arc of rotation is checked (with a ruler or suture) and closure of the donor site is checked with a pinch technique. Common flaps are the rhomboid, paramedian nasal, and bilobe flaps.

In performing a rhomboid flap, the excision is performed as a parallelogram. A rhomboid flap is transposed into the defect, first making sure the donor site will close with a pinch test (C–C_1 in Fig. 9.10). Rhomboids are commonly used on the forehead and cheek (Fig. 9.11).

The tripier flap is elevated off the opposite eyelid as a pedicle flap based laterally in the canthal region (Fig. 9.12). The flap is elevated including the underlying preseptal orbicularis muscle. It is a useful flap in preventing ectropion.

The bilobe flap is an elegant flap that is useful for nasal defects. The first flap is made the same size or slightly smaller than the defect. The second flap closes the first and is about half the width of the first. The donor site of the second flap is closed primarily (Figs. 9.13 and 9.14). This flap transports the excess mobile nasal dorsa or sidewall skin into the defect in stages.

The paramedian forehead flap can close medial canthal and large nasal defects (Fig. 9.15). The base of the flap is designed 2–3 cm in width to capture branches of the supratrochlear artery and the rich periorbital vascular arcade. The tip of the flap is thin, elevated in the subdermal plane. This is made deeper toward the base, progressively including frontalis muscle and then perichondrium 2–3 cm from the base. The base is divided as a second stage after 2–3 weeks. If necessary, the flap can be re-elevated in a third stage for thinning.

Potential Pitfalls

When considering flap closure, margin control should be ensured to avoid closing over residual cancer. Should positive margins occur, it is usually best to reexcise the cancer rather than adopting a "wait-and-see" posture. This possibility of re-excision for positive margins should be discussed with the patient *before* the initial excision.

Contracture can be a problem around the eyelids, causing ectropion (Fig. 9.16). Flaps and grafts should be generous and tension free. Management is by contracture release and

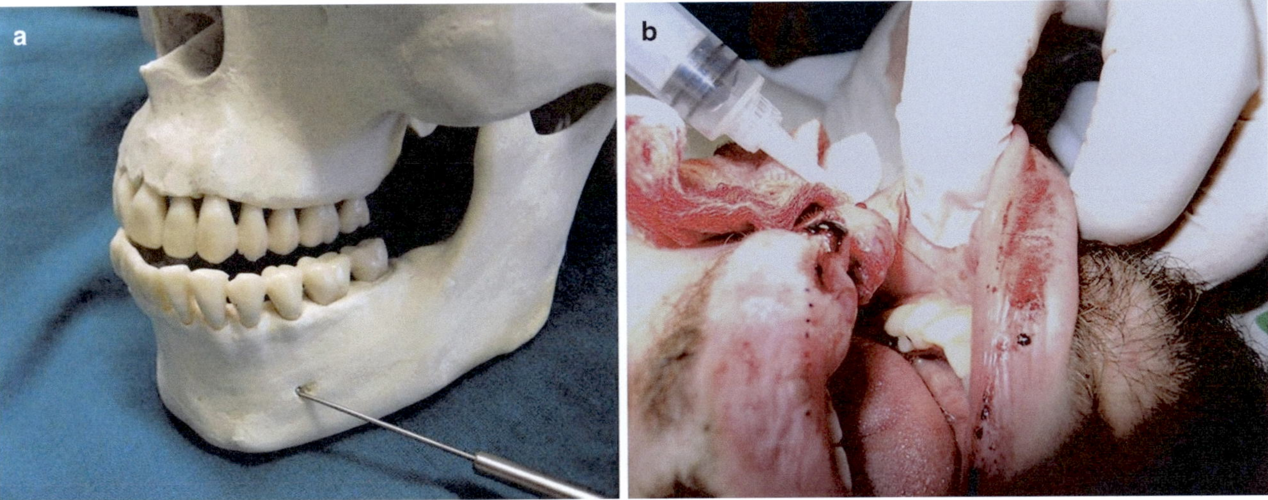

Fig. 9.9 Blocking the mental nerve. The mental nerve exits the mental foramen at the level of the first bicuspid (**a**). The injection can be placed just beneath the mucosa in the labiobuccal sulcus at the level of the first bicuspid and advanced toward the foramen (**b**)

Fig. 9.10 Rhomboid flap. Multiple rhomboid flaps can be planned around a defect (**a**). The optimum rhomboid flap is chosen by testing the line of maximum (line C–C_1) with a pinch test (**b**) to ensure closure (**c**)

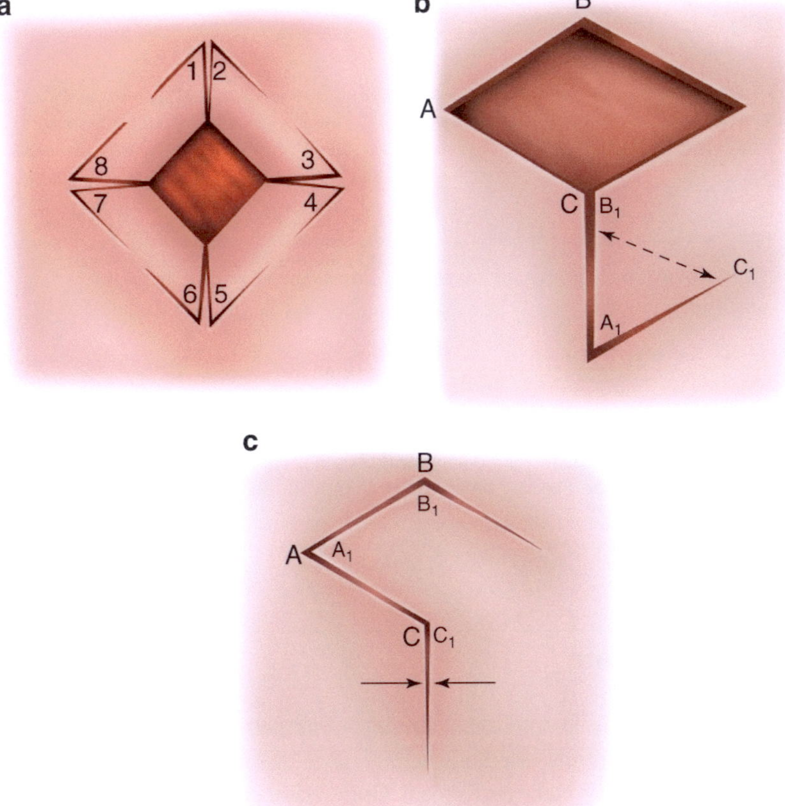

full thickness grafting or flap (Tripier) closure. Canthopexy is often included.

Facial nerve damage is a possibility, most likely involving the frontal branch. The possibility should be discussed with the patient if the lesion lies near the course of the nerve (Fig. 9.17). The course of the frontal branch lies along a line from the inferior tragus to one centimeter above the lateral brow.

Unexpectedly deep invasion can occur, particularly at the medial canthal region, alar base, and with long-standing nasal lesions. Sometimes, *palpation* of deep induration will raise clinical suspicion of such a lesion.

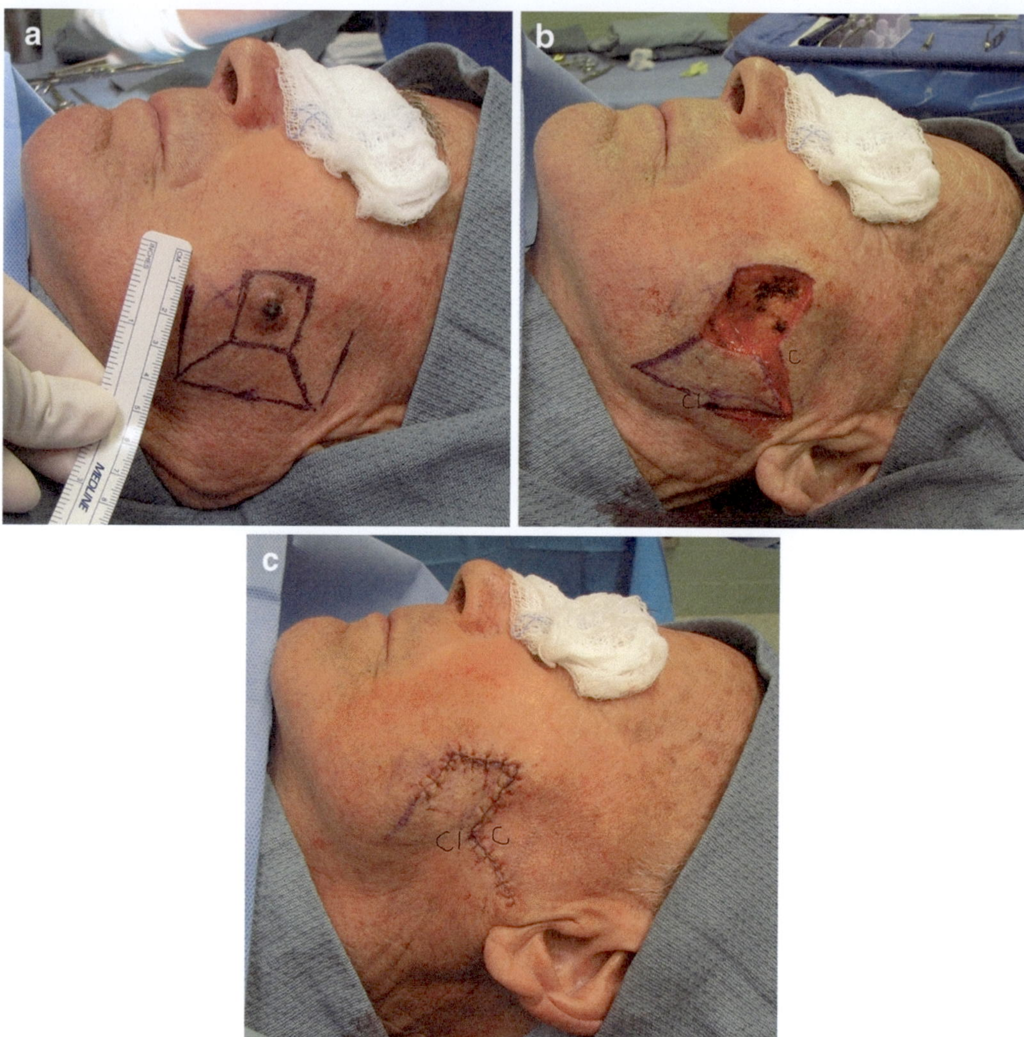

Fig. 9.11 (**a**) Multiple rhomboid flaps are considered in planning closure of the defect. (**b**) The rhomboid flap that is chosen is based on a "pinch test," choosing the flap that closes point $C–C_1$ with the least tension. (**c**) The final closure coapts point $C–C_1$ and has, in effect, transposed the excess, lax tissue in the upper neck into the defect

Postoperative Care

Postoperative care is simple. Moisturizing ointments are used for 2–3 days. Sutures are removed at 6 days, assuming a layered closure has been performed. Graft bolsters are removed at 5 days and the patient may shower and moisturize the graft with a thin layer or Vaseline. Scar creams are not effective on normal scars but sunscreen is recommended as long as the scar is pink to avoid hyperpigmentation. Scar massage is instituted after 10 days.

Common Complications

Flap ischemia is uncommon. Even flap that are blanched and under mild to moderate tension will become "pink" due to the phenomenon of skin creep. Should ischemia persist, sutures are removed and the flap is then inset in a delayed fashion in 2–3 days. Frank necrosis is rare. Most defects will heal well by secondary intention after demarcation and delayed debridement.

Hematomas of significance should be aspirated or drained to prevent skin or flap necrosis.

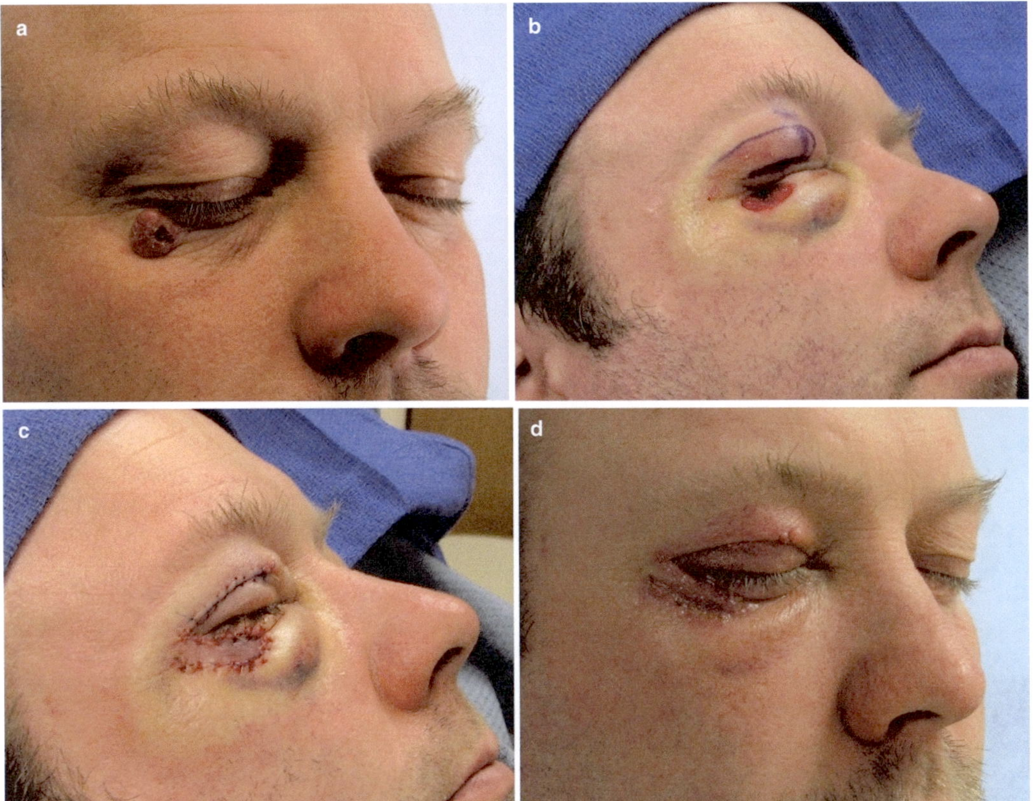

Fig. 9.12 Tripier flap. (**a**) A basal cell cancer of the lateral lower eyelid. (**b**) A tripier transposition flap is planned from the upper lid as a musculocutaneous flap based on the lateral canthal region. (**c**) The flap is transposed and inset, closing the donor site primarily. (**d**) Final result. Note the absence of ectropion

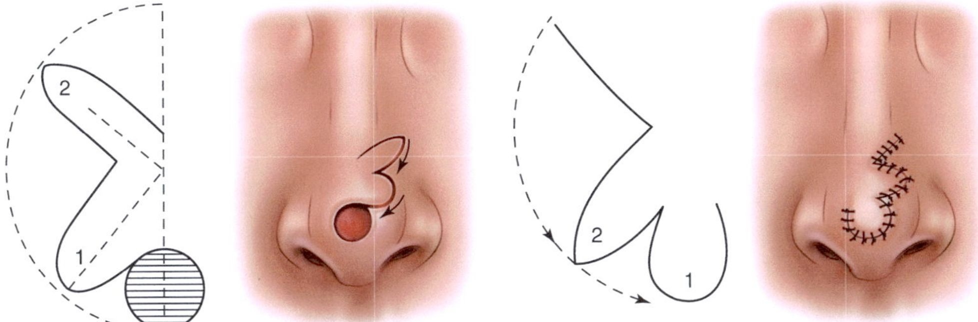

Fig. 9.13 Bilobe flap. The flap is elevated so that the first flap closes the primary defect. The defect from the second flap is closed primarily, taking advantage of excess, distensible skin on the upper nasal dorsum or nasal sidewall. A pinch test is used to ensure that this second donor area will close

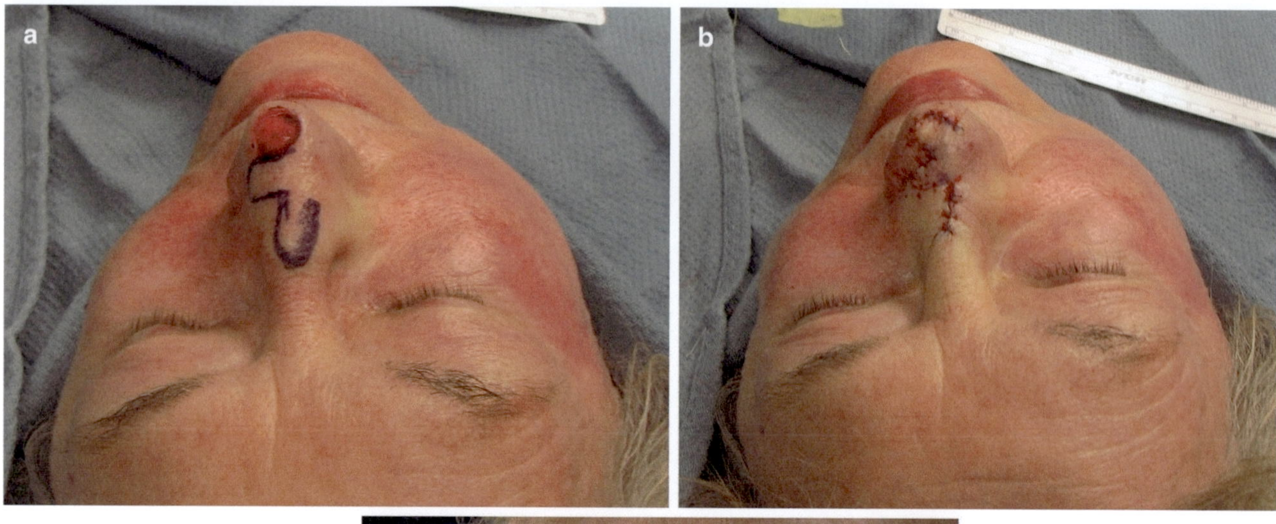

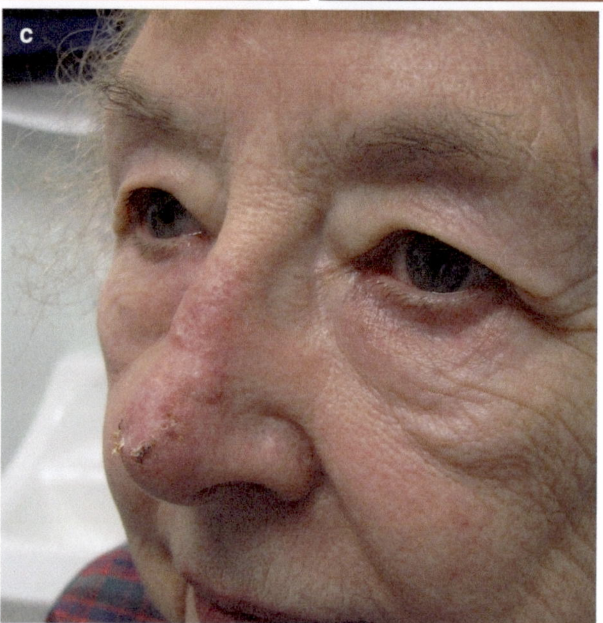

Fig. 9.14 Bilobe flap. (**a**) In this case, the distensible, "excess skin" of the upper dorsum or sidewall is recruited and rotated through 90° using a series of two flaps. (**b**) Flap 1 closes the defect. Flap 2, which is slightly smaller than flap 1, rotates to close the defect of flap 1. The resultant defect at the nasal dorsum is closed primarily. (**c**) Results are good because the flap matches the thick sebaceous skin of the nasal tip. The flap does not tend to heap up ("pin-cushion")

Positive margins on permanent section should be reexcised rather than adopting a "wait-and-see" posture. This is particularly true if a flap has been used for closure. It is helpful to explain to the patient up front that sometimes the reexcised specimen may return with no cancer. In very special situations, radiation may be considered.

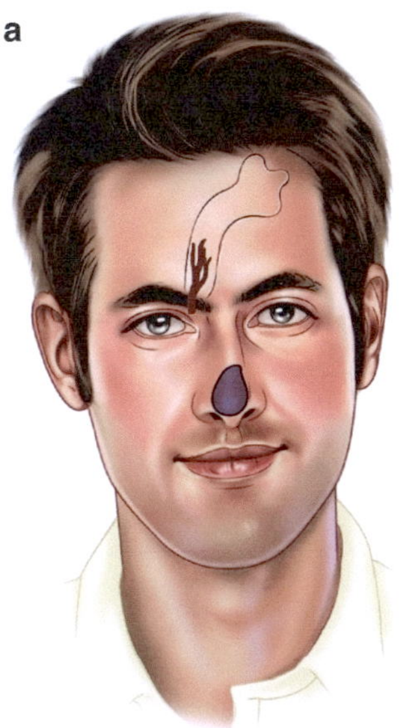
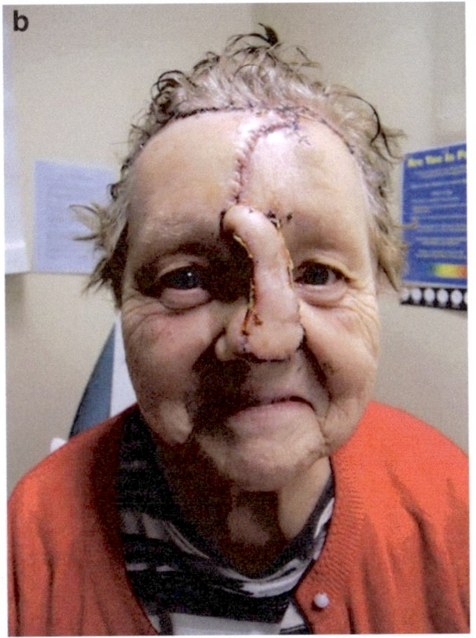
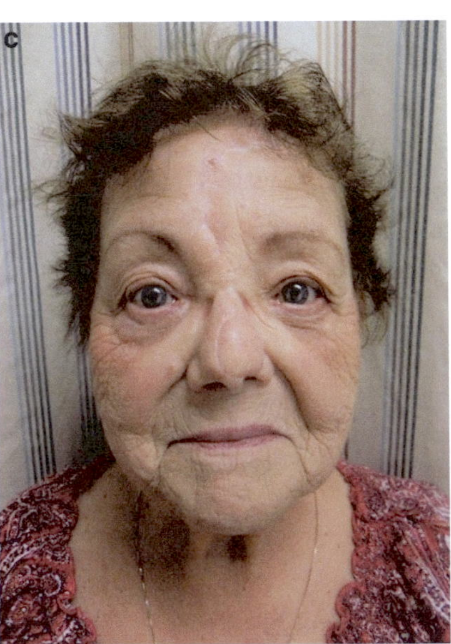

Fig. 9.15 Paramedian forehead flap. (**a**) The flap is based on the supratrochlear "watershed" vessels. (**b**) A flap is rotated to cover a defect at the tip of the nose. The flap can cover the entire nasal dorsum as needed. The forehead is closed primarily by wide undermining, aided by anterior hairline incisions. (**c**) Final result after division and inset. The flap was thinned at the time of inset

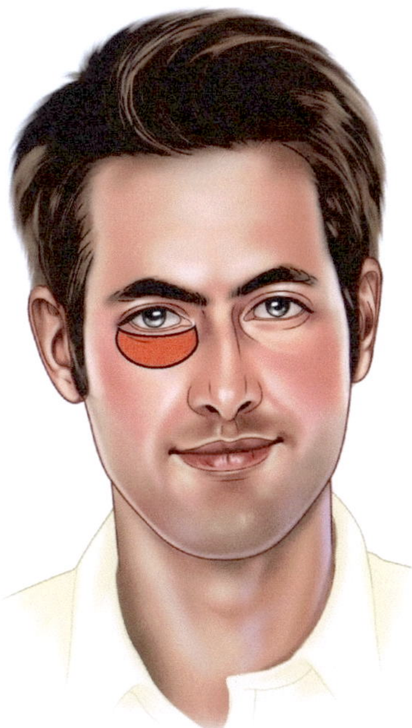

Fig. 9.16 Danger zone for contracture and ectropion

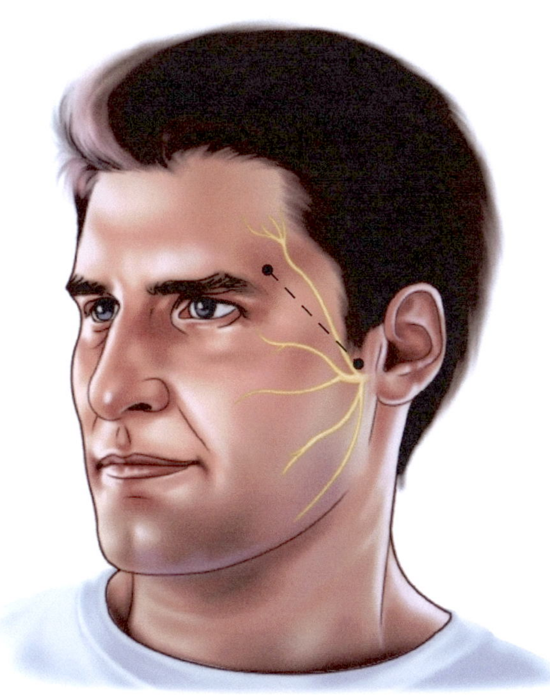

Fig. 9.17 Course of the frontal nerve

When to Transfer

Patients may require Mohs surgery in high risk lesions such as recurrent lesions, lesions in risk zones (medial canthus, alar base), or those arising in an irradiated field. Poorly defined lesions may also require Mohs surgery.

Suggested Reading

Jackson IT. Local flaps in head and neck reconstruction. 2nd ed. St. Louis: Quality Medical Publishing; 2007.

Defect Closure After Lesion Excision of the Face

Kent Lam and Douglas M. Sidle

Indications

The reconstruction of soft tissue defects is an inherent part of the resection of benign and malignant cutaneous lesions of the face. Because the face serves essential functional and aesthetic roles in daily human activities and interactions, surgeons must pay meticulous attention to the repair of facial defects in order to achieve optimal patient outcomes. The ultimate goal of facial reconstruction is twofold: (1) to preserve the functional abilities of the face and (2) to restore cosmetic shape and structure following soft tissue excision.

Preoperative Preparation

The ability to complete a successful reconstruction of a facial defect involves adequate planning prior to the surgical procedure. Preoperatively, surgeons should carefully assess the size, depth, and location of the cutaneous lesion that requires surgical resection. Large and deep soft tissue defects tend to necessitate more complex reconstructive options than small and superficial wounds. Likewise, the involvement of certain anatomical facial aesthetic subunits, including the eyes, nose, and lips, oftentimes involves a higher level of reconstructive complexity due to regional differences in skin quality and risk for asymmetry and distortion following repair. Figure 10.1 illustrates the various facial aesthetic subunits, which are based upon the skin thickness, color, texture, and underlying structural contour of the region. A working knowledge of the facial aesthetic subunits and their boundaries aids the surgeon in excisions and cosmetic repairs. Better cosmetic outcomes can be achieved if the surgeon is able to keep an excision within a specific subunit. Better yet, the surgeon may be able to hide an excision in one of the subunit boundaries.

The preoperative evaluation additionally provides valuable details regarding patient-related variables that may affect the successful repair of a facial defect. Patient comorbidities, for example, is an important consideration for choosing the most appropriate options for wound repair. Patients who have significant comorbidities may benefit from a simple reconstructive effort, even though this technique may result in a less desirable cosmetic outcome. For patients who are active smokers, smoking cessation can be encouraged preoperatively in order to promote improved wound healing following facial reconstruction. Most importantly, at the preoperative evaluation, surgeons should have an open discussion with patients about specific expectations with the facial reconstruction. This preoperative discussion, combined with characteristics of the facial defect and surrounding soft tissue, allows surgeons to formulate an individualized surgical plan that is not only feasible and acceptable from a surgical perspective, but also compatible with patient priorities and desires.

Facial defect closures may occur in either the outpatient setting or the operative suite, depending on the extent of facial soft tissue resection, complexity of reconstruction, patient comorbidities, and the preferences of surgeons and patients. The use of local anesthesia, intravenous sedation, or general anesthesia also varies according to the specific patient-related factors and surgeon preferences. The use of local anesthesia or intravenous sedation offers certain advantages in medically complex patients, including decreased postoperative recovery time and overall operative cost. On the other hand, healthy patients and their surgeons may opt for the use of general anesthesia if there are concerns for airway monitoring, if the planned facial reconstruction is complex and complicated, and if patients anticipate significant anxiety during the procedure.

K. Lam, M.D. • D.M. Sidle, M.D., F.A.C.S. (✉)
Department of Otolaryngology, Northwestern University Feinberg School of Medicine, 676 North Saint Clair Street, Suite 1325, Chicago, IL 60611, USA
e-mail: dsidle@nmff.org

A.L. Halverson and D.C. Borgstrom (eds.), *Advanced Surgical Techniques for Rural Surgeons*,
DOI 10.1007/978-1-4939-1495-1_10, © Springer Science+Business Media New York 2015

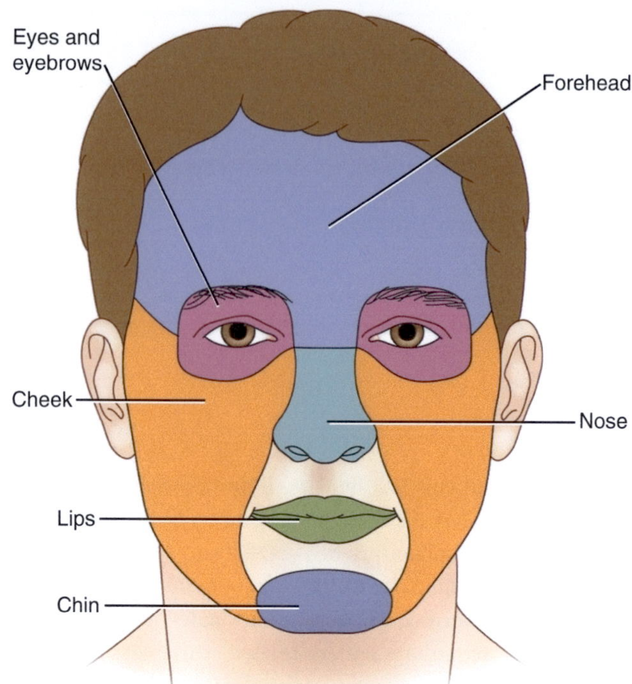

Fig. 10.1 Major aesthetic facial subunits. The six major subunits of the face includes (a) the forehead, (b) eyes and eyebrows, (c) nose, (d) cheek, (e) lips, and (f) chin

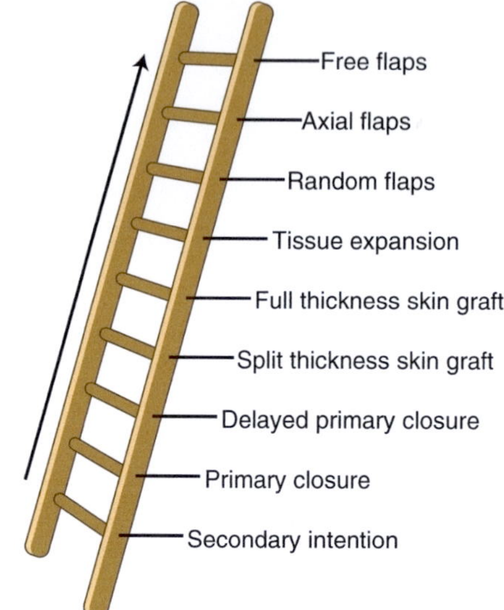

Fig. 10.2 The reconstructive ladder. The basis for reconstructive efforts of soft tissue defects is conceptualized on a continuum that places techniques along a range of complexities

Operative Strategy

The reconstructive ladder is used to conceptualize the variety of options used to close facial defects as a continuum of increasing levels of complexity (Fig. 10.2). These options range from closure by secondary intent, which is the simplest of techniques in the reconstructive ladder, to a microvascular free flap, which sits at the highest rung of complexity in the reconstructive ladder. Consideration of reconstructive options for cutaneous facial defects generally start with the simplest options, but move up the reconstructive ladder as needed in order to achieve a functionally and cosmetically adequate outcome for patients. Along this gradient of options, the use of linear primary closures on the face is oftentimes a sufficient and reliable technique for most soft tissue defects encountered by surgeons.

The merits of primary closures with bilateral advancement flaps are reflected in the ability of surgeons to repair soft tissue defects using simple primary wound closures while attaining adequate and cosmetically acceptable results. By closing wounds primarily, surgeons are more likely to maximally preserve healthy tissue and effectively match skin texture, color, and thickness. Primary wound closure also avoids the risks that are associated with more advanced reconstructive techniques, including wound contracture with skin grafts and tissue necrosis due to compromised vasculature with local flaps. While other advanced reconstructive techniques may be indicated in facial soft tissue defects that are extensive in size and involve more complex facial aesthetic subunits, these cases are more commonly executed with the consultation of a facial plastic surgeon. Other reconstructive techniques, specifically flap repair, are discussed extensively within the literature.

As is the case for all rungs of the reconstructive ladder, the successful execution of a plan to repair a facial defect with primary closure is based upon general principles of aesthetic reconstruction. First, soft tissue should be handled delicately to reduce excessive trauma and crush injury. Second, a primary wound closure should be completed with the eversion of skin edges and minimizing of wound tension. Wound tension increases the risk for wound dehiscence and widening scarring, and may be reduced through undermining of skin flaps adjacent to the wound and through a layered closure of the soft tissue defects. Third, closure of soft tissue defects along the relaxed skin tension lines most effectively hide scars from the facial repairs. Incision lines at the boundaries of the facial aesthetic subunits are also effectively camouflaged by the light reflections and shadows of facial contours at these locations (Fig. 10.3).

Operative Technique

Soft tissue defects of the face may be repaired sequentially after excision of cutaneous lesions or several days after the excision. In either case, the wound should be thoroughly

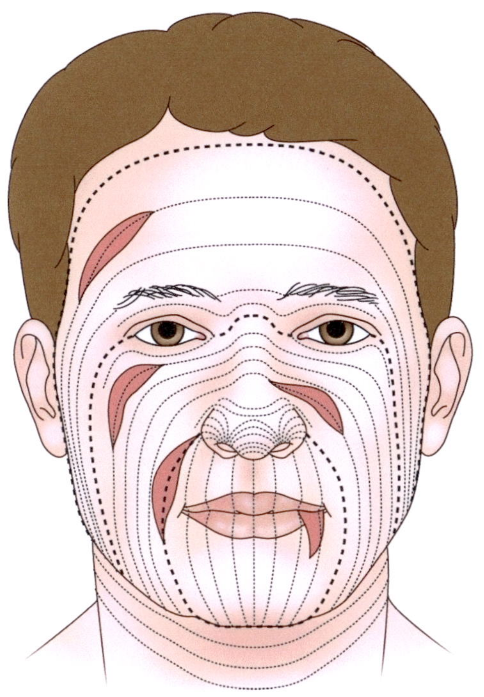

Fig. 10.3 Relaxed skin tension lines (RSTL) of the face. Repairs are best hidden by aligning incisions with the RSTLs of the face

cleaned prior to the reconstruction. Wound preparation includes removing contaminants and bacteria within the wound through the use of mild disinfectants. Once the wound has been appropriately prepped, areas of nonviable tissue should be debrided to optimize wound healing and to prevent infectious complications.

Local anesthesia, routinely 1 % lidocaine with 1:100,000 epinephrine, is administered prior to the process of cleansing and debriding the wound. The injection of local anesthesia into the wound bed also provides vasoconstrictive effects, tumescence, and hydrodissecton of adjacent tissue planes. The hydrodissection achieved by the injection of local anesthesia assists with the undermining of adjacent skin for bilateral advancement flaps.

Facial defects following the resection of cutaneous lesions are routinely fashioned in a circular fashion, given the need to perform the excision with a margin of healthy tissue. A vertical line closure can be created for these circular facial defects by converting the wound bed into long elliptical defects. The ratio of the short axis of the ellipse to the long axis should be appropriately 1:3. The long axis of the elliptical wound should be oriented such that the linear line closure follows along the relaxed skin tension lines (Fig. 10.4).

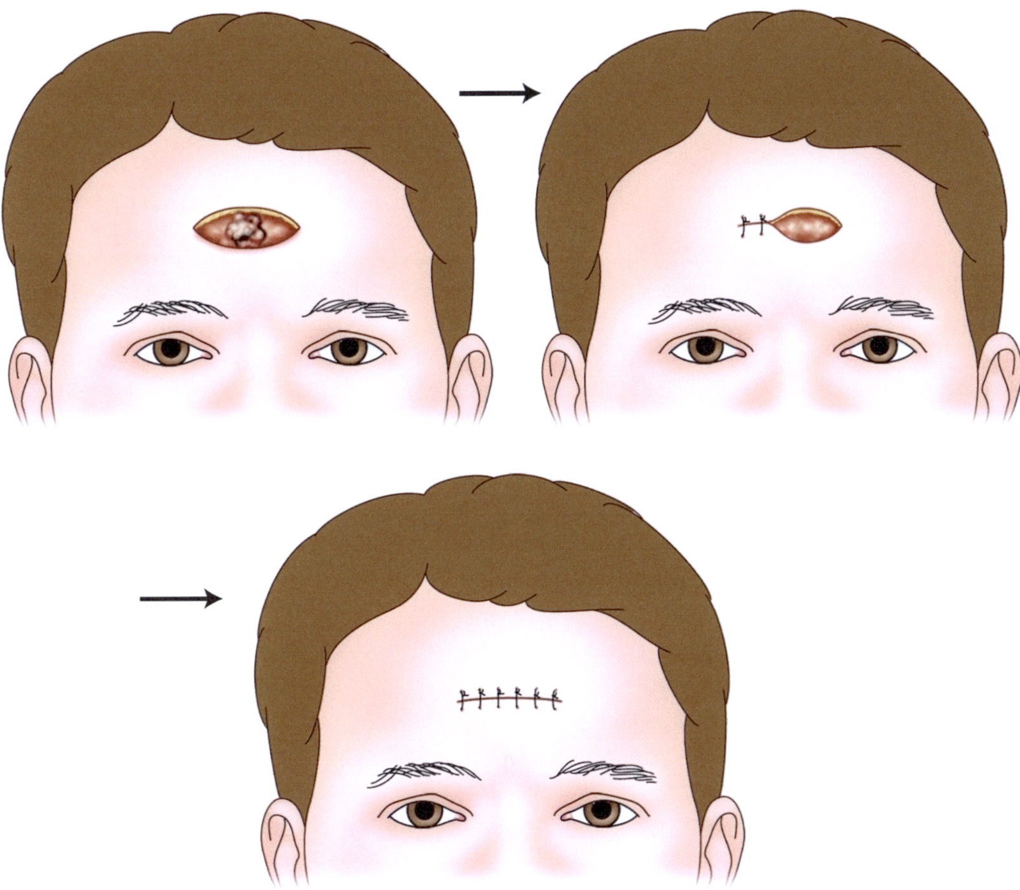

Fig. 10.4 Fashioning of an elliptical-shaped wound. The conversion of a soft tissue defect from a round shape to an elliptical shape allows for improved linear primary closure of the wound

Table 10.1 Common suture materials used on the face and neck

Suture material	Biodegradation: absorption time	Retention of 50 % original tensile strength (days)	Physical configuration	Primary uses	Special characteristics
Percutaneous sutures					
Prolene—synthetic	Nonabsorbable	Indefinite	Monofilament	• Percutaneous facial closure	• Best for prolonged tensile strength • Lowest tissue reactivity • High plasiticity to accommodate wound swelling
Nylon—synthetic	Nonabsorbable	Indefinite	Monofilament	• Percutaneous facial closure	• Good for prolonged tensile strength • Minimal tissue reactivity • Difficult to handle and tie
Fast-absorbing gut—natural	Absorbable: 21–42 days via proteolytic enzymatic digestion	4–6 days	Monofilament	• Percutaneous facial closure • Ideal for use in pediatric wound closure	• Low tensile strength • High tissue reactivity • Does not require suture removal—low tensile strength
Dermal sutures					
Vicryl—synthetic	Absorbable: 56–70 days via hydrolysis	30 days	Multifilament	• Dermal closure of deep soft tissue lacerations • Closure of intraoral mucosa or tongue lacerations	• Improved tensile strength compared to catgut sutures • Minimal tissue reactivity
Polydioxanone (PDS)—synthetic	Absorbable: 180–200 Days via slow hydrolysis	45–60 days	Monofilament	• Dermal closure of deep soft tissue lacerations • Ideal for contaminated wounds	• Best tensile strength compared to other absorbable sutures • Least tissue reactivity

Following the creation of an elliptical defect, the surrounding loose tissue planes are undermined with blunt dissection using sharp scissors. The undermining within the subcutaneous planes creates advancement flaps that minimize wound tension and trapdoor formation. Meticulous hemostasis during this dissection is performed with electrodessication to minimize the risks of hematoma formation. Excision of dog-ears or standing cone deforming at the ends of the reapproximated skin edges may be necessary to eliminate pincushioning and to improve cosmetic outcomes.

The wound is closed in layers first using buried deep dermal layers using absorbable sutures (i.e., vicryl) with #4-0 or #5-0 caliber. The purpose of these deep dermal stitches for primary closure is to relieve wound tension and to eliminate dead space within the defect. Percutaneous sutures using nonabsorbable sutures (i.e., Prolene) or absorbable sutures (i.e., fast-absorbing gut) with #5-0 or #6-0 caliber are thereafter placed along the surface of the wound edge with attention paid to ensure good wound eversion. While simple interrupted percutaneous suture may generally be used to provide strong reapproximation of the wound edges, a running percutaneous closure may be used to provide even distribution along the wound length. Table 10.1 highlights several of the commonly used sutures for wound closure.

Potential Pitfalls

For primary closures of facial soft tissue defects, acceptable functional and cosmetic outcomes require the closure to be completed with minimal wound tension. Insufficient undermining of the skin edges, failure to perform a layered closure, and patient inability to minimize straining after wound closure may all result in elevated wound tension. If soft tissue defects cannot be repaired primarily with minimal wound tension, surgeons should move higher on the reconstructive ladder to choose another surgical technique to adequately repair the facial defect.

Postoperative Care

Meticulous wound care is essential for optimal healing of soft tissue wounds. A nonadhesive dressing may be applied immediately following the soft tissue repair in order to provide gentle compression and promote reepithelialization of the wounds. Beginning on the first postoperative day, gently removing the crusting over the reapproximated skin edges with small amounts of hydrogen peroxide improves the process of reepithelization. This may be followed by application of a thin layer of antibiotic ointment, which moisturizes the wound and also contributes to the prevention of wound infections. Patients are generally advised to not shower until at least 24 h following the repair. For primary closures of soft tissue defects on the face, sutures are usually removed 5–7 days following the reconstruction.

Common Complications

Common complications in the closure of facial soft tissue defects vary according to the method of reconstructive technique selected for use. For primary closures, common complications are divided into early and late types. Early problems include wound dehiscence, bleeding, hematoma formation, and infections. Late complications include cosmetic deformity and functional loss, such as the development of ectropion and entropion following the repair of soft tissue defects near the eyelid. Hypertrophic scar formation as a late complication can be treated with triamcinolone injections and topical application of silastic sheeting.

When to Transfer

Given the importance of achieving a good functional and cosmetic outcome with the repair of facial defects, consultation of facial plastic surgeons is recommended if the defect is expected to be complex. Complicated cases resulting from lesions of larger size or in more complex locations with reduced skin laxity should be directed to specialists who are more experienced with performing more complex procedures along the reconstructive ladder.

Suggested Reading

1. Fazio MJ, Zitelli JA. Principles of reconstruction following excision of nonmelanoma skin cancer. Clin Dermatol. 1995;13(6):601–16. Epub 1995/11/01.
2. Poulsen M, Burmeister B, Kennedy D. Preservation of form and function in the management of head and neck skin cancer. World J Surg. 2003;27(7):868–74. Epub 2003/09/26.
3. Soliman S, Hatef DA, Hollier Jr LH, Thornton JF. The rationale for direct linear closure of facial Mohs' defects. Plast Reconstr Surg. 2011;127(1):142–9. Epub 2011/01/05.

Kyle R. Miller and Jeffrey D. Wayne

Indications

While melanom a accounts for only 4 % of all skin cancers, it contributes to almost 80 % of skin cancer deaths. The recommended therapies for melanoma differ significantly from that of basal cell carcinoma and squamous cell carcinoma. When faced with a suspicious pigmented lesion, thought must be given to the ultimate therapy, should the lesion in fact be a malignant melanoma. We therefore recommend full thickness biopsy, including punch biopsy or narrow-margin (1–2 mm) excisional biopsy, if the lesion is greater than 8 mm in diameter. For lesions on the trunk or proximal extremity, primary closure of the biopsy site is preferred. It is crucial that all biopsy specimens be reviewed by a qualified Dermatopathologist, with expertise in the diagnosis of melanoma. An appropriate wide local excision includes the previous scar along with the tumor bed while obtaining appropriate margins per current NCCN guidelines, which are based on the depth of the lesion (Table 11.1). Under appropriate circumstances, consideration should be given to performing a sentinel lymph node biopsy at the same operative setting (Table 11.2).

Preoperative Preparation

Most lesions can be excised using an elliptical, longitudinal excision of the scar and tumor bed following Langer's lines on the trunk and proximal extremities (Fig. 11.1). The Breslow depth is used to determine the margins of the resection. In situ lesions are routinely resected with margins of 0.5–1.0 cm. T1 melanomas, with a Breslow depth of less than or equal to 1.0 mm, are excised with 1 cm margins. T2 lesions, 1.01–2 mm in depth can be safely excised in most locations with a 1–2 cm margins. An exception may be the scalp, where consideration should be given to perform a 2 cm wide local excision, due to the higher rate of local recurrences in this location. T3 lesions (2.01–4 mm in depth) should be excised with 2 cm margins. Thick, T4 (>4.0 mm) lesions are also excised with a 2.0 cm margin.

Thin melanomas with a Breslow's depth of ≤0.75 mm (and especially those with no ulceration and no mitotic figures) have a low likelihood to metastasize to regional lymph nodes (<5 %). Patients with lesions ≤0.75 mm thick are usually not offered a sentinel lymph node biopsy, unless they have a lesion with one or more adverse prognostic indicators. Such factors include ulceration, lymphovascular invasion, a high mitotic count, or Clark's level >III (if the mitotic count cannot be determined). All patients with a measured Breslow thickness ≥0.76 mm, with clinically negative nodes (clinical Stage I and II), are appropriate candidates for sentinel node biopsy. Almost all procedures are performed an outpatient basis. We prefer a single dose of a first generation cephalosporin, or clindamycin in the setting of a penicillin allergy, as prophylaxis. As per current Surgical Care Improvement Project (SCIP) guidelines, the perioperative antibiotics should be administered prior to creation of the incision.

Operative Strategy

Lymphoscintigraphy should be performed in every case in which sentinel lymph node biopsy is performed. Preoperative lymphoscintigraphy helps identify the number and relative location of the sentinel lymph node(s) in a particular basin. The mapping may also identify in transit sentinel nodes that may be a source of regional or distant metastasis if not recognized and excised. The lymphoscintigraphy is typically done on the morning of surgery, 1–2 h prior to the excision.

K.R. Miller, M.D., M.B.A. • J.D. Wayne, M.D., F.A.C.S. (✉)
Department of Surgery, Northwestern University,
Feinberg School of Medicine, 676 North Saint Clair Street,
Arkes 650, Chicago, IL 60611, USA
e-mail: jwayne@northwestern.edu

A.L. Halverson and D.C. Borgstrom (eds.), *Advanced Surgical Techniques for Rural Surgeons*,
DOI 10.1007/978-1-4939-1495-1_11, © Springer Science+Business Media New York 2015

Table 11.1 Surgical margins for wide excision of primary melanoma (NCCN guidelines)

Tumor thickness	Recommended clinical margins
In situ	0.5 cm
≤1.0 mm	1.0 cm (category 1)
1.01–2 mm	1–2 cm (category 1)
2.01–4 mm	2.0 cm (category 1)
>4 mm	2.0 cm (category 1)

Margins may be modified to accommodate individual anatomic or functional considerations

Table 11.2 Indications for sentinel lymph node biopsy (clinically node negative patients)

Discuss and consider:
Breslow depth ≥0.76 mm, no ulceration, no ulceration, mitotic rate <1 per mm^2
Discuss and offer:
Breslow depth ≥0.76 mm, and any of the following:
Ulceration
Mitotic rate ≥1 per mm^2
Lymphovascular invasion
Breslow depth >1 mm (any)

Operative Technique

The patient is seen in nuclear medicine the morning of the surgical excision. A four-point intradermal injection technique is used to inject 0.5–1 mCi of 99m-technetium sulfur colloid into the lesion. Early and frequent images using a gamma camera are then obtained in anterior and lateral views in order to identify the sentinel lymph nodes to be biopsied. At surgery, just prior to prepping and positioning the patient, 1–3 mL of 1 % isosulfan blue dye (Lymphazurin) is injected in a sterile fashion in the area around the lesion or biopsy scar. 1 cc of 1 % plain lidocaine may be added to the lymphazurin for patient comfort.

The patient is prepped and draped in the usual sterile fashion including the nodal basins from which the sentinel nodes will be harvested. The patient should be positioned to allow for nodal biopsy along with excision of the malignant lesion if at all possible. The patient can always be repositioned if needed between the sentinel node biopsy and the wide local excision. A time out is performed with the side and site of the surgery verified.

Attention is first turned toward the sentinel node basin(s). A handheld gamma probe is brought on the field with the use of a sterile sheath (Fig. 11.1). After injection of a local anesthetic, a #15 blade is used to make a focused 2–3 cm incision directly over the highest point of radioactivity. Careful sharp and blunt dissection should then be performed to identify the blue channels leading to the first sentinel node. (Meticulous hemostasis can be achieved using electrocautery and absorbable ties, as necessary. The channels are traced down

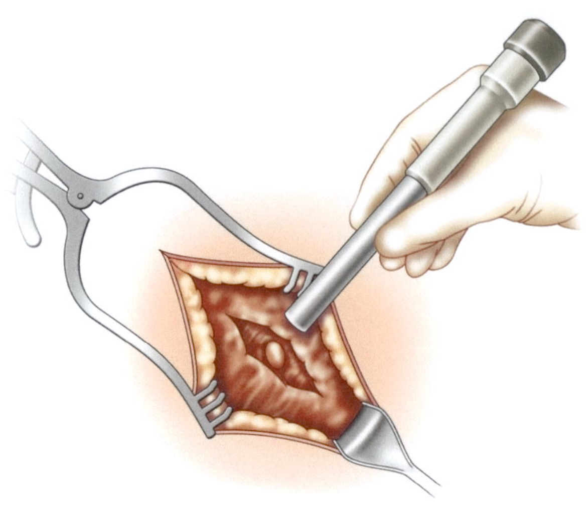

Fig. 11.1 Identification of a sentinel lymph node with a sterile gamma probe

with careful dissection to identify the blue nodes, which are then isolated and excised. Upon excision, the sentinel node is scanned ex vivo with the maximal radioactivity (counts per second) recorded. The basin is then rescanned and all blue nodes, and any node with an ex vivo count within 10 % of the hottest node should be removed. In addition, any node which is abnormal to palpation should be harvested and sent as a non-sentinel node to pathology. The nodes are individually identified, marked, and sent for permanent histology and immunohistochemistry. Frozen section analysis should not be performed. Immunohistochemistry with a panel of melanoma-specific markers, often including s-100, HMB-45, and Melan-A, is required to confirm that the sentinel nodes are positive for micrometastatic disease. After the wound is irrigated with sterile saline and hemostasis is achieved, the wound is closed in two layers. Deep dermal sutures using 3-0 undyed, absorbable suture are used with a 4-0 monofilament suture used for the skin. Steri-strips or 2-Octyl Cyanoacrylate (Dermabond) is then placed over the incision.

After excision of the sentinel nodes, attention should then be turned toward the primary site. A sterile ruler is used to mark out the planned margins from all edges of the lesion of biopsy scar. Local anesthetic (typically 1 % lidocaine with or without epinephrine and 0.5 % marcaine in a 1:1 mixture) is used in the areas of the skins to be resected. The excision is then typically extended along the long axis of the extremity (Fig. 11.2a). The length of the excision should be at least three times the measured width of the planned excision for a tension-free closure and to avoid redundant skin at the ends of the excision. An initial incision is performed using a #15 blade. The incision is then carried down to the investing muscular fascia using electrocautery. The dissection should be performed in a perpendicular fashion, until the specimen is cleared from the underlying fascia.

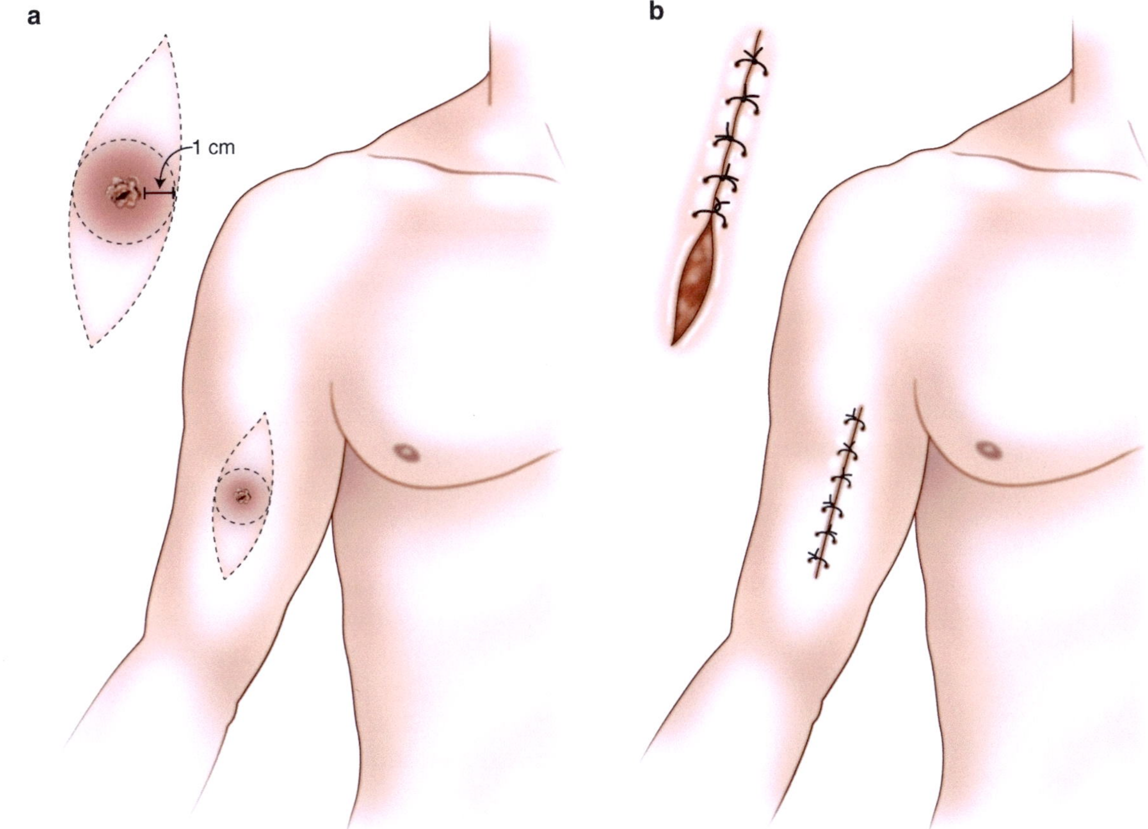

Fig. 11.2 (**a**) Wide local excision with 1 cm margins. (**b**) Preparation of a melanoma defect for closure

The specimen should be marked with silk sutures for orientation and sent for permanent sections. Irrigation with normal saline should then be performed followed by hemostasis with electrocautery, as necessary. At this point, single skin hooks are used at each end of the incision to align the wound so that 1 cm interval lines can be placed in order to approximate the deep dermal sutures (Fig. 11.2a). With a deep soft tissue defect, a closed-suction drain may be placed in the wound bed prior to closure to prevent the development of a seroma postoperatively. The deep dermis is then re-approximated using interrupted 3-0 undyed, absorbable sutures at 8–10 mm intervals as previously marked. The skin is then closed with either interrupted 3-0 nylon sutures or a running 4-0 monofilament, subcuticular stitch. Preference should be given to interrupted suture placement if there is a concern for excessive tension along the excised area.

Potential Pitfalls

A primary concern is achieving histologically negative margins. Emphasis thus remains on a perpendicular dissection down to the underlying fascia. This is especially true for lentigo maligna melanoma, where there may be sub-clinical extension of disease well beyond the biopsy site. An option here would be to perform the excision and closure at separate settings, waiting for negative margins on permanent sections, prior to proceeding with the final closure. Another pitfall would be the inability to close the incision primarily with a tension-free closure. Thus, careful consideration should be given to enlisting the aid of a plastic surgeon for areas that may require a skin graft or rotation flap for ideal closure. This is often the case with areas of the body with minimal skin laxity, such as the distal extremities, scalp, or face.

Postoperative Care

Most patients are discharged home on the day of surgery and educated on the potential for complications. Drain care teaching with instructions on how to record the outputs done prior to discharge if appropriate. If a drain is left in place, the patient is instructed to return to clinic for removal if total output is less than 20 cc per day for two consecutive days. Sutures are typically removed approximately 10 days to 2 weeks postoperatively with subsequent placement of steri-strips. A 2-week initial follow-up also allows time for the return of the pathology including the margins and sentinel lymph node results in order to facilitate further management and follow-up.

In follow-up, all patients should be examined with a full head-to-toe skin survey with examination of all lymph node basins every 3–12 months. There is no role for routine LDH levels or chest radiographs in the follow-up for patients with Stage I-IIA disease.

Should a sentinel node be positive, completion lymph node dissection remains the standard of care. For positive inguinal nodes, the patient should undergo a superficial and possible deep ilio-inguinal lymph node dissection. For a positive axillary node, the patient requires a level III axillary lymph node dissection with complete surgical clearance of the level III nodes above the axillary vein and medial to the pectoralis minor. For a positive neck node, a modified radical neck dissection is performed to gain regional control of the disease. In general, these complex operations should be performed by a surgeon with advanced oncologic training, who performs several such operations each year. Alternatively, the patient may consider entry onto a clinical trial, which randomizes patients to either completion nodal dissection or observation with ultrasound at 3-month intervals. Alternatively, the patient may consider entry onto a clinical trial.

Common Complications

Seroma

Hematoma

Cellulitis

Wound infections

Wound edge dehiscence

Subcuticular closure in a high-tension wound or from premature suture removal

Lymphedema

($\leq$5 %) all patients undergoing a sentinel node biopsy should be counseled regarding the risk of lymphedema

When to Transfer

Melanomas of the head and neck can be challenging. Almost all require the assistance of a plastic surgeon for closure with acceptable function and cosmesis. Similarly, subungual melanomas of the digits will require, in most cases, amputation in addition to surgical staging of the nodal basin. If an orthopedic or plastic surgeon is not available to assist, the patient should be transferred to a regional center with expertise in the care of melanoma patients. Finally, if a patient presents with grossly palpable nodal disease, metastasis should be confirmed with an FNA of the node in question. Transfer of the patient to a multidisciplinary melanoma center is then warranted to determine if the patient should be treated with neoadjuvant therapy, or undergo excision of their primary with regional node dissection at the same setting. Finally, patients with substantial regional recurrence, who may benefit from an isolated limb infusion or perfusion, should be transferred to a center with experience with such procedures.

Suggested Reading

Grotz T. Preservation of the deep muscular fascia and locoregional control in melanoma. Surgery. 2013;153(4):535–41.

Fincher T. Patterns of recurrence after sentinel lymph node biopsy for cutaneous melanoma. Am J Surg. 2003;186(6):675–81.

Morton D. Overview and update of the phase III Multicenter Selective Lymphadenectomy Trials (MSLT-1 and MSLT-II) in melanoma. Clin Exp Metastasis. 2012;29:699–706.

National Comprehensive Cancer Network. NCCN guidelines v.20013.2. 2013. http://www.nccn.org/professionals/physician_gls/pdf/melanoma.pdf

Sladden MJ, Balch C, Barzilai DA, Berg D, Freiman A, Handiside T, Hollis S, Lens MB, Thompson JF. Surgical excision margins for primary cutaneous melanoma. Cochrane Database Syst Rev. 2009;4: CD004835.

Wasif N, Gray RJ, Bagaria SP, Pockaj BA. Compliance with guidelines in the surgical management of cutaneous melanoma across the USA. Melanoma Res. 2013;23(4):276–82.

Jennifer E. Cheesborough, Michael Gart, and Mohammed Alghoul

Introduction

Repair of any skin defect is determined primarily by the size of the defect and the laxity of the surrounding skin. Approximating the edges of any defect with reasonable tension depends on the mobility of the neighboring tissue, which varies according to the location. For instance, closing an abdominal defect primarily is easier than closing a sternal defect or one over the shoulder area. Similarly, as a general rule, the more distal an extremity wound is, the more challenging the reconstruction becomes. Primary skin closure is the simplest method of repair on the reconstructive ladder. It is relatively straightforward, easy to perform, and avoids a donor site. By applying a gentle pinch on the wound edges, one should be able to judge whether primary closure is feasible. If tension is excessive, then other strategies such as skin grafting or closure with local flaps must be considered.

Tissue recruitment is a key concept in reconstructive surgery. Recruitment is achieved with tissue mobilization or transfer while preserving vascularity since recruiting nonviable skin will complicate the problem further. Mobilization is achieved with undermining in primary closure and/or making specifically designed cuts to rotate, transpose, or advance tissue into the defect. It is also an important concept to achieve an aesthetic repair that preserves body contour and minimizes scarring. Using the relaxed skin tension lines as a guide to design incisions, excising any standing cones (dog-ears) at the end of a closure and avoiding skin grafts in cosmetically sensitive areas are all consistent with this concept.

This chapter will discuss the basic principles and technical steps of post-excisional defect closure of the trunk and extremities.

J.E. Cheesborough, M.D. • M. Gart, M.D. • M. Alghoul, M.D. (✉)
Division of Plastic and Reconstructive Surgery, Northwestern University, 675 North St. Clair Street, Suite 19-250, Chicago, IL 60611, USA
e-mail: malghoul@nmh.org

Indications

- Excisional biopsy wound
- Clean wound under tension
- Wound that is either too large for primary closure, or would significantly distort the surrounding tissue architecture if closed primarily

Preoperative Preparation

- Confirm that the lesion has been completely excised (await final margins from pathology if necessary)
- Administer appropriate systemic antibiotics prior to skin incision (if not performed concurrent with excision of lesion)
- Determine and administer appropriate anesthesia (local anesthesia such as lidocaine 1 % with 1:100,000 epinephrine with or without IV sedation)

Pitfalls and Danger Points

- Incomplete excision of the lesion prior to closure
- Incomplete debridement of wound if closure is delayed
- Skin necrosis due to excessive tension or devascularization of skin edges
- Shearing injury or hematoma preventing skin graft take
- Injury to surrounding blood vessels, nerves

Operative Strategy

The first step in any reconstructive procedure is to define the defect fully. While the dimensions of the defect are important, one must also consider the quality of the skin and subcutaneous tissue, the type of tissue at the base of the wound,

A.L. Halverson and D.C. Borgstrom (eds.), *Advanced Surgical Techniques for Rural Surgeons*,
DOI 10.1007/978-1-4939-1495-1_12, © Springer Science+Business Media New York 2015

and the surrounding structures. If reconstruction has been delayed from the initial excision, gentle debridement of all granulation tissue must be performed prior to closure. After careful inspection of the clean wound, consideration of the closure options begins. Many wounds can be closed primarily provided that sufficient undermining is performed to allow for minimum tension on the skin edges. Other wounds may require tissue recruitment from the surrounding skin in the form of rotation or advancement flaps, or skin grafting from distant donor sites.

Operative Technique

Primary Closure

Elective incisions or excisions on the trunk should be planned so that they lie parallel to the relaxed skin tension lines (Fig. 12.1) to allow for low- or no-tension closures. In the extremities, incisions should lie parallel to the longitudinal axis of the limb. For lacerations and local trauma, it is important

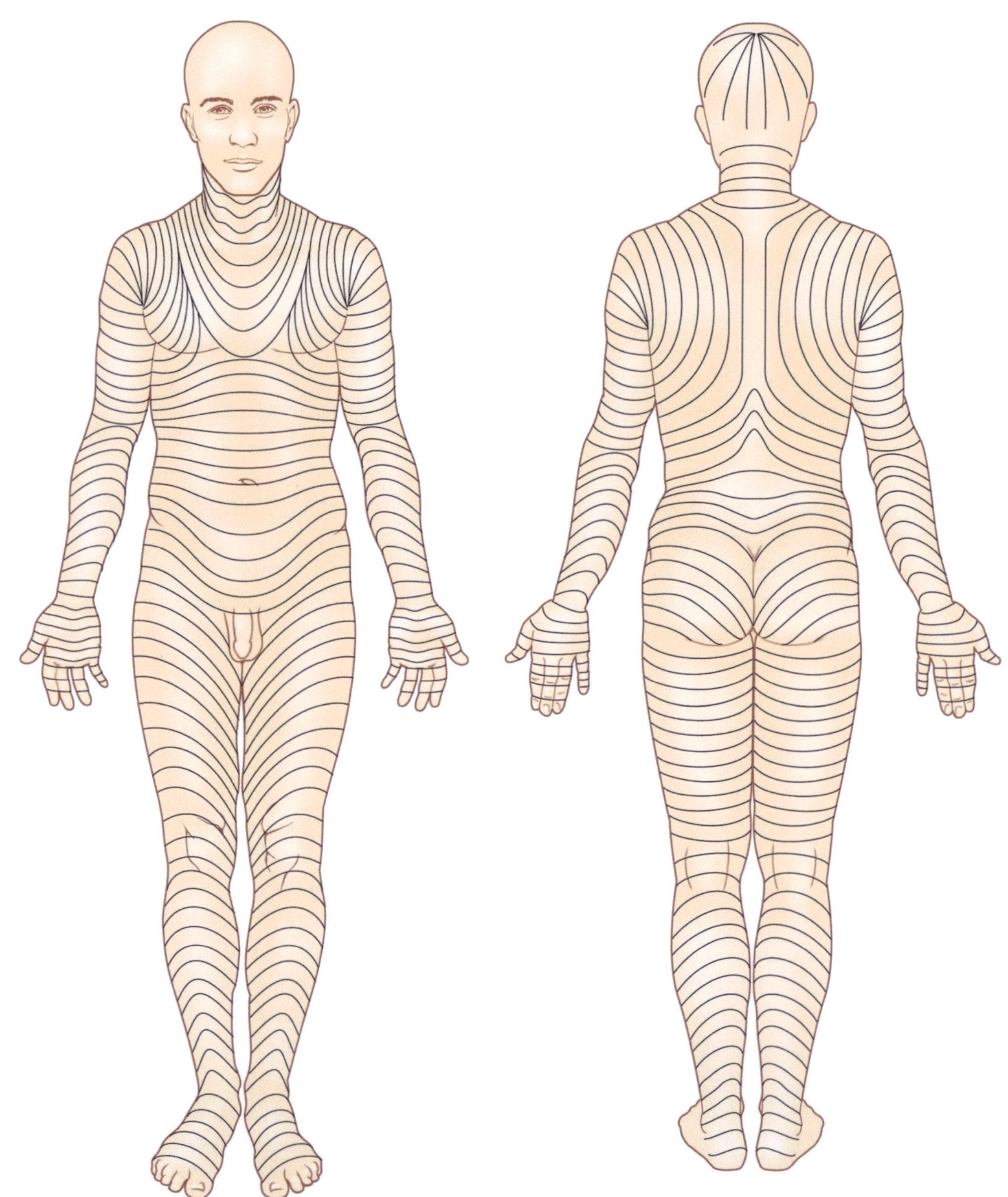

Fig. 12.1 Incisions should be designed so that they lie in parallel to the depicted relaxed skin tension lines to minimize tension upon closure

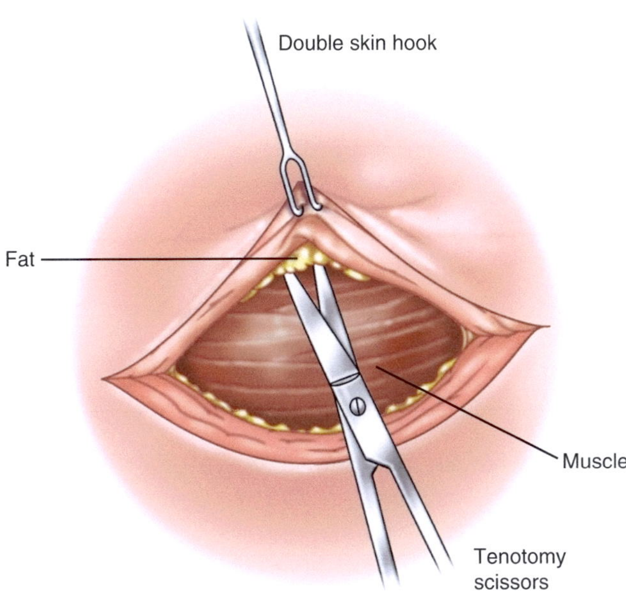

Fig. 12.2 Proper dissection technique involves the use of double skin hooks to minimize damage to the skin edges (forceps cause a crush injury), and blunt dissection in the avascular plane using tenotomy scissors

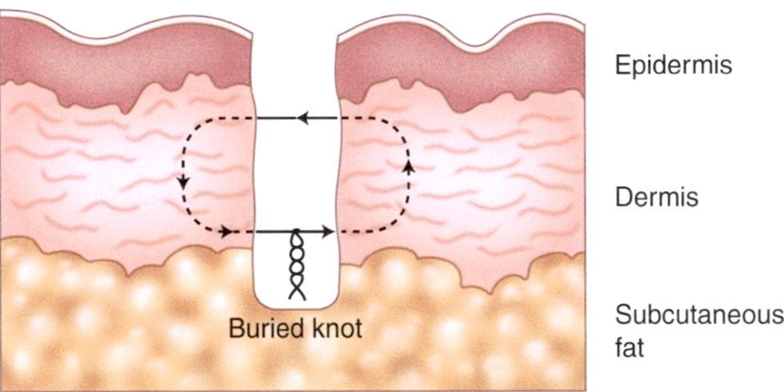

Fig. 12.3 Deep dermal sutures are interrupted sutures with a buried knot designed to take tension off the final layer of closure. It is important to enter and exit the skin at the same level on each side in order to bring the skin edges together properly

to excise crushed and nonviable tissue to provide clean wound edges for approximation.

After performance of any necessary debridement, care should be taken to minimize any crush injury to the skin edges. Double skin hooks are used to elevate the skin edges, not toothed forceps. The defect should be undermined sufficiently to allow for a low or no tension closure. Undermining is performed in the avascular plane just superficial to the underlying fascia using tenotomy scissors in a spreading motion (Fig. 12.2). A low current monopolar electrocautery can also be used. Attention is given to preservation of perforating vessels of significant size and avoidance of injury to superficial sensory nerves. This is particularly important in the extremities as injury to a major superficial vein, such as the saphenous or cephalic vein, or a sensory nerve can easily occur. A surgeon must anticipate and avoid these structures in their predictable anatomic locations. Once the skin edges lie in close approximation with application of gentle pressure, attention is turned to closure of the wound.

A layered closure is always employed on the trunk and extremities. If the underlying superficial fascia (Scarpas's fascia) can be identified, then it should be reapproximated using interrupted 2-0 or 3-0 absorbable suture. Dead space, although unusual in straightforward primary closures, must be eliminated to prevent formation of a seroma and eventual dehiscence of the wound. The placement of "quilting sutures," between the deep undersurface of the undermined skin and the deep fascia can be very helpful in obliterating the dead space. Placement of a closed suction drain, such as a Jackson-Pratt drain is also acceptable.

The skin edges should then be approximated using 3-0 absorbable interrupted buried deep dermal sutures (Fig. 12.3). Remember that buried dermal sutures provide strength to allow the external sutures to be removed early, but they do not prevent eventual widening of the scar as they are absorbable sutures. The skin edges should be everted to obtain the best result, as a wound that is precisely brought together tends to widen whereas a wound with everted skin edges will flatten over time into a narrower scar. The final layer of closure everts the skin.

There are several techniques for skin closure. The most commonly utilized is the simple interrupted suture. In order to evert the skin edges, the suture needle pierces the skin at an angle away from the incision so that the deeper aspect of the suture is further apart than the superficial aspect thus creating a parallelogram (Fig. 12.4). As with all techniques, the depth of the suture on opposite sides of the wound should be equal to prevent the edges from overlapping. Horizontal or vertical mattress sutures may be employed in areas of thicker skin (the back and glabrous tissue on the hands and feet) to maximize eversion of the skin edges and to distribute tension in areas of mobile skin. Both of these techniques are best performed using a 3-0 or 4-0 nonabsorbable monofilament suture.

Subcuticular (intradermal) sutures prevent suture marks in the skin and therefore are often preferred in areas of cosmetic importance. In this running dermal closure, horizontal bites through the superficial dermis approximate the skin edges. A 4-0 nonabsorbable or absorbable monofilament may be employed. Nonabsorbable suture should be removed in approximately 10–14 days regardless of closure type.

Staples may save time for long incisions. The skin edges should be gently everted using toothed forceps prior to placement of each staple, as there is a tendency for the skin to invert otherwise. Staples must be removed early (by postoperative day 7) to prevent "train track" scars.

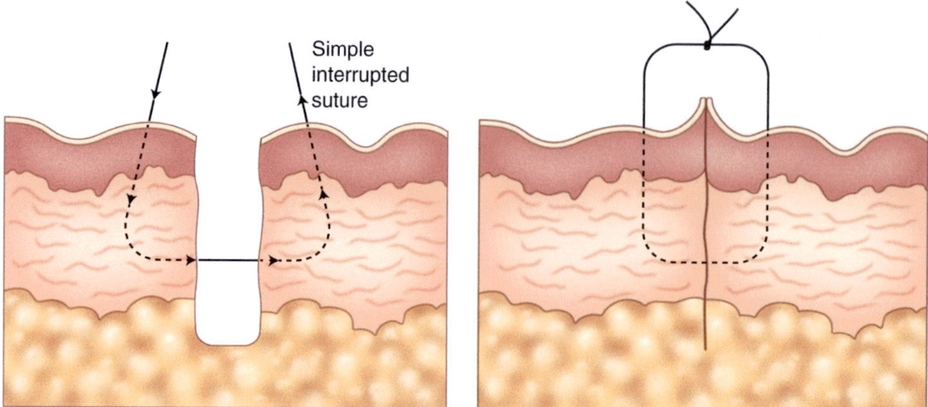

Fig. 12.4 Simple interrupted sutures are very useful for small wounds and can provide excellent skin eversion

Skin adhesives can be used as a primary skin closure only if the deeper layer of sutures has already everted the skin edges and the wound is under no tension. Skin adhesive can also be used to "seal" the skin overlying a subcuticular suture if application of dressings in this area would be difficult or if the wound is at risk for contamination (e.g., the perineum).

Dressings should remain in place for 24–48 h after surgery. If skin adhesive has been employed, they may not be necessary. Dry gauze dressings with an overlying ABD pad are held in place with paper tape on the trunk. On the extremities, the dry gauze dressings are held in place with a gauze wrap followed by a non-constricting cotton elastic dressing.

Postoperative Care

Two days after closure, the patient may remove the dressings and cleanse the wound gently with soap and water. Showering is encouraged but the patient may not soak the wound (tub bathing, swimming pool, hot tub, lake, ocean). Dressings should be reapplied and changed daily if there is any residual fluid egress from the wound or if the patient will be in an environment that risks infection to the wound.

Sutures should be removed at 10–14 days and staples by 7 days. Steristrips should be applied especially on areas with high tension and constant movement. Scar care may be initiated at this time. Gentle pressure massage of the scar in a circular motion for a few minutes 2–3 times daily can significantly soften and flatten scars. Silicone gel or sheets have been shown to improve the appearance of scars over time. If a patient appears to develop a keloid scar, intralesional steroid injection may be considered.

Skin Grafting

Skin grafts can be performed as full-thickness grafts (containing the entire thickness of the dermis) or split-thickness grafts (containing only a small portion of the dermis), with advantages/disadvantages and specific indications for each.

Important Facts About Skin Grafts

As skin grafts do not carry their own intrinsic blood supply, and, therefore, rely on recipient bed tissues for survival, they *cannot* be used to cover areas with exposed (denuded) cartilage, bone, or tendon. If perichondrium, periosteum, and/or paratenon are intact, skin grafting can be performed; however, these situations are often better addressed with tissue transfer techniques, discussed later.

Contracture

All skin grafts undergo two processes of contracture: primary (immediate) and secondary (delayed). Primary contracture refers to the diminution of graft size immediately after its removal from the donor site, and is directly proportional to the dermal content of the graft, which contains elastic connective tissue. Since the dermis is completely removed with a full-thickness skin graft, the donor site must be designed in such a way that it can be closed primarily. This limits the size of full-thickness skin available for grafting, but will vary from patient to patient based on skin laxity.

Secondary contracture is due to scarring of the recipient site as the graft heals over time, and is inversely proportional to the dermal content of the graft. Therefore, in areas where minimal long-term scar contracture is favored (eyelids, across joints, etc.) a full-thickness graft would be preferred. Similarly, a split-thickness graft would be preferable to cover large areas where secondary contracture is less problematic (chest, back, abdomen, perineum, thighs, upper arms, etc.).

Skin Graft Physiology

Understanding the physiology of skin graft survival is critical to preventing postoperative complications, discussed below. In the first 24–48 h, skin grafts adhere to the recipient bed through fibrin deposition and survive through simple diffusion, often referred to as *serum imbibition*. Following this initial stage, the capillaries remaining in the dermal element of the graft begin to align with those in the recipient site through a process called *inosculation*. The third stage of skin graft healing is revascularization through true angiogenesis.

Because they initially survive primarily through simple diffusion, which is distance-limited, skin grafts can be compromised by any fluid accumulation between the graft and recipient site, including blood (hematoma) or serous fluid (seroma). Similarly, any mechanical process that could interrupt the delicate alignment of vessels that occurs during inosculation, such as shear force, can impair graft survival.

Preoperative Preparation

Unless a very large surface area is planned for split-thickness grafting (i.e., large total-body surface area burns), in which case blood loss could be significant, routine preoperative lab work should not be necessary for these procedures. As with all wound healing interventions, every effort should be made preoperatively to optimize the patient's nutritional status, cessation of tobacco use, etc.

Operative Technique

Recipient Site Preparation

The best wound to graft is an acute excisional wound that needs no preparation. If a defect is not repaired immediately, in case of positive margins and re-excision, then the wound has to be appropriately prepared, cleaned of any necrotic material or fibrinous exudate, and washed thoroughly to remove bacteria that may be harbored in the crevasses of the wound. Several techniques exist for achieving a clean bed, and include mechanical debridement with the back of a forceps or curette, gentle scraping with a blade, or pressurized water systems, including pulse lavage or VersaJet™. Regardless of how the bed is prepared, *the most important step in the entire procedure is obtaining meticulous hemostasis prior to application of the graft*. Hematoma formation beneath a graft is the most common reason for graft failure.

Full-Thickness Skin Grafts

Once a wound has been appropriately selected and prepared for closure with a full-thickness skin grafts (FTSG), the first step is to select a donor site. The inguinal crease provides a large amount of full-thickness skin while still allowing primary closure, and harvest can be performed bilaterally if additional graft is needed. The medial surface of the arm and upper thigh are alternative donor sites if a thinner skin graft is desired.

Once the dimensions of the wound bed are known, an FTSG can be designed—it should be oversized approximately 15–20 % to account for primary contracture. Regardless of the location, donor sites should be excised in

an elliptical fashion, with a 3-4:1 length: width ratio oriented to place a linear scar in the relaxed skin tension lines (Fig. 12.1). The ability to close the donor site primarily can be verified with the "pinch test" before committing to the final graft dimensions.

After marking the donor site, the tissues are infiltrated with local anesthetic containing epinephrine to optimize hemostasis. Once this has taken effect, the area is sharply incised through the level of the dermis, and elevated from the underlying subcutaneous tissues using either a knife or electrocautery. Once the graft has been harvested, it is kept in saline-moistened gauze for later use while the donor site is closed. With larger grafts, the donor site wound margins may require slight undermining to allow closure without tension.

To maximize graft take, all remaining subcutaneous tissues should be removed from the dermal surface of the graft so that only dermis and epidermis remain. This is done sharply with curved scissors, e.g., curved Iris, mayo or face-lift scissors (Fig. 12.5). In order to allow egress of any fluid which may build up beneath the graft, it may be "pie-crusted," by cutting small slits in the graft with a scalpel blade.

Once the graft is prepared, it is placed onto the wound bed, dermis side down, and trimmed to fit the wound bed. The graft can be secured in a number of ways, most often with running or interrupted nonabsorbable suture around the periphery. Bacitracin ointment is applied to the graft before

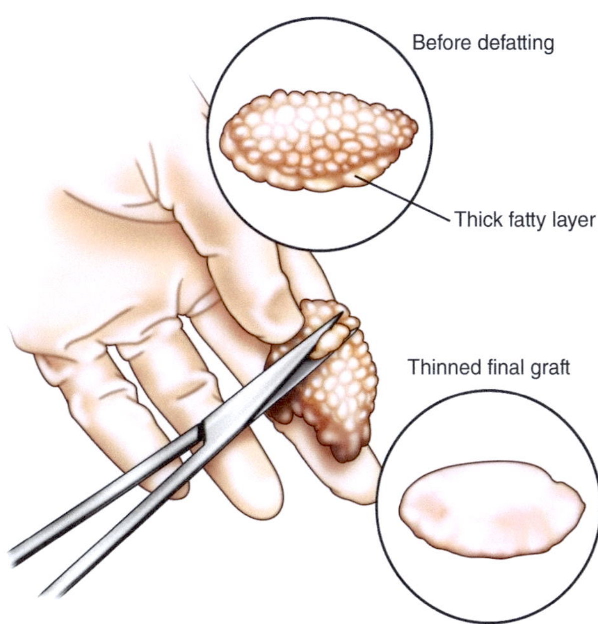

Fig. 12.5 Preparation of a full-thickness skin graft. After harvest of the full-thickness skin graft, a variable amount of subcutaneous tissues will remain adherent to the underside of the dermis. This excess tissue must be removed in order to maximize contact of the dermis to the recipient bed. Curved scissors should be used to cut away the subcutaneous fat and fibrous tissue until only dermis remains (the epidermal side of the graft is untouched)

securing to the wound bed with a tie-over bolster of nonstick dressing or a negative pressure wound therapy dressing (see below for postoperative care).

Split-Thickness Skin Grafts

Donor sites for split-thickness skin grafts (STSG) should be hidden, when possible, as the donor site will heal with a noticeable scar. Common areas of harvest include the lateral and anterior thigh. In order to increase the surface area an STSG can cover, the graft can be meshed. Meshing is most commonly performed in a 1.5:1 ratio. However, with increasing meshing, there remains a greater proportion of open wound and a correspondingly longer time to wound healing. Moreover, a meshed skin graft will heal with a cobblestone appearance and may not be cosmetically acceptable in certain areas of the body, such as the dorsum of the hands or face, where an intact ("sheet graft") is preferred.

Once the donor site has been selected, the area to be harvested should be shaved (if necessary) and cleansed with colorless or removable surgical prep solution to allow for post-transplant graft vascularity to be accurately assessed. Betadine is commonly used to prepare the donor site as this is easily washed off intraoperatively. Infiltration of the harvest site with saline or dilute lidocaine with epinephrine solution should be considered, as this will minimize blood loss and increase tissue turgor, which may facilitate graft harvest. The area to be harvested is then marked, taking into account any post-harvest meshing that will occur. Split-thickness grafts are most often harvested with a dermatome, but can be harvested manually using a Humby (or Watson) knife (Fig. 12.6). Based upon the area to be harvested, the appropriate dermatome blade guard and/or Watson knife is selected.

Set the dermatome to the desired graft thickness, usually 12/1,000th inch or thicker if a thicker graft is desired. Liberally apply mineral oil to the donor site as well as the gliding surface of the dermatome, if used, to allow for frictionless harvest of the skin graft. Using the nondominant hand (or an assistant), place traction on the proximal and/or distal harvest site to provide tension and counter tension. This will facilitate a smooth and uniform harvest. If using a dermatome, turn the power on before contacting the skin and apply to the skin at a 45° angle, with constant, firm pressure, allowing the dermatome to glide across the surface of the skin (Fig. 12.7). Upon reaching the distal extent of the harvest site, gently lift the dermatome off in a gradual fashion with the power still *on* to remove the graft completely (think of a plane taking off from the runway).

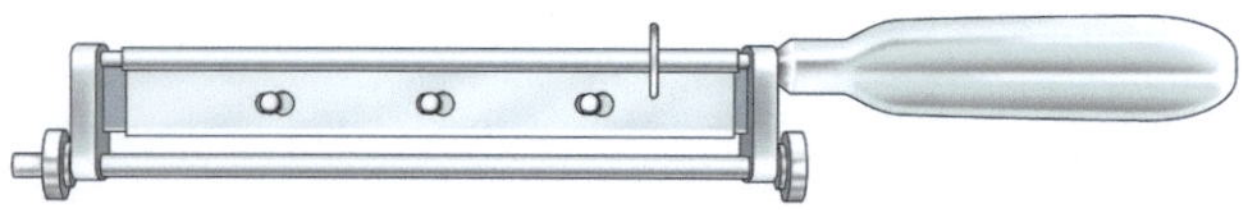

Fig. 12.6 Humby (Watson) knife used for harvest of split-thickness skin grafts

At this point, it is important to orient the graft, particularly in fairer-skinned individuals, so that the surgeon is certain which side contains the epidermis (Fig. 12.8). Once a graft has been removed from its vascular supply (and particularly

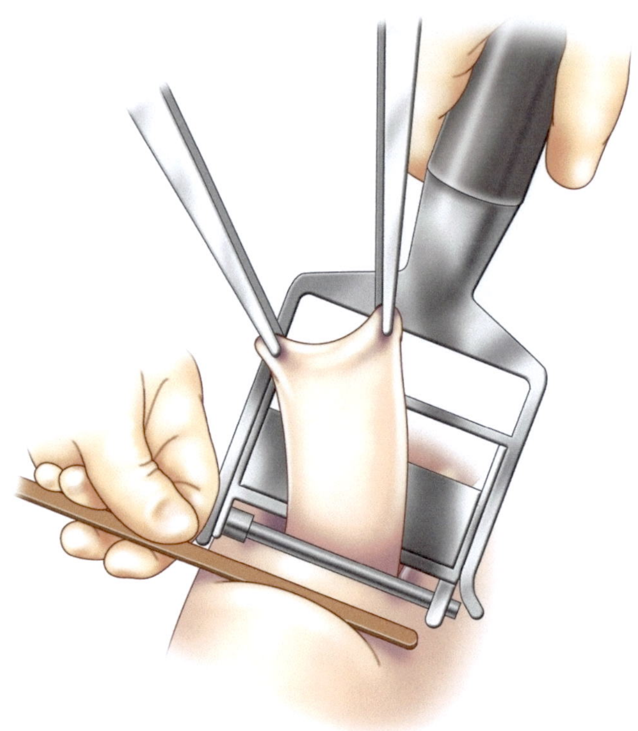

Fig. 12.7 A dermatome may be used to harvest a split-thickness skin graft from a relatively flat surface such as the anterior or lateral thigh. The dermatome should be held at an angle while tension is applied to the donor site surrounding tissues

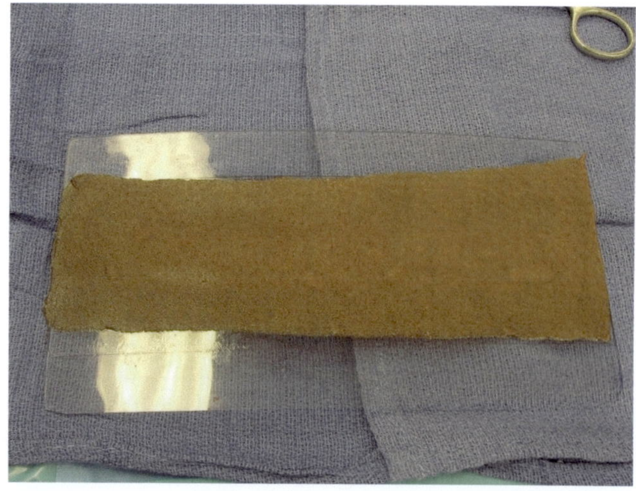

Fig. 12.8 This photograph demonstrates the split-thickness skin graft oriented with the epidermal side up in preparation for meshing. Note that the graft appears matte instead of the shiny appearance of the dermal side

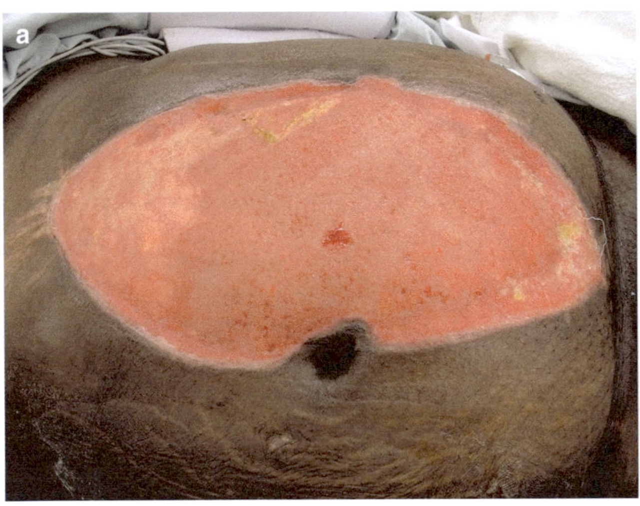
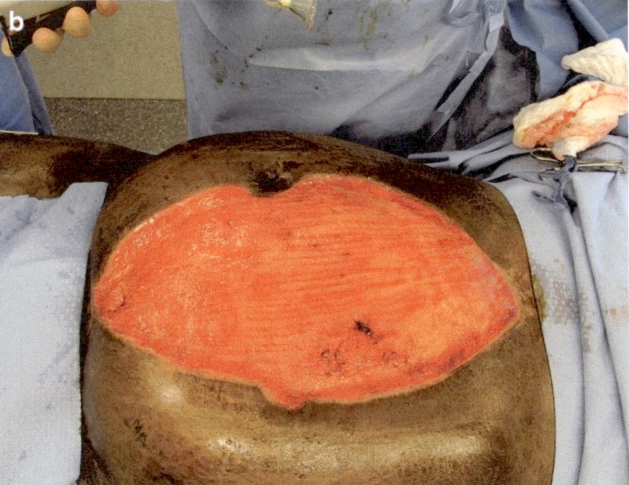

Fig. 12.9 (**a**) For delayed skin grafting, the recipient site should appear clean and to have granulation tissue present. (**b**) However, prior to placement of the skin graft, the tissues must be gently debrided until punctate bleeding is present

once it has been meshed), it can be very difficult to determine this orientation. If meshing is planned, this will proceed based upon which system is available.

Once the recipient site has been prepared (Fig. 12.9a, b), the graft is placed *dermal side down* (epidermis side up) onto the recipient site and spread to fit the wound bed as needed. If there is confusion, the dermal element is often shinier in appearance. The skin graft is secured into the contours of the wound bed using absorbable suture (chromic or fast gut), usually 5-0, and secured around the wound periphery using a similar running suture or surgical stapler (Fig. 12.10). Care should be taken to ensure the graft is in contact with the entirety of the wound bed, and not "tented" as close approximation is essential to graft survival. This can be done with judicious use of absorbable "quilting" sutures. Moreover, care must be exercised when trimming "excess" graft from the wound margins, as tucking the graft into the wound crevasses will often require more skin than anticipated. Measure twice, cut once.

Postoperative Care
Donor Sites

A common method of dressing the donor site immediately after harvest, while the graft is inset, is to place an epinephrine-soaked Telfa™ over the harvest site to stop any ongoing blood loss. Donor sites for STSG will heal by re-epithelialization from the periphery and the remaining dermal appendages in the donor bed. This process will usually take between 2 and 3 weeks, depending on the thickness of the graft. A skin graft taken at 10/1,000th in. will take approximately 1 week to heal completely. The optimal dressing for skin graft donor sites is a subject of considerable research and attention. The two most common ways include

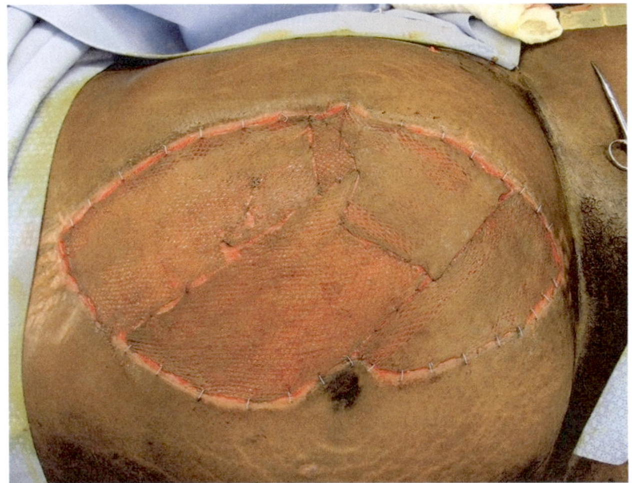

Fig. 12.10 The split-thickness skin graft has been meshed, secured at the periphery using staples, and secured in the central portion using chromic-gut sutures

placing a Xeroform gauze over the site and allowing it to dry onto the site as a "scab" which will slowly peel off the bed as it re-epithelializes. This must be kept dry until healed. More current research has suggested that wounds re-epithelialize faster in a moist environment, which has led to a preference for dressing these sites with a semiocclusive dressing such as Tegaderm™ or OpSite™. These should be sufficiently overlapped onto adjacent, normal skin and adhesive such as tincture of benzoin or Mastisol™ should be considered to promote long-term adherence. This dressing is left in place for 1 week, after which patients should clean the area with daily showers and apply petroleum jelly-based ointment to the wound until fully healed. This dressing, which can get wet, is often better tolerated and less painful for patients.

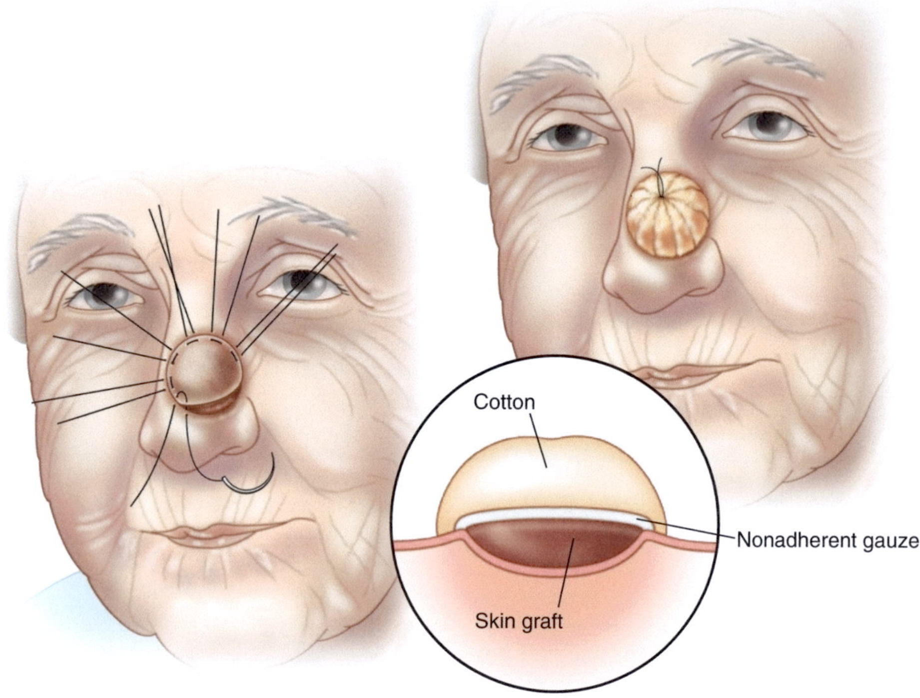

Fig. 12.11 Bolster dressings should be applied in areas of the body where a circumferential dressing cannot be employed. A non-adherent layer is applied over the secured skin graft. A bulky dressing is then secured in place using tie-over sutures. This dressing is left in place for 5 days

Recipient Site

To avoid the complications of fluid accumulation beneath the graft and minimize shear forces, the recipient sites of either full-thickness or partial-thickness skin grafts are dressed with bolster dressings or negative pressure wound therapy dressings. Directly atop the graft, a layer of non-adherent gauze (Owen's gauze, Xeroform, or Adaptec™) is placed and may be stapled in place to minimize motion across the graft. This is bolstered with layered gauze followed by Reston™ foam, which is secured with staples or a tie-over bolster (Fig. 12.11). A useful alternative, which will actively remove any fluid that might accumulate beneath the graft, is application of a Wound Vac device. The negative pressure maintains the graft in contact with the recipient bed, while the suction removes any fluid that accumulates and would otherwise compromise graft survival. These dressings are also quite resistant to shear forces. In situations where skin grafting is performed on a distal extremity, immobilization in the form of a splint or cast is critical to protect the graft from shear forces resulting from ambulation.

Regardless of bolster method, this dressing is left in place for 5 days, after which the graft should show excellent take. The graft can then be dressed with daily nonstick gauze dressings until the graft appears fully adherent to the wound bed in approximately one additional week. At this point, lotion or petroleum jelly-based products can be applied to the graft site without dressings to moisturize the graft until fully healed.

Local Flap Closure

When primary closure would put excessive tension on the skin edges, consider local flap options. This chapter will only cover skin flaps that carry both the skin and subcutaneous tissue. The flap will bring its own blood supply into the defect either through a random pattern or an axial pattern of blood supply. Flaps are most often indicated for coverage of a defect with poor blood supply, exposed vital structures such as tendons and blood vessels, or a bony prominence that needs cushioning.

Proper preoperative planning is vital for local flap closure. There are many different types of local flaps that employ rotation, advancement, and/or transposition of donor skin into the defect. The challenge arises in choosing the best flap for each defect.

Rotation Flap

A rotation flap is a crescent-shaped flap of skin and subcutaneous tissue based upon a pivot point that rotates into the defect site (Fig. 12.12). The donor site is usually closed primarily, but may also be closed using a skin graft. It is

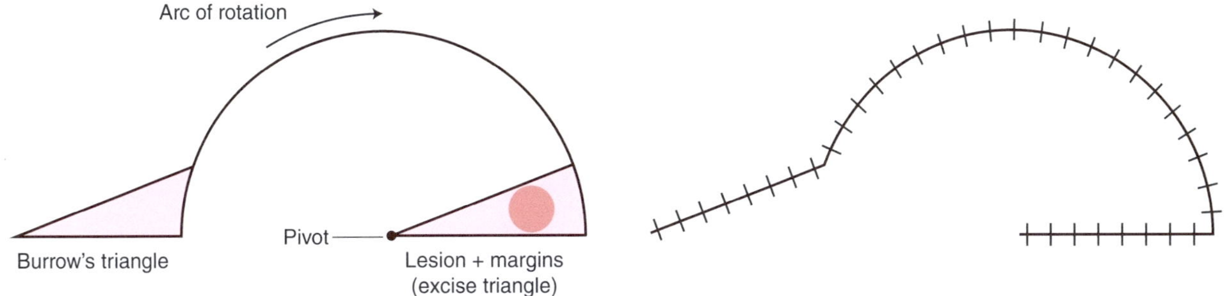

Fig. 12.12 The rotation flap is designed around a pivot point and employs a large amount of tissue elevation and rotation to close a defect. The shaded areas indicate tissue to be discarded as these will become dog-ears

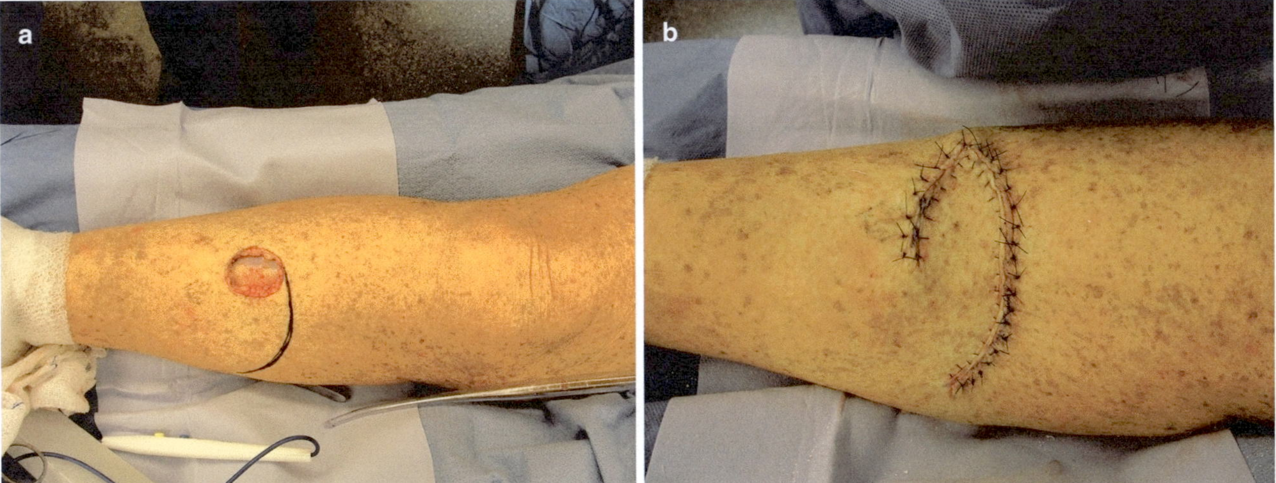

Fig. 12.13 This patient underwent rotation flap closure of a wide local excision site on the forearm: (**a**) demonstrates the planning while (**b**) reveals the inset of the flap

important to realize that the flap diameter becomes effectively shortened with increasing rotation. The arc of the flap should be approximately 4–5 times longer than the base width of the defect. In general, whenever a local flap, whether rotational, transposition, or advancement, is mobilized to cover a given defect, buckling of adjacent tissue may occur at the base of the flap. This buckling or tissue crowding, also known as standing cone or dog-ear, makes it difficult to inset the flap into the defect while maintaining a smooth flat surface. Excising a triangle of tissue in this area solves the problem; this triangle is known as Burow's triangle. Usually, excising two small triangles adjacent to either side of the base of the flap will facilitate mobilization and a smooth closure. Excising two triangles is not always necessary and in some situations only one triangle is removed. Additionally, backcut may be made to facilitate donor site closure A Burow's triangle does not compromise the flap blood supply, but a backcut does and therefore should be made cautiously until the skin tension is relieved. One should not commit to removing Burow's triangles or backcuts until the flap is mobilized

into the defect. It is only then when tissue tension and/or standing cones reveal themselves.

These flaps are elevated along the avascular plane deep to the subcutaneous fat, immediately superficial to the underlying fascia. The entire flap should be undermined to allow maximal rotation with the understanding that the blood supply to this flap comes from the dermal plexus, not from perforating blood vessels (Figs. 12.13, 12.14, and 12.15).

Transposition Flap

A transposition flap is similar to a rotation flap as they both rotate about a pivot point; however in this case, the rectangular flap of skin and subcutaneous tissue is elevated and transposed into the defect along the line of greatest tension (Fig. 12.16). Again, as the flap rotates, the effective length is reduced—planning for this shortening is absolutely necessary. An OR towel may be used to simulate flap movement and to predict the amount of flap shortening. The skin and subcutaneous fat flap is, again, elevated off of the underlying fascia to allow for transposition into the defect. The donor site may be skin grafted if it cannot be closed primarily.

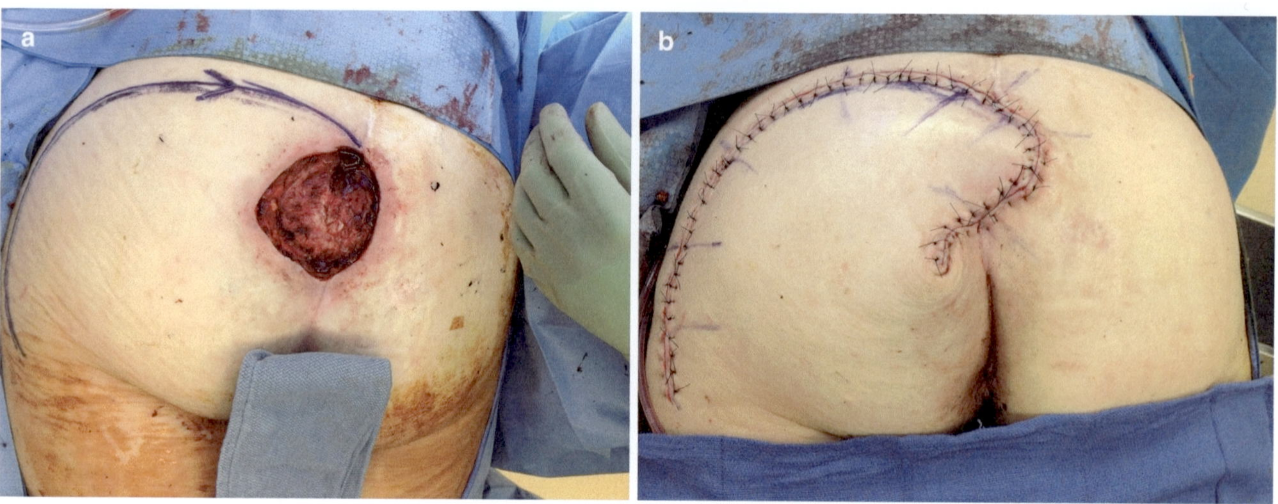

Fig. 12.14 This clinical example of a sacral wound closure is included to demonstrate that very large fasciocutaneous flaps may be safely rotated in to close larger defects on the trunk (**a**) Sacral defect and the design of a rotation flap marked (**b**) Final closure after flap rotation

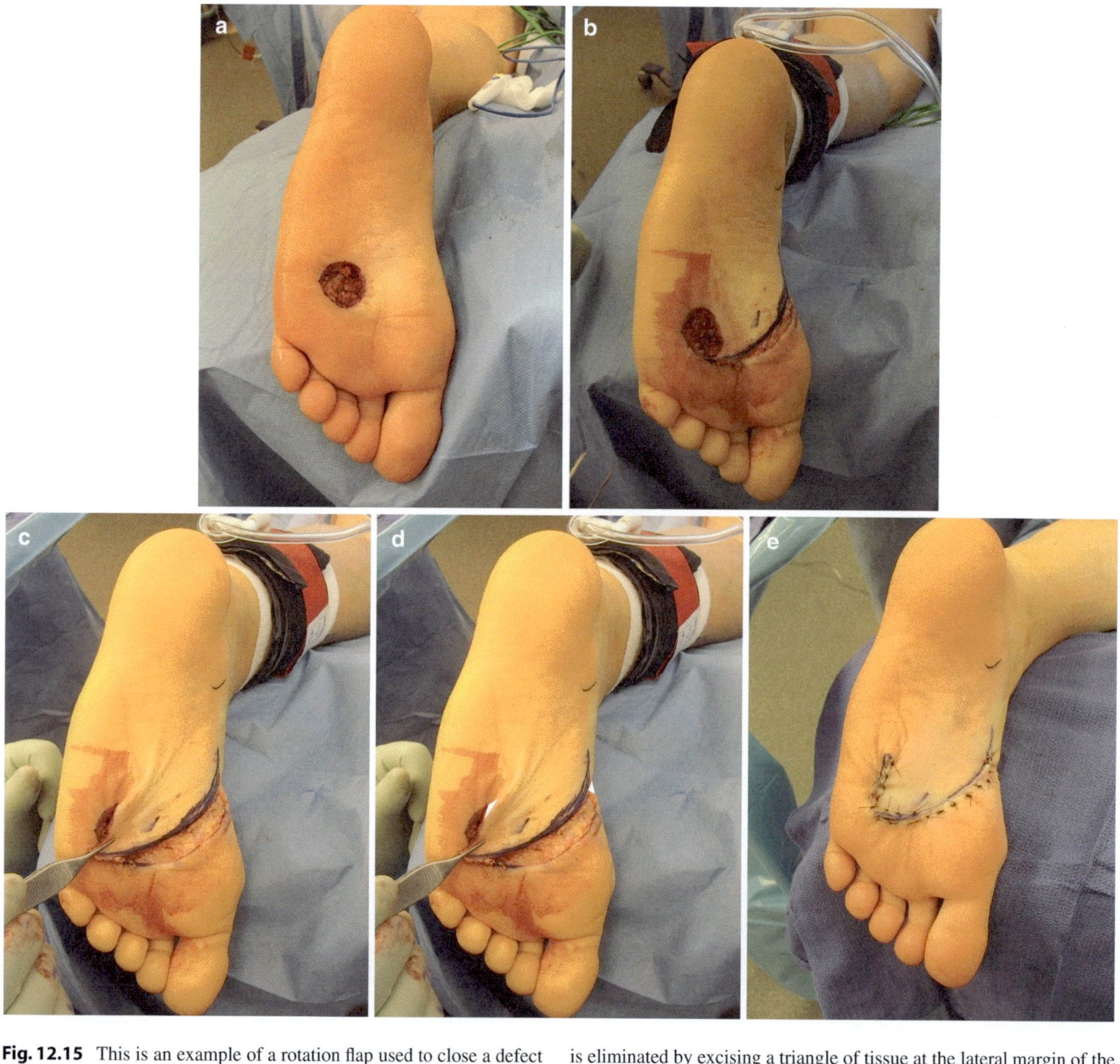

Fig. 12.15 This is an example of a rotation flap used to close a defect on the sole of the foot (**a**). After incision (**b**), note how rotation of the flap results in a dog-ear at the lateral portion of the flap (**c**). The dog-ear is eliminated by excising a triangle of tissue at the lateral margin of the flap and tension is released by excising a triangle of tissue at the medial margin of the flap (**d**). The flap is completed (**e**)

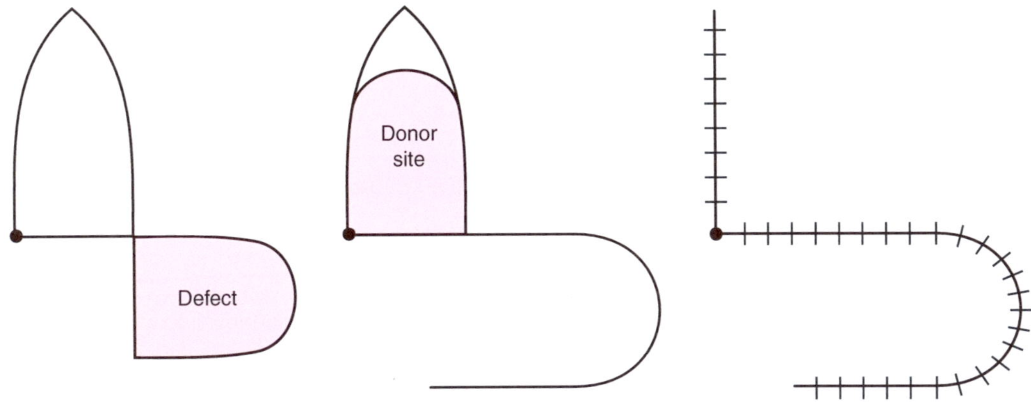

Fig. 12.16 The transposition flap is best utilized when the donor site is at a 90° angle to the recipient bed as closure of the donor site then facilitates a tension-free closure of the recipient site

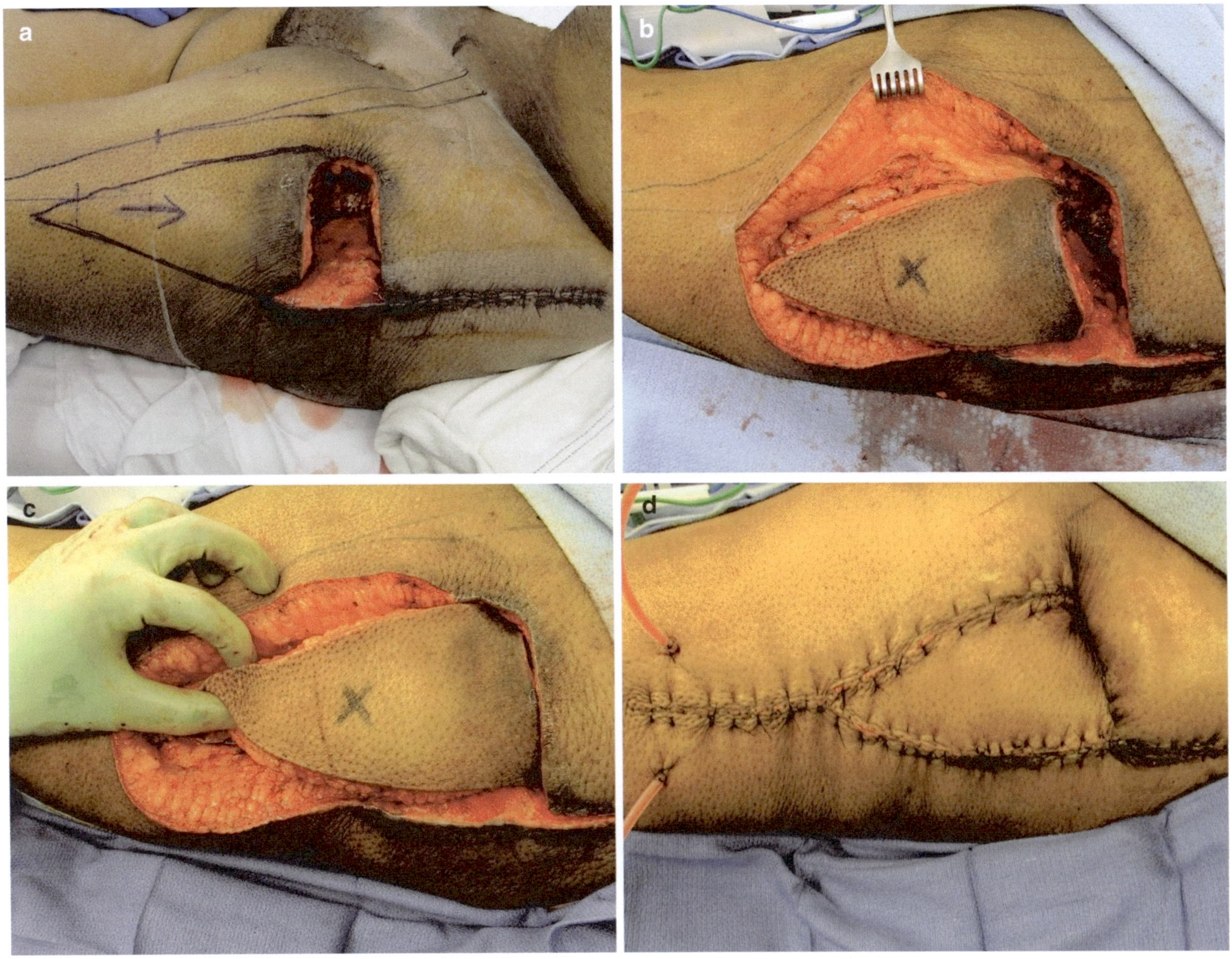

Fig. 12.17 The V-Y advancement flap does not involve undermining of the flap, unlike other rotation and transposition flaps (**a**) Full thickness defect in the anterolateral left proximal thigh (**b**) V-Y advancement flap after making the cuts, no undermining is performed (**c**) Flap is advanced into the defect (**d**) Final closure, notice the resulting Y shape, hence the V-Y terminology

Advancement Flap

An advancement flap moves forward into a defect without rotation. The inherent elasticity of skin enables a certain amount of forward stretch of the skin and subcutaneous tissue.

While rectangular flaps may be advanced into the donor site, the most commonly utilized type of advancement flap is the V-Y flap. A V-shaped incision is designed with the apex furthest away from the defect (Fig. 12.17). An incision is made

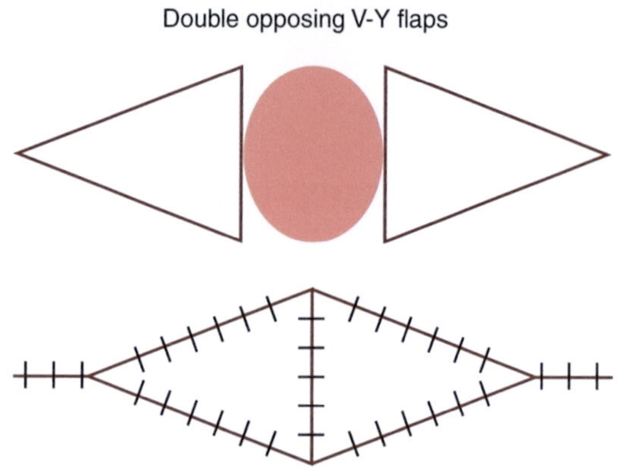

Fig. 12.18 Double opposing V-Y Flaps may be employed to cover very large defects

through the skin, subcutaneous tissue, and deep fascia along the V, but there is no undermining of the flap performed. This is because the blood supply to a V-Y flap is from perforators through the subcutaneous fat as the entire dermis has been incised. The flap is advanced into the defect site and the donor site is closed primarily resulting a Y-shaped incision. Incising muscle fibers under the deep fascia along the V is often necessary to "slide" the flap into the defect. Two opposing V-Y flaps may be employed to close larger defects (Fig. 12.18).

Each of these types of flaps should be closed in layers utilizing deep dermal sutures to set the position of the flap followed by either simple interrupted, simple running, or horizontal mattress sutures as described above. Dry gauze dressings are usually sufficient for coverage of these wounds.

Postoperative Care

For postoperative care, see primary closure.

Complications

- Wound dehiscence
- Wound infection
- Partial flap necrosis

- Hypertrophic scar or keloid
- Incomplete take or complete loss of the skin graft
- Skin graft donor site pain and hypopigmentation

When to Transfer

- Large defects not amenable to primary closure, skin grafting, or small local flap coverage.
- Defects with exposed joint, tendon, cartilage, or bone not amenable to primary or local flap closure.
- Defects with exposed bone fracture or hardware.
- Defects involving aesthetic sensitive areas like the breast especially in younger females.
- Complex defect involving the hand and weight bearing areas should be referred to a hand or plastic surgeon.
- Large total-body surface area burns requiring management by a regional burn center.

Suggested Reading

Ahuja RB. Mechanics of movement for rotation flaps and a local flap template. Plast Reconstr Surg. 1989;83(4):733–7.

Capla JM, et al. Skin graft vascularization involves precisely regulated regression and replacement of endothelial cells through both angiogenesis and vasculogenesis. Plast Reconstr Surg. 2006;117(3): 836–44.

Converse JM, Uhlschmid GK, Ballantyne Jr DL. "Plasmatic circulation" in skin grafts. The phase of serum imbibition. Plast Reconstr Surg. 1969;43(5):495–9.

Goldman GD. Rotation flaps. Dermatol Surg. 2005;31(8 Pt 2):1006–13.

Hynes W. The early circulation in skin grafts with a consideration of methods to encourage their survival. Br J Plast Surg. 1954;6(4): 257–63.

Paletta CE, Pkorny JJ, Rombolo P. Skin grafts. In: Mathes SJ, editor. Plastic surgery. 2nd ed. Philadelphia: Saunders; 2006. p. 293–316.

Thorne CH. Principles and techniques in plastic surgery. In: Thorne CH et al., editors. Grabb & Smith's plastic surgery. 6th ed. Philadelphia: Lippincott Williams & Wilkins; 2007. p. 7–9.

Voineskos SH, et al. Systematic review of skin graft donor-site dressings. Plast Reconstr Surg. 2009;124(1):298–306.

Weisberg NK, Nehal KS, Zide BM. Dog-ears: a review. Dermatol Surg. 2000;26(4):363–70.

Mary J. Milroy

Ultrasound is an accurate, noninvasive, cost-effective, portable modality for both evaluation and intervention of the breast. Within a short period of time, rural surgeons can be successful in incorporating breast ultrasound into routine clinical practice.

Indications

1. Evaluation of abnormal or indeterminate findings on clinical breast exam
2. Evaluation of abnormal or indeterminate findings on breast imaging including mammography, MRI, or PET/ CT
3. Minimally invasive biopsy of abnormal or indeterminate breast findings
4. Evaluation of axillary lymph nodes
5. Nonoperative management of breast abscess
6. Guidance for preoperative wire localization for lumpectomy
7. Intraoperative guidance instrumentation such as balloon placement for accelerated partial breast irradiation (APBI)

Preoperative Preparation

Surgeon

Breast ultrasound provides a dynamic study and is quite operator dependent. Therefore, it is imperative to obtain a good fundamental knowledge of the physics and techniques of breast ultrasound. It is very helpful to take a course with both didactic and hands-on components in basic ultrasound and advanced ultrasound techniques for the breast. Become familiar with normal and abnormal breast anatomy as seen by ultrasound. Practice, practice, practice! Routinely use your ultrasound to compare the findings on your clinical breast exam with the images you see by ultrasound. Ultrasound will rapidly become an extension of your clinical breast exam. Partner with your local radiologists and ultrasound technologists and they will prove to be an invaluable resource as you develop your ultrasound skills.

Learn your ultrasound machine. A high-quality ultrasound machine is essential to producing quality images, eliminating artifactual shadowing, and allowing the appropriate tissue penetration. Correct probe selection is also vital. High frequency probes 7.5–15 MHz are best to increase resolution. Gain control adjusts amplification and affects the brightness of the image. The time gain component enhances imaging of deeper structures. Depth of signal and focus should also be adjusted. Harmonics can help determine cystic characteristics and color Doppler may be used to evaluate blood supply.

Careful, gentle treatment of the ultrasound and probes combined with regular maintenance will maintain high-quality images and avoid complications such as malfunction of probe or electrical shocks.

Patient

Minimal patient preparation is required for breast ultrasound. Obtain information as to allergies and coagulation status before any interventions. Patients do not need to be NPO.

Operative Strategy

In diagnostic breast ultrasound, the goal is to obtain high-quality images of the breast and to correlate them with clinical exam and other images available to form a clinical

With appreciation and gratitude to the excellent ultrasound team at the Yankton Medical Clinic: Dr. Will Eidsness, Pam Cokeley, Todd Lange, Deb Lehl, Janet Schrempp, Sarah Smith, and Judy VanHeek.

M.J. Milroy, M.D., F.A.C.S. (✉)
Associate Clinical Professor, Department of Surgery, Sanford School of Medicine, Yankton Medical Clinic, 1104 West 8th Street, Yankton, SD 57078, USA
e-mail: mary.milroy@gmail.com

diagnosis and determine whether intervention is indicated. In breast intervention, the goal is to allow accurate, safe placement of needle for aspiration, biopsy, wire or balloon placement.

Operative Procedure

Diagnostic Breast US

Begin by carefully identifying and documenting the patient and the date of the procedure. The patient is usually positioned supine with the ipsilateral arm elevated above the head in order to best disperse the breast tissue over the chest wall (Fig. 13.1). For lateral or axillary tail evaluation, a wedge placed under the patient will help to raise the lateral aspect of the patients and allow for improved visualization. Use plenty of gel. It is important for quality image so don't scrimp on it. Adjust your machine for optimal image. During clinical breast exam, ink marking the skin helps target the areas for ultrasound scanning and helps you correlate your clinical breast exam findings with the ultrasound images. Use firm pressure, scan slowly and be alert for findings that may be artifacts. Carefully obtain and save images transverse and longitudinal or radial and antiradial. If necessary, additional modalities such as harmonics or color Doppler may be applied to aid in evaluation.

Many benign and malignant lesions can be visualized by ultrasound. The differentiation is made by utilizing several criteria.

Margin Analysis

Smooth, sharp margins are more likely to represent a benign finding while irregular, poorly defined margins are more suspicious.

Echogenicity

Anechoic or the complete absence of echoes represents fluid as would be found in a benign breast cyst. Uniform internal echoes represent a solid lesion but are more likely to be benign while very mixed echo patterns are more likely to be malignant.

Acoustic Shadow

The shadow cast may be enhanced, decreased, or unchanged. Benign cysts and fibroadenomas have posterior enhancement while carcinomas often have posterior shadowing. Unchanged patterns are indeterminate.

Growth Pattern

Horizontal growth with a wider than tall pattern is often benign while vertical growth with a taller than wide pattern is often malignant.

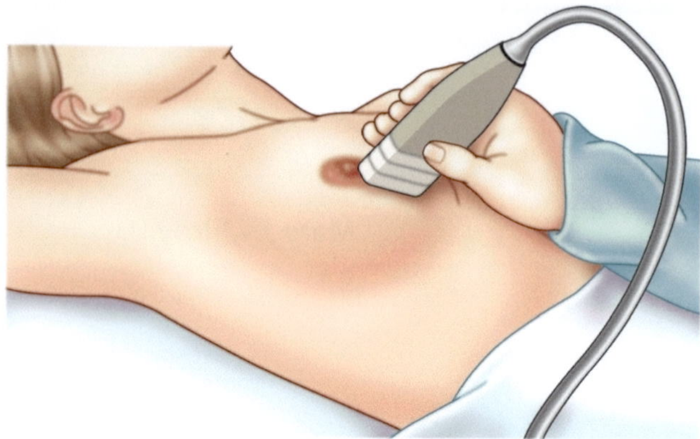

Fig. 13.1 Artist generated drawing of patient in position for breast ultrasound

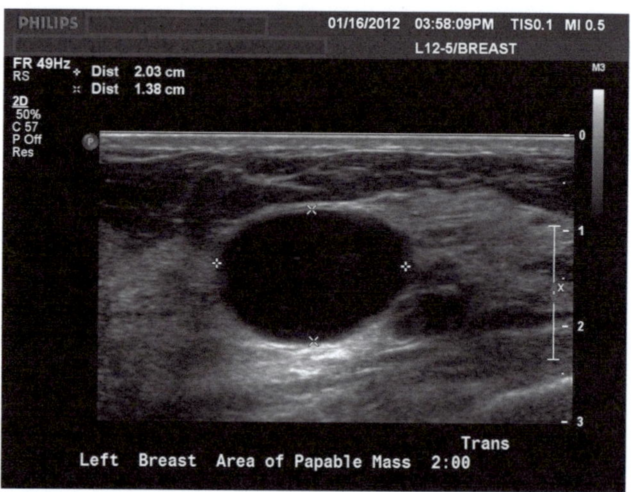

Fig. 13.2 Typical breast cyst with sharp margins, posterior enhancement, horizontal growth pattern, and absence of internal echoes

Compressibility

Carcinomas are usually hard and resist compression while cysts containing fluid may be compressed. Therefore, varying the pressure on the transducer indicates compressibility and aids in evaluation.

Lymph Nodes

Lymph nodes may be axillary or intramammary, and when benign usually have a distinct image with sharp margins, fatty hilum, side notch, and thin cortex.

After carefully reviewing the ultrasound images and correlating with patient history, clinical breast exam, and other images, a clinical diagnosis is made and a course of management discussed with the patient. Be careful to strictly adhere to criteria for benign lesions. Failure to meet all the criteria may mask a carcinoma. Benign conditions can be followed while indeterminate findings should be aspirated or biopsied. Abscesses may be aspirated, irrigated, and cultures obtained.

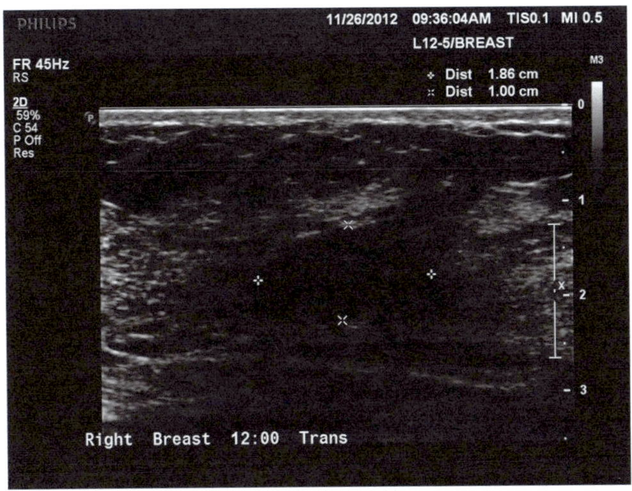

Fig. 13.3 Indeterminate lesion with partially sharp margins, horizontal growth pattern, internal echoes, and absence of posterior enhancement. This lesion was a benign fibroadenoma on core needle biopsy

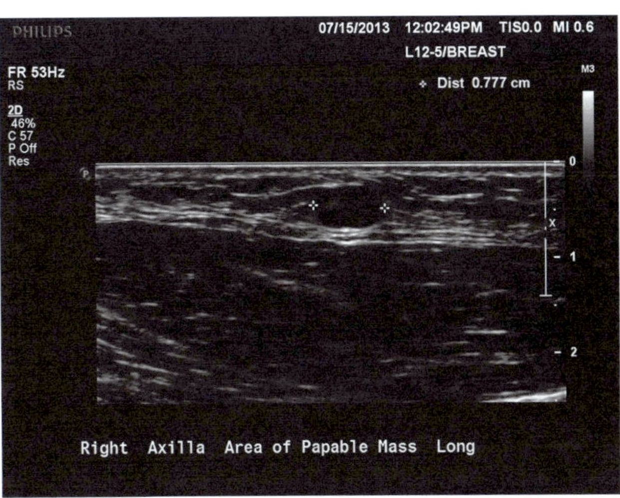

Fig. 13.5 Axillary lymph node with sharp margins, horizontal growth pattern, central hilum, and posterior enhancement

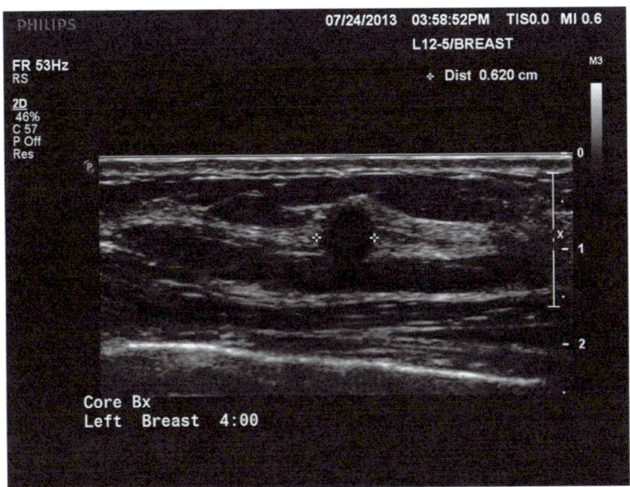

Fig. 13.4 Suspicious lesion with sharp margins, vertical growth pattern, internal echoes, and absence of posterior enhancement. This lesion was a carcinoma on core needle biopsy

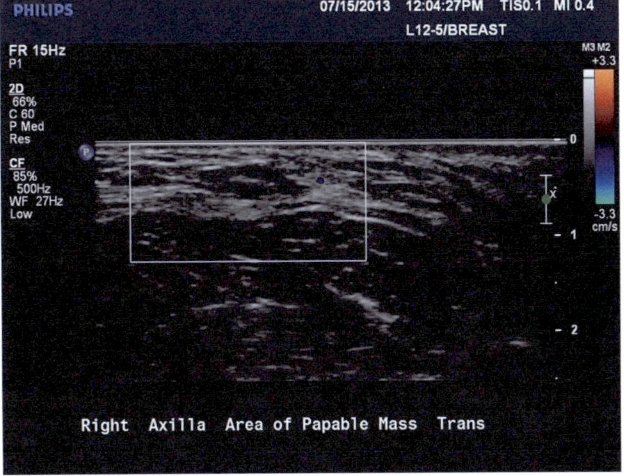

Fig. 13.6 Color Doppler visualizes blood flow in hilum and confirms lymph node

Suspicious lesions can be evaluated either by FNA, large core, or vacuum-assisted large core biopsy with the guidance of the ultrasound in a minimally invasive manner. This may occur immediately following the diagnostic ultrasound obviating the need to set up a separate time for the procedure.

US Images

(Figs. 13.2–13.7).

Breast Intervention

The patient is identified, documented, coagulation status reviewed, and consent obtained. The patient is positioned as in diagnostic ultrasound. The lesion is imaged and a path

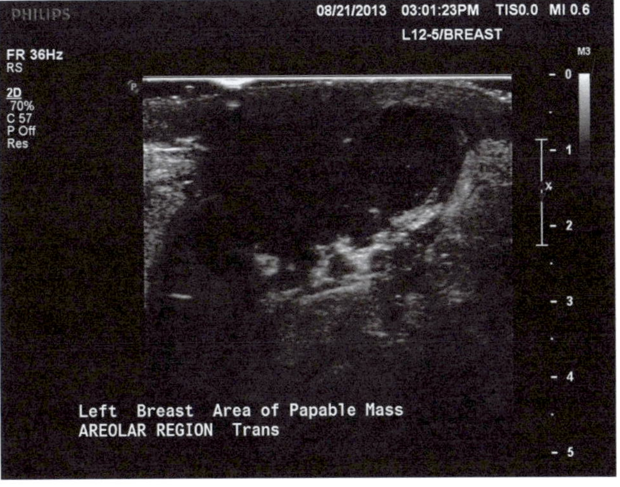

Fig. 13.7 Breast abscess

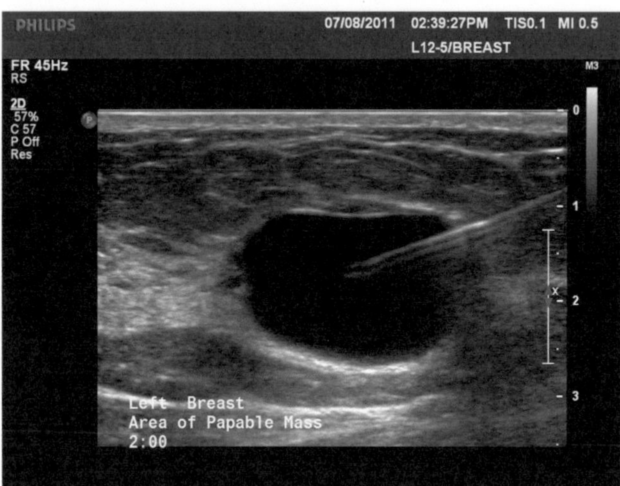

Fig. 13.8 Needle visualized entering cyst

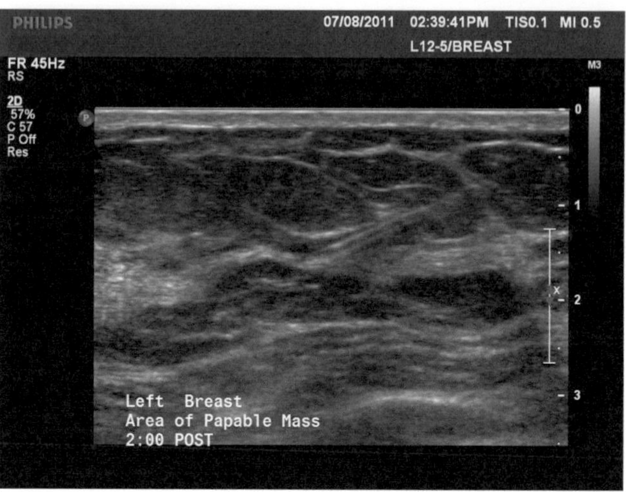

Fig. 13.9 Complete disappearance of cyst visualized

shortest from skin to spot is chosen. In preoperative wire localization, the wire location can be planned to be placed in a site that allows for optimal surgical incision. The breast is scrubbed with an antiseptic and local anesthetic placed in the skin immediately adjacent to the probe and along the path to the lesion. Remember the ultrasound beam is linear and the needle must be kept parallel to the beam. Placing the index finger of your nondominate hand on the probe in the direction of the ultrasound while your dominate hand guides the needle will help the needle stay parallel. Stabilizing the lesion with the transducer or by your ultrasound technologist can help keep the area taut so the breast tissue does not move during needle placement. During procedures if the transducer is held by an assistant, it will free both your hands for the procedure which will be advantageous. Carefully watch the needle tip to be certain that the target lesion does not move, and that needle does not inadvertently enter undesired nearby tissue such as chest wall or cavity. Gently wiggling the needle will often help you locate the needle tip on the screen and then be sure to keep the needle tip in sight while you advance the needle.

Aspiration

No incision is required. For aspiration a small gauge needle such as a 22-gauge is placed under real-time direct visualization into the lesion (Fig. 13.8). Gently aspirate as you enter the cyst. Simple benign cysts should be completely aspirated (Fig. 13.9). Complex cysts may be more difficult to aspirate and switching to a larger gauge needle may be helpful. Lesions that cannot be aspirated are indeterminate and FNA for cytology or large core biopsy for histology should be obtained. Breast abscess fluid is very thick and a large gauge needle such as an 18- or 16-gauge will be necessary. Aspirated purulent fluid confirms abscess and can be sent for culture. The needle can be left in place and a new normal

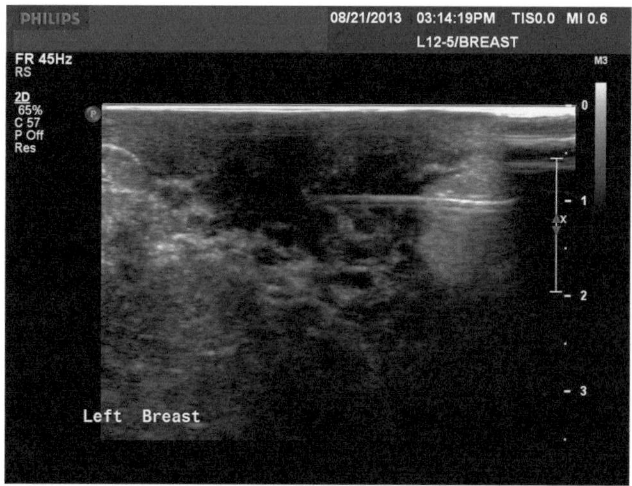

Fig. 13.10 Abscess with needle in place

saline filled syringe can then be placed in order to accomplish repeated irrigations of the abscess cavity (Fig. 13.10).

Core Biopsy

Incision is required for ease of needle placement. Therefore, sterile setup with gloves and probe cover is utilized. A sterile tray with 15 or 11 blade scalpel, 4 by 4 s, local anesthetic, biopsy device, and clip applicator should be prepared prior to procedure and placed at hand. Biopsy devices can be obtained from a number of manufacturers and are usually large core from 8- to 14-gauge and may be vacuum assisted. It is helpful to trial several until you find the core biopsy device that suits your practice. Once the breast is scrubbed and the local anesthetic placed a small incision just large enough to permit entry of the biopsy device is made. The biopsy device is placed and core biopsies are obtained. Be careful, most needles have a solid tip and the sample is obtained from a side

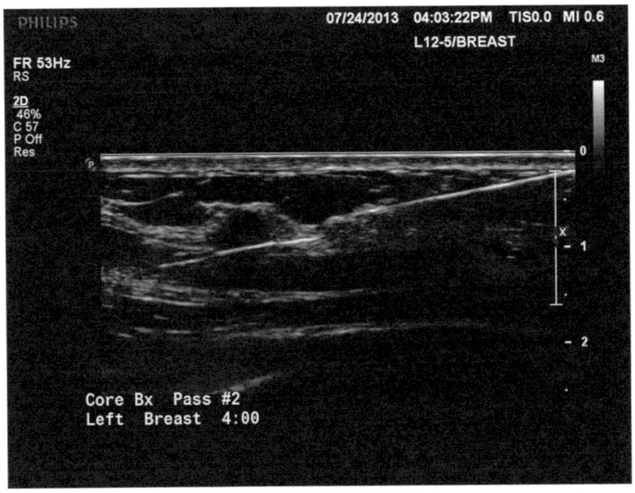

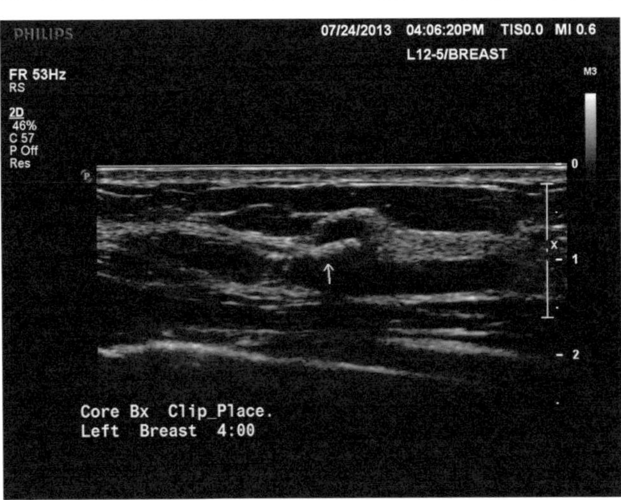

Fig. 13.11 Lesion visualized in the sample notch of the core biopsy needle

Fig. 13.12 Lesion visualized with clip in place

opening a distance behind the tip. Most needles are spring loaded and when fired the needle projects through the lesion. This can be very helpful in entering firm, dense tissue but be sure to evaluate where the anticipated needle throw will go. If not careful, nearby structures could be injured. For small lesions or those close to other structures such as chest wall, an alternate method, if your device permits, is to open the side sample notch prior to placing the needle into the lesion and then close the notch to obtain the biopsy (Fig. 13.11). This eliminates the risk of tissue damage from the needle throw. Evaluate the tissue obtained. Good solid cores will usually sink in the formalin and indicate an adequate sample. Fatty, floating cores are often inadequate and additional cores should be obtained. When adequate tissue sample is obtained a marker clip can be placed to document which lesion was evaluated and to make relocating the lesion easier if necessary for surgical removal. Marker clips are commercially available in needle introducers and can be placed down the biopsy path and deployed under direct ultrasound vision into the lesion (Fig. 13.12).

Wire Localization

No incision is required. Many commercially available wire localization needles are available. Select whichever one you prefer in surgery. The localization can be done preoperatively in the ultrasound department or in the operating room. Select the optimal site for your incision. Position the ultrasound probe in order to both locate the lesion and to allow you to place the localization wire at the site of the future surgical incision. The better you place your wire, the easier you will make the operation. Once the needle has traversed the lesion, the wire can be stabilized and the needle removed. Repeat ultrasound will confirm the wire in place and often even visualize the stabilization hook. The surgical excision can then proceed in standard fashion.

Intraoperative or Post-lumpectomy Balloon Catheter Placement for APBI

APBI is a technique whereby intracavity irradiation can be delivered twice a day for 5 days rather than external beam whole breast radiation which is delivered 5 days per week for 6–7 weeks and which can be an obstacle for breast conservation in rural patients who may live long distances from the radiation center. This option may be considered in carefully selected early stage breast cancer patients in consultation with Radiation Oncology. The balloon catheter may be placed at the time of the original lumpectomy or may be placed postoperatively. Introperatively a cavity evaluation device (CED) is often placed as both a sizer and a space holder until the pathology report on the cancer margins and the axillary lymph node status is available. At that time, a swap of the CED for the radiation balloon catheter may be done in the ultrasound department. Postoperative balloon placement may also be done at the request of either the patient or the radiation oncologist usually depending on patient preference and the timing of the radiation treatments. If a sufficient post-lumpectomy seroma remains, a trocar can be placed with ultrasound visualization and the radiation balloon catheter placed.

Intraoperative Placement of CED

After completion of standard lumpectomy, a CED may be placed under direct vision and skin and subcutaneous tissue closed. The intraoperative ultrasound can then be used to check balloon conformance, size, and measure surrounding distances, especially balloon to skin distance. In several days, after the pathology report is reviewed and decision to proceed with APBI is made, the patient can return to the ultrasound department. The balloon position and distances can be rechecked. If all looks acceptable, the skin is scrubbed and the CED is deflated and removed and the radiation-

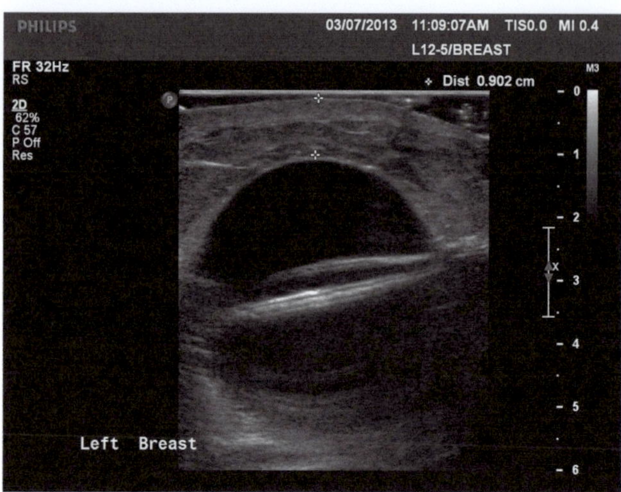

Fig. 13.13 Radiation balloon catheter in place

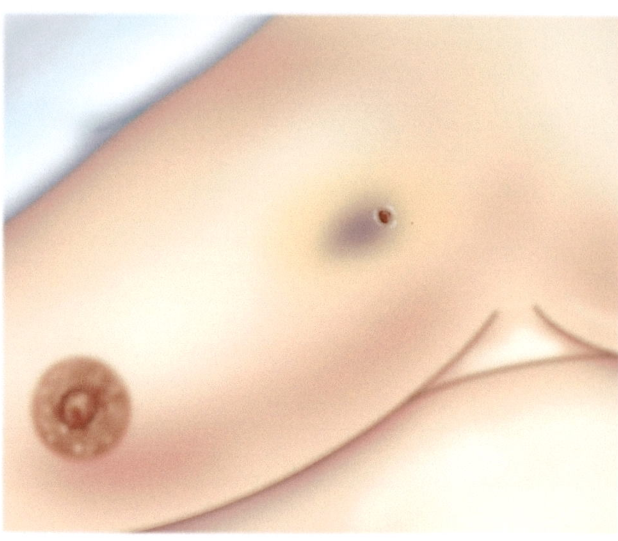

Fig. 13.14 Biopsy site post procedure

capable balloon catheter is tested and then under direct ultrasound visualization placed down the tract. The balloon is inflated and conformance and distances reevaluated. APBI can then begin.

Postoperative Placement of Balloon Catheter

Within several weeks of standard lumpectomy while the seroma cavity is still visible by ultrasound, an APBI balloon catheter can be placed. The patient is positioned and the lumpectomy seroma is visualized and evaluated for suitability. If felt adequate, the breast is scrubbed and local anesthetic placed in the skin and along the path to the seroma. An incision is made and the trocar is placed into the seroma under direct ultrasound visualization. The balloon catheter can then be inflated and tested for symmetry and absence of leak, deflated and placed through the trocar and the trocar removed. The balloon can then be reinflated and the ultrasound image of the balloon conformance and tissue distances can be evaluated and if felt adequate, APBI can then begin (Fig. 13.13).

The rural surgeon can provide all the surgical care and placement of the balloon catheter locally and only have the patient receive their radiation at another facility if their rural facility does not have radiation oncology facilities. This can greatly decrease the amount of time the patient needs to be away from home and family.

Potential Pitfalls

It is vital to remember that false negative images can occur because not all cancers can be seen by ultrasound. Palpable or image-detected abnormalities not visualized by ultrasound must still be evaluated and either carefully followed or biopsied.

Inadequate or sample errors can occur. Be sure to carefully correlate the pathology/cytology findings with the entire clinical picture. A suspicious exam with a negative ultrasound-guided biopsy should be reevaluated and rebiopsied.

Be very careful to keep all needles parallel to the chest wall to avoid entering the chest wall or cavity and causing pneumothorax. Never point the needle at the chest wall.

Many core biopsy devices are spring loaded and fire with a significant throw beyond the end of the needle at time of placement. Be sure to adequately assess the tissue beyond the tip of the needle in the throw distance to prevent inadvertent injury to surrounding or deeper tissues.

Post-procedure Care

Minimal post-procedure care is usually required. Following the procedure, 5 min of firm manual pressure is used. Needle puncture sites may just have a bandage placed. Core biopsy incisions rarely require a stitch (Fig. 13.14). The edges are brought together with a surgical closure tape and an occlusive dressing is placed. The patient may shower the following day and the dressing may be removed in 4–5 days. Ice is often placed the first few hours post procedure. Findings and pathology report are discussed with the patient as soon as available. Clinical follow-up is arranged with reevaluation including repeat clinical breast exam and imaging in 3–6 months.

Common Complications

Ecchymosis and small hematomas are common and usually self-limited. Large hematomas are infrequent and rarely require drainage or aspiration. Infection is infrequent and usually responds to oral antibiotics. Pneumothorax is very rare.

Breast ultrasound is easily incorporated into rural surgical practice because it is accurate and reproducible. Ultrasound becomes an extension of the clinical breast exam and rapidly becomes the "stethoscope" to the breast. Ultrasound is well tolerated and portable and can be brought to the patient, to the operating room and even to very rural outreach clinics. Ultrasound has a wide variety of clinical indications in both the diagnosis and management of breast disorders and allows minimally invasive diagnostic and therapeutic procedures. Breast ultrasound is truly an indispensable tool in the armamentarium of today's rural surgeon.

Oncoplastic Techniques for Breast Conservation

14

Rachel D. Wooldridge

Indications

Oncoplastic breast surgery techniques have been developed over the past several years, allowing for improved cosmesis and bilateral symmetry in the setting of an oncologically sound procedure. Techniques including the combination of a partial mastectomy with a reduction mammoplasty, lateral or medial approaches, parenchymal rearrangement surgery, and flexible pedicle-based reconstructions are all appropriate for a general surgeon to master. There is no primary tumor size restriction for these techniques, but there must be sufficient breast volume remaining to allow for acceptable cosmesis relative to breast size. Oncoplastic surgery is not appropriate for multicentric disease. Consideration of neo-adjuvant chemotherapy to decrease/eliminate primary tumor volume is an increasingly common practice.

Broadly, breast conserving surgery should be followed by postoperative radiation therapy. Unique to oncoplastic breast conserving surgery is the likely indication for a symmetry procedure for the contralateral breast. This is commonly a reduction procedure, and technique may be tailored to allow for scar symmetry in addition to matching volume. This may be performed at the time of the cancer surgery (immediate) or following radiation therapy (delayed).

Preoperative Preparation

Multicentric cancer is a contraindication to oncoplastic breast conserving surgery. Standard two-view bilateral mammograms should be performed, augmenting with MRI if extensive calcifications are seen or a discrepancy exists between clinical exam and imaging. Defining the extent of the primary tumor is paramount in the success of oncoplastic techniques in breast surgery. Preoperatively, the patient should be marked in an upright position (sternal notch to nipple distance, upper breast border, inframammary fold, anatomic midline, planned nipple position). Patients should be positioned supine, with arms extended at a 90° angle. Both breasts should be marked and prepped into the field, with the prep extending down to the bed to include the lateral chest wall.

Operative Strategy

Each approach is dependent on the location of the tumor, and discussed separately below. Peri-areolar incisions remain favorable if operatively feasible and no contouring of the breast is necessary. Generally, any incision on the breast should be made in a curvilinear fashion, as this has been shown to decrease overall deformity of the breast (especially in the superior quadrants).

Basic Principles

The tumor bed should be marked with clips following excision to aid radiation oncologists in treatment planning. If pectoralis major fascia is taken with the surgical specimen (as is recommended by this author), the deep tissue should be closed over the pectoralis major muscle to prevent dimpling and formation of a divot. The specimen should be in one piece, including overlying skin, breast tissue, and pectoralis fascia to allow for correct margin interpretation and assessment. Sentinel node biopsy (or axillary dissection) can be performed through the inframammary fold if it is part of the planned procedure or through a separate incision. For operations that involve relocation of the nipple, the ideal nipple position is in the mid-clavicular line at the level of the inframammary fold (8–10 cm below the upper breast border).

R.D. Wooldridge, M.D. (✉)
Division of Surgical Oncology, UT Southwestern Medical Center, 5323 Harry Hines Boulevard, Dallas, TX 75390, USA
e-mail: rachel.wooldridge@utsouthwestern.edu

A.L. Halverson and D.C. Borgstrom (eds.), *Advanced Surgical Techniques for Rural Surgeons*, DOI 10.1007/978-1-4939-1495-1_14, © Springer Science+Business Media New York 2015

Operative Techniques

1. Upper outer/upper inner quadrant: inferior pedicle reduction mammaplasty (Multiple variations of the Wise pattern—the three incision "anchor" technique). Best approach for patients with large, ptotic breasts who are interested in substantial reduction. (Fig. 14.1)
   (a) Preoperative marking is imperative (Fig. 14.1a)
       i. Mark the sternal midline, the inframammary fold (IMF), the sternal notch to nipple distance, and the breast meridian in the sitting position. The breast meridian is the midpoint of the clavicle through the midline of the breast—this usually bisects the nipple-areolar complex. The new location of the nipple-areolar complex is based on the intersection of the breast meridian and the inframammary fold. Mark all distances.
   (b) With an inferior pedicle technique, the nipple is usually moved 8–10 cm cranially, and derives its blood supply from the breast tissue along the natural inframammary fold—the inferior pedicle. It is vital that this pedicle not be too narrow, or undercut in any way, as this could lead to nipple ischemia or loss. (Fig. 14.1b)
   (c) Inscribe the nipple-areolar complex with a round metal "cookie cutter," aiming for a 4 cm diameter in most reductions, at the level previously marked and measured in pre-op (Fig. 14.1b).
   (d) Incise the pedicle along the markings, and de-epithelialize from the nipple to the inframammary fold, taking care to preserve the subdermal plexus. (Fig. 14.1c)
   (e) Flaps of at least 1 cm in thickness are developed up to the clavicle with electrocautery. Several large vessels are usually encountered and addressed with targeted electrocautery.
   (f) The medial and lateral margins of the inferior pedicle are defined with electrocautery, and then sharply divided with a Watson blade (taking care not to bevel into the pedicle) down to the chest wall. This enables all tissue medial and lateral to the pedicle (below the inframammary fold) to be resected. With an inferior pedicle, the tissue resected is usually superior and lateral. Take care not to apply tension or torque to the pedicle. Preserve pectoral attachments within the pedicle. (Fig. 14.1c)
   (g) Place a 0-silk suture through the nipple-areolar complex (in situ on the inferior pedicle).
   (h) Breast parenchyma is re-approximated, starting with a buried 3-0 absorbable suture placed to define the new midpoint of the inframammary fold—the "triangle corner stitch"—to incorporate the medial and lateral flaps with the center of the inframammary fold. (Fig. 14.1d)
   (i) Close the remaining dermal layers with interrupted buried 3-0 absorbable suture.
   (j) De-epithelialize the skin from the new nipple-areolar complex location. (Fig. 14.1e)
   (k) Remove any dermal sutures needed to allow for use of the previously placed 0-silk suture to deliver the nipple into the new location (previously delineated with the "cookie cutter"). (Fig. 14.1e)
   (l) Close the entire incision with a running 4-0 monofilament suture.
   (m) Tack the areola in place using buried interrupted 3-0 absorbable suture, placed first at the cardinal points, and then with sutures in between, until the areola is secure.
   (n) Finish the areolar closure with a running baseball 5-0 fast-absorbing suture. (Fig. 14.1f)
   (o) All tissue from any breast reduction should be sent for pathologic evaluation. Drains may be left at the discretion of the surgeon.
2. Retro-areolar or lower outer/lower inner quadrant tumors (Fig. 14.2):
   (a) Incise the inframammary fold sharply. Dissect through the parenchyma perpendicular to the chest wall until the pectoralis fascia is encountered using electrocautery, taking care to maintain grossly negative margins (aim for at least 1 cm circumferentially around tumor). De-epithelialize the nipple-areolar complex sharply with a 15-blade. Preserve the subdermal plexus, the blood supply to the nipple. (Fig. 14.2a, b)
   (b) Place the nondominant hand through the inframammary incision and elevate the breast anteriorly; mobilize the breast off of the chest wall moving from inferior to superior, (including pectoralis fascia) using electrocautery. Stop at the level of the nipple.
   (c) Complete the preoperatively marked incision sharply.
   (d) Minimally grasp the inferior border of the de-epithelialized nipple-areolar complex with Allis clamps. Create a superiorly based 5 mm thick flap, elevating the nipple-areolar complex sharply with Metzenbaum scissors and obtaining hemostasis as needed, underneath the de-epithelialized area. (Fig. 14.2c)
   (e) Dissect the specimen free posterior to the superior border of the flap (full thickness), moving in a perpendicular fashion to the chest wall using electrocautery.
   (f) Mark the specimen for orientation and perform specimen radiography. Irrigate and confirm hemostasis. Place 5 mm clips at the superior, infero-medial, and infero-lateral borders of the tumor bed.
   (g) Place a 2-0 silk suture through the superior edge of the nipple.

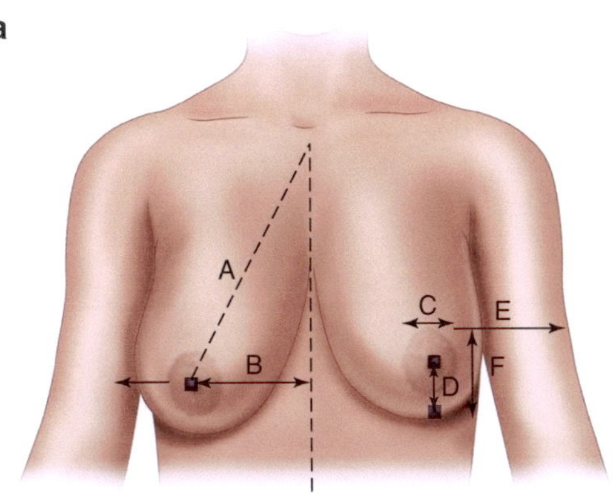

A: Notch to nipple distance (19-21 cm)
B: Nipple to midline distance (9-11 cm)
C: Areolar diameter (4.5 cm)
D: Nipple to inferior breast border (5-8 cm)
E: Inframammary fold
F: Equal to D minus E (0-2 cm)

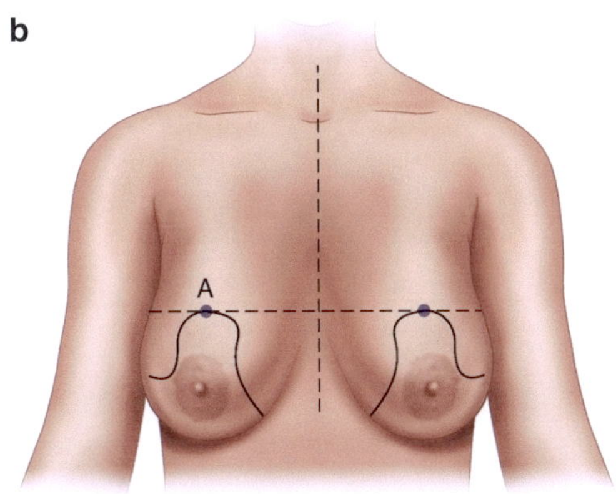

A: New location of the nipple areolar complex

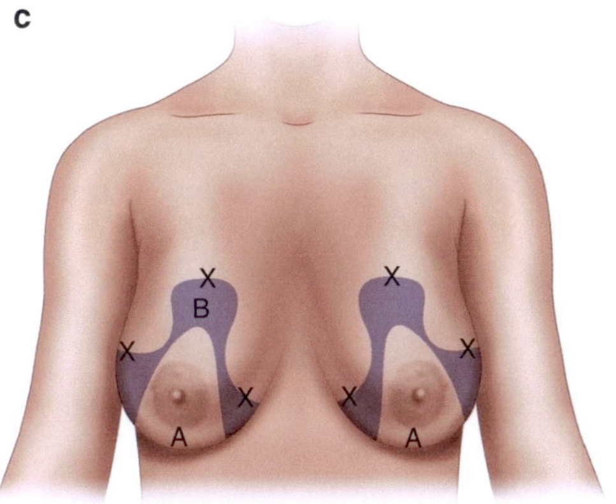

A: Inferior pedicle, de-epithelialized
B: Tissue to be resected
X: Marks incisions

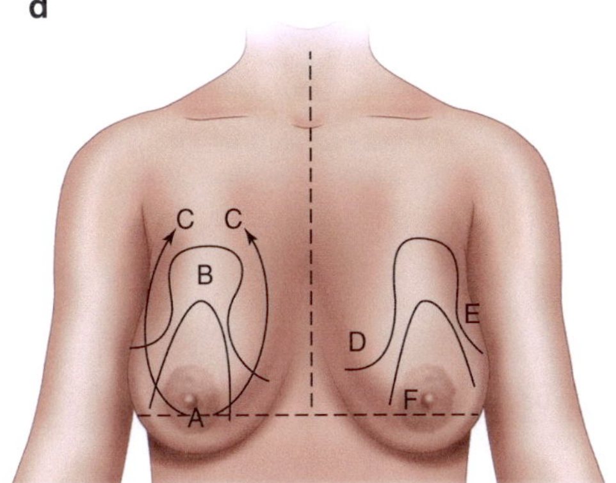

A: Inferior pedicle
B: Defect
C: Superior/cranial advancement of the inferior
pedicle underneath the superior flap
D - F: "Triangle" corner stitch to bury the
pedicle and attach flaps from medial and lateral
to the inframammary fold

Fig. 14.1 (**a**) Standard markings for oncoplastic surgery. (**b**) Standard wise pattern markings. (**c**) Isolating the inferior pedicle. (**d**) Creating the breast mound. (**e**) Relocation of the nipple-areolar complex. (**f**) Final appearance of the breast

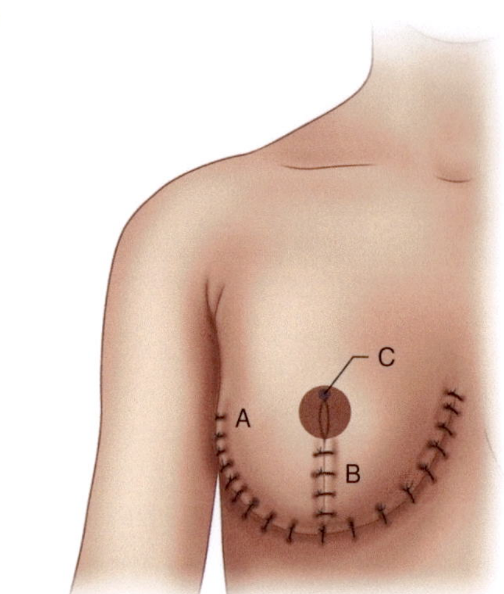

A: Breast re-approximated at the inframammary fold
B: Breast re-approximated in the midline
C: New nipple-areolar complex location, de-epithelialized

Final appearance of the breast

Fig. 14.1 (continued)

(h) Re-approximate the breast parenchyma along the lateral/medial pillars with figure of eight 2-0 absorbable suture. This should be achieved without tension. (Fig. 14.2d)

(i) Place a single buried 3-0 absorbable suture at the superior border of the nipple. This will mark the inferior border of the new nipple location. (Fig. 14.2d)

(j) Use the silk suture to deliver the nipple into the appropriate spot.

(k) Tack the nipple into place using buried interrupted 4-0 absorbable suture at the cardinal points, and close with a 4-0 subcuticular absorbable suture.

(l) The remaining incision should be closed in layers with absorbable suture. (Fig. 14.2e)

3. Lateral/medial quadrant tumors
   (a) Radial ellipse (Fig. 14.3)
       i. Incise sharply (specimen will include skin).
       ii. Resect entire segment sharply down to the pectoralis fascia, switching at that point to electrocautery
       iii. Mark the specimen for orientation and perform specimen radiography.
       iv. Irrigate and confirm hemostasis.
       v. Place 5 mm clips at the superior, infero-medial, and infero-lateral borders of the tumor bed.
       vi. Advance surrounding tissue with deep figure of eight 2-0 absorbable suture to cover the pectoralis major muscle
       vii. The remaining tissue should be closed in layers with absorbable suture.
   (b) Medial pedicle vertical breast reduction:
       i. This pattern is a modified pedicle-based reduction mammoplasty technique using modified Wise markings, and is too detailed for this chapter. Basically, breast parenchyma is removed as a vertical wedge inferiorly, and a lateral flap is created. The parenchyma remains attached to the superior skin flaps, and the nipple is supplied by the medial flap.

4. Central tumor necessitating removal of the nipple-areolar complex
   (a) Batwing technique (Fig. 14.4)
       i. Measure the height of the skin resection both in preoperative marking and again on the operating table (Fig. 14.4a).
       ii. The two triangles, or "wings," must have identical heights (Fig. 14.4a). The base of the triangles should be vertical to allow for the opposition of the medial corners.
       iii. The tip of each triangle should be at most 4 cm away from the base (Fig. 14.4a).
       iv. De-epithelialize the triangles to increase perfusion of the flap.
       v. Pull the nipple and tumor anteriorly; dissect to macroscopically negative margins with electrocautery. (Fig. 14.4b)
       vi. Incise the superior leg of each triangle 1 cm in depth.
       vii. Rotate the de-epithelialized triangle underneath the upper border of each triangle. Suture the inferior leg into place using a 2-0 absorbable suture under minimal tension. (Fig. 14.4c)
       viii. The remaining tissue should be closed in layers with absorbable suture (Fig. 14.4d).

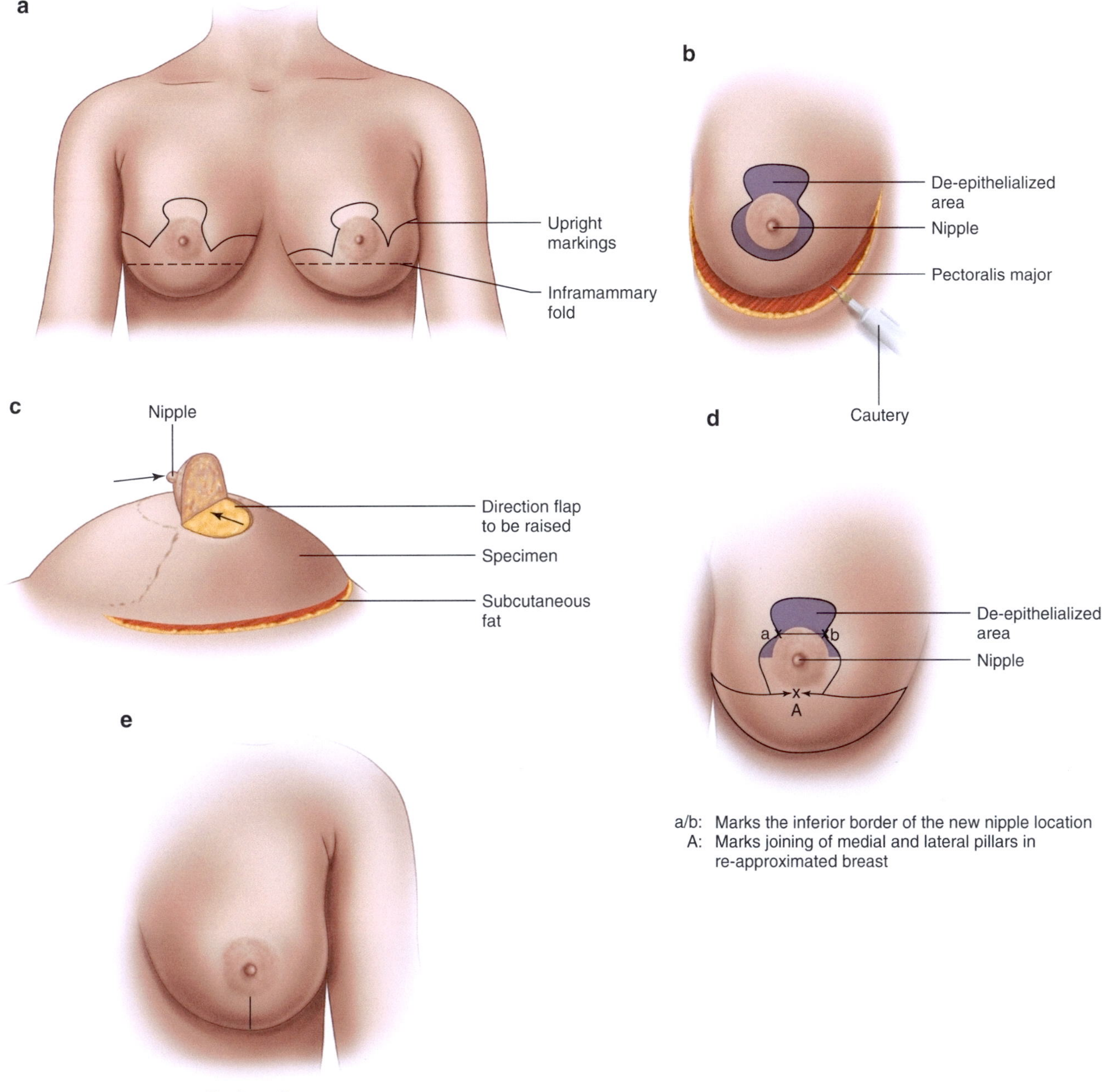

Fig. 14.2 (**a**) Standard markings for oncoplastic approach to lower quadrant tumors. (**b**) Mobilization of the specimen. (**c**) Creation of the nipple flap. (**d**) Re-approximation of the breast. (**e**) Final appearance of the breast

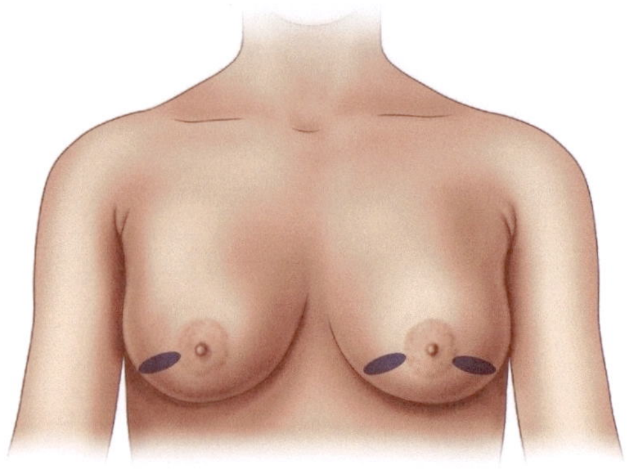

Fig. 14.3 Common locations for radial ellipse Incision—always below the 3:00 position and the 9:00 position The nipple-areolar complex is rarely distorted

Potential Pitfalls

Positive margins after complex tissue rearrangement, hematoma, seroma, flap necrosis, nipple ischemia or loss, unexpected malignancy in a procedure performed for symmetry.

Postoperative Care

Drain at the discretion of the surgeon and extent of flap mobilization. The patient should wear a supportive slightly com pressive garment for at least 72 per this author's recommendation. No heavy lifting or aggressive exercise for 7 days.

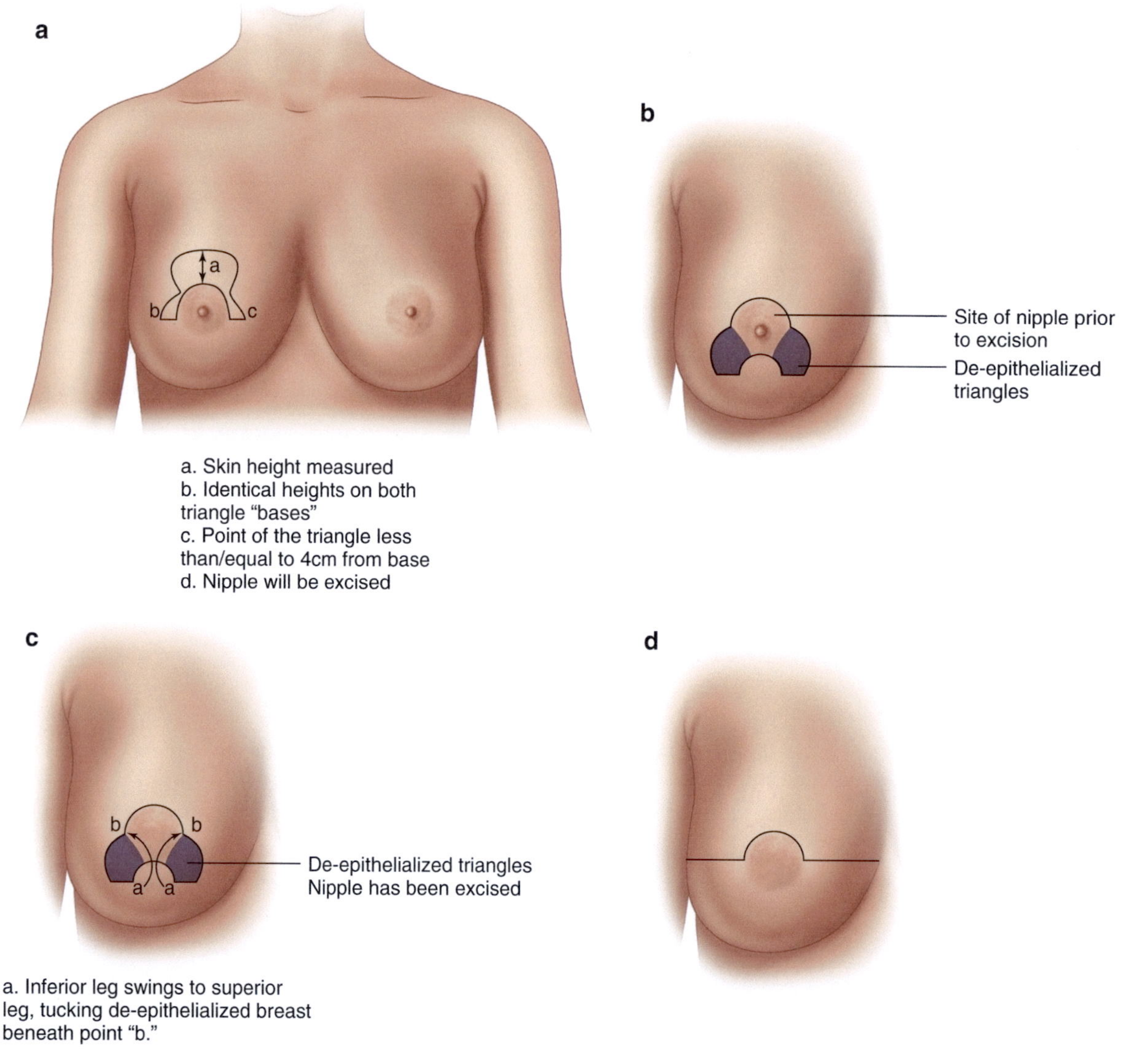

Fig. 14.4 (**a**) Standard markings for oncoplastic approach to central tumors. (**b**) Defect after excision. (**c**) Filling the defect. (**d**) Final appearance of the breast (nipple has been excised)

Common Complications

Seroma is uncommon; may observe or aspirate if symptomatic. Techniques that involve mobilization of the nipple may rarely result in nipple necrosis or loss. Sensation to the nipple may be affected and should be discussed preoperatively. Positive margins, symptomatic hematoma, and flap and/or nipple necrosis may result in a return to the OR.

When to Transfer

Plastic surgery availability for complex reconstruction, re-do operations, prior breast reduction, symmetry concerns, or nipple reconstruction. The techniques described here are fairly straightforward. Variations on a pedicle reduction mammoplasty can be very complex technically, and may not be appropriate in some settings. The remaining described operative strategies, however, should be amenable to a standard general surgery practice.

Suggested Reading

Clough KB, Lewis JS, Couturaud B, Fitoussi A, Nos C, Falcou M-C. Oncoplastic techniques allow extensive resections for breast-conserving therapy of breast carcinomas. Ann Surg. 2003;237(1): 26–34.

Fitoussi A, Berry MG, Couturaud B, Salmon RJ. Oncoplastic and reconstructive surgery for breast cancer—the Institut Curie experience. Heidelberg: Springer; 2009.

Fitzal F, Schrenk P. Oncoplastic breast surgery: a guide to clinical practice. Vienna: Springer; 2010.

Nahabedian MY. Oncoplastic surgery of the breast. London: Elsevier; 2009.

Lauren Smithson and Krista M. Bannon

Indications

1. DCIS requiring total mastectomy
   (a) Large involved area preventing cosmetic result with lumpectomy alone
   (b) True multifocal DCIS not amenable to lumpectomy
   (c) Multicentric disease (more than one quadrant affected)
   (d) Contraindication to radiation therapy or patient preference to forgo radiation therapy after breast conservation therapy
2. Stage 0–II invasive breast cancer, or those down-staged to 0–II after neoadjuvant chemotherapy
   (a) No central tumor involvement or at least 2 cm from the nipple-areolar complex
3. Prophylactic surgery for genetically high risk patients (BRCA1 or BRCA2)
4. Patient preference

Preoperative Preparation

Although the total skin-sparing mastectomy (TSSM) was introduced in 1962, which preserved the nipple-areolar complex (NAC), skin-sparing mastectomies (SSM), where the NAC is sacrificed, became more prevalent in the treatment of breast cancer after 1991. SSM and TSSM have emerged as the treatment of choice in select cases, once a detailed work-up and discussion with the patient have been completed.

L. Smithson, M.Phil., M.D. (✉)
Department of Surgery, Providence Hospital and Medical Centers, 16001 W. Nine Mile Road, Southfield, MI 48075, USA
e-mail: lauren_smithson@yahoo.com

K.M. Bannon
General Surgery, Providence Hospital and Medical Centers, 16001 W. Nine Mile Road, Southfield, MI 48075, USA

Preoperative Imaging and Laboratory Testing

In keeping with the standard of care, mammogram and ultrasound often accurately predict invasive masses. These modalities, however, are not as successful in the evaluation of noninvasive lesions. Despite mammography diagnosing 80 % of DCIS lesions, the microcalcifications that are the hallmark of this disease can often be missed. Ultrasound is even less useful in the diagnosis of this disease presentation, although it may serve in the dense breast to rule out any masses. Once a diagnosis is made, further mammographic imaging is required to evaluate suspicious lesions, including compressive mammography and magnification views.

Currently under debate is the routine employment of MRI, which has been increasingly used for breast imaging. It is not, however, the standard of care due to high false positive rate and elevated cost of routine use. It is not the most practical modality for the rural surgeon, considering availability and expense. It is recommended in the genetically high risk patients or in unusual clinical presentations. Previous unclear imaging or women with a history of multiple biopsies may also benefit from an MRI, but this is not as well supported in the literature. Certainly MRI has a role in the pregnant patient with breast cancer. To date, no literature presents high level evidence to support the use of MRI in routine screening in women with early stage breast cancer. Although some studies suggest that the enhanced sensitivity of MRI may alter surgical planning from lumpectomy to mastectomy, especially in patients with multifocal or multicentric disease, evidence showing that MRI improves surgical care, reduces the number of required surgeries, or reduces local recurrence after surgery, is still lacking.

Also important in the preoperative assessment of patients with early stage breast cancer or DCIS is the evaluation for distant disease. A chest roentgenogram and a full set of labs, including complete blood count, electrolytes with calcium, pregnancy testing, and coagulation studies, are important. A hepatic panel, including AST, ALT, and alkaline phosphatase, is recommended to evaluate for any liver abnormalities.

A.L. Halverson and D.C. Borgstrom (eds.), *Advanced Surgical Techniques for Rural Surgeons*,
DOI 10.1007/978-1-4939-1495-1_15, © Springer Science+Business Media New York 2015

Bone scans, PET scans, and other full body imaging are currently not recommended for early stage disease where SSM or TSSM are treatment options.

Tissue Diagnosis and Multidisciplinary Discussions

The next important preoperative principle is a well-executed needle biopsy for diagnosis. Accurate tumor localization is an imperative principle when planning surgical removal of a tumor. Communicating with radiologic imagers allows accurate preoperative identification of lesions and defines the goals of resection. Also, collaboration in a multidisciplinary approach will aid in achieving a single stage surgical removal of the tumor. Once the lesion has been accurately imaged and histologically proven by biopsy, the discussion on appropriate surgical approach can be held with the patient.

Ductal Carcinoma In Situ and Invasive Ductal Carcinoma

When considering the indications for SSM or TSSM, the nature of the identified lesion becomes paramount. While lumpectomy, quadrantectomy, or other forms of breast conserving therapy (BCT) are indeed possible with DCIS or early invasive cancers, mastectomy remains an option. In DCIS, determining the extent and histologic nature of disease helps to determine the appropriate surgical approach. Multicentricity, with more than one quadrant of the breast involved, was originally thought to occur in 30 % of patients. More recently it has been noted that large DCIS lesions, rather than appearing as two isolated lesions, often extend continuously between quadrants. Multifocal DCIS is due to separate foci within the same ductal system, but this is more likely to be artifact secondary to biopsy technique. Despite the debate over accurate terminology, both presentations fall into the category of extensive disease, and mastectomy offers a solution that lumpectomy might fail to address. The type of DCIS also raises questions regarding treatment options. DCIS presents as comedo and non-comedo type. From a clinical standpoint, non-comedo DCIS may be more appropriately treated with SSM as the lesions are harder to see on mammography and more difficult to follow. Calcifications also do not always map the full extent of the disease. Non-calcified sections of DCIS may be left behind with BCT. Local recurrence has been quoted as 1–2 % with BCT and radiation versus 0–0.5 % with mastectomy.

In the case of invasive cancer, staging becomes important, as the recommendation for SSM includes invasive cancer to stages 0–II. Neoadjuvant therapy for more advanced stages of breast cancer can reduce the size of the lesion to meet the

criteria for SSM or TSSM. What must also be addressed in breast cancer surgery is the need for axillary node biopsies and/or axillary node dissections. Neither are contraindications for SSM.

Considerations for SSM and TSSM

Preoperatively, the natural history of the lesion should be discussed and all surgical options presented. In a majority of cases, SSM or TSSM becomes a question of patient preference. To help determine the best surgical option, preoperative discussion should include any associated follow-up such as radiation, antiestrogen therapy and/or chemotherapy. In terms of treatment for DCIS, BCT with radiation is an option, as is antiestrogen therapy. SSM offers an alternative, such that, if all margins are negative, radiation therapy can be avoided, and antiestrogen therapy becomes a matter for discussion. With invasive cancer, even stage I and II, radiation becomes a mainstay in therapy if any breast tissue remains. SSM offers an alternative without radiation, as long as axillary nodes are negative. Positive nodal disease, especially if >4 positive nodes, indicates a need for radiation therapy and often adjuvant chemotherapy. Hormone therapy in these patients, if they are receptor positive, should be expected and discussed preoperatively. These treatments help, even in the cases of mastectomy, to reduce local recurrence. Discussing radiation should include the patient's perspectives on cosmesis and reconstruction. For example, certain procedures, like SSM, are more difficult to perform after radiation, and should therefore factor into the pretreatment discussions.

With SSM or TSSM, the cosmetic goals of the procedure run in tandem with the oncologic goals. Tumor size to breast size ratio is the key factor to bring into the discussion. Large tumors in a small breast might lead a patient to choose mastectomy for cosmetic reasons. Previous surgery, including mastopexy or other circumareolar incision, is not a contraindication for SSM. If SSM is the appropriate choice for the treatment of the disease, exploring surgical approaches preoperatively with the patient will assist in determining the type of incision that is appropriate for the nature of the cancer, and the cosmetic and psychological outcomes desired by the patient. Preservation of the nipple-areolar complex, if possible based on tumor location and stage, should be addressed. Preservation of the nipple results in a more natural cosmetic outcome, and has added psychological benefits for the patient. Currently, the literature does not definitively address how much risk is conferred by leaving the nipple-areolar complex dermis, but data does report that <10 % of invasive cancers are found in the NAC, with less invasive tumors found in nipple duct tissue. Regardless of the decision for SSM or TSSM, patient preference, especially in the case of prophylaxis, must be carefully determined, with the patient well-informed preoperatively of all possible options and outcomes.

Operative Strategy

With a skin-sparing approach, the skin envelope of the breast is protected and retained. The nipple-areolar complex (NAC), previous biopsy sites, and skin overlying a superficial tumor are resected with all breast parenchyma. Multiple options exist to preserve the native breast skin and inframammary fold without compromising the oncoplastic outcome of the procedure. Other options for preservation and reconstruction have been described, including the nipple-sparing mastectomy, where part, or all, of the NAC is retained. Postoperative complications and recurrences are similar as long as the retained portion of the NAC is far enough away from the tumor to meet oncologic principles. Little local recurrence is found if the tumor was more than 1 cm from the nipple and the retro-areolar area is histologically negative, even after chemoradiation or with advanced tumors. If choosing to spare the NAC, avoid a periareolar incision as there is an increased risk of nipple necrosis.

A sentinel lymph node biopsy can be performed through a separate curvilinear axillary incision, and if the frozen section is positive, then an axillary dissection can be performed prior to starting the reconstruction of choice. Some reconstructive surgery is manageable in a rural setting, but should be performed with the assistance of a plastic surgeon until the general surgeon is comfortable with the technique and cos-mesis of the procedure. Those without formal plastic surgery training should identify complex patient cases which may warrant referral to a tertiary center where a formal plastic surgery consultation can achieve a satisfactory cosmetic result.

Operative Technique

Determine the Best Skin Incision

Determining the best skin incision should be performed in clinic and finalized in ink in the preoperative area while patient can be seated upright and the appropriate lines drawn and measured. The type of incision will be based on SSM versus TSSM, where the NAC is preserved. The periareolar incision includes the entire areola (Fig. 15.1a). A "tennis-racquet" incision not only encircles the areola but also extends laterally (Fig. 15.1b). The modified elliptical incision is similar to the incision made for a simple mastectomy, only smaller, removing the NAC with an ellipse of skin at least 5 cm in length (Fig. 15.1c). A reduction mammoplasty is appropriate if the contralateral breast is also to be reduced (Fig. 15.2a). To help reduce the risk of necrosis, the flap can be deepithelialized (Fig. 15.2b). If indicated, previous biopsy sites can be incorporated into the initial incision or separately excised. The TSSM incisions include inframammary, lateral radial, and mastopexy. The inframammary incision is an incision along the inframammary fold of a least 10 cm, which allows access to all borders of the breast tissue and is safer to use in women with smaller breasts so that the supe-

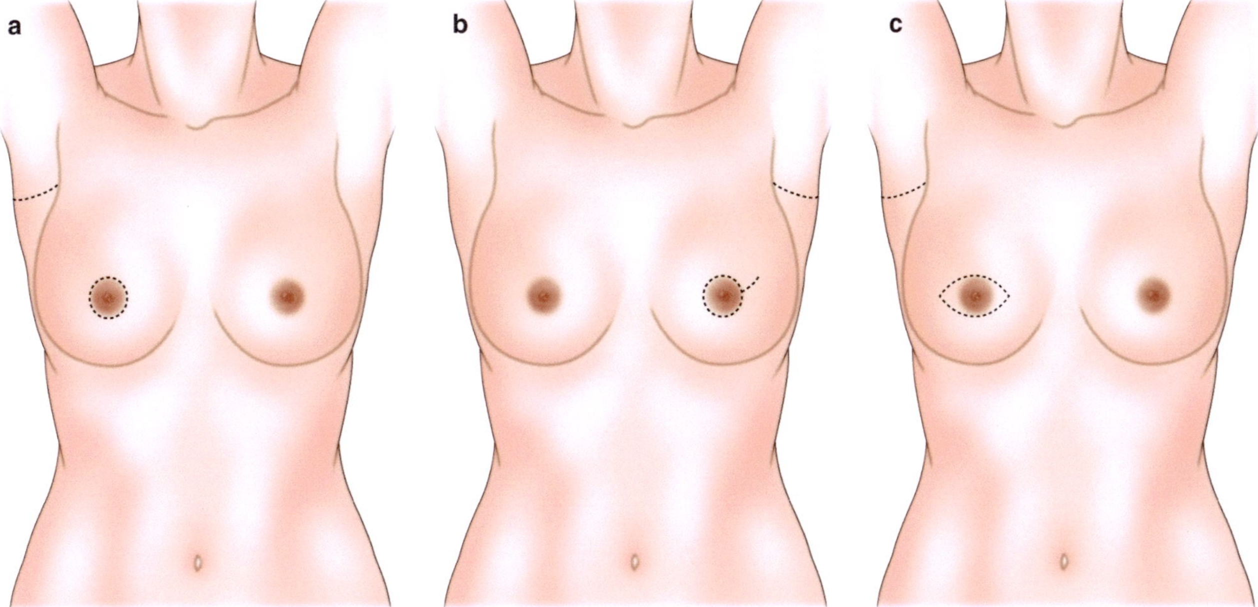

Fig. 15.1 (**a**) Periareolar incision. Note the separate axillary incision for SLNB or dissection. (**b**) Tennis-racquet incision. Note the separate axillary incision for SLNB or dissection. (**c**) Modified elliptical incision, excising the NAC with 5 cm or skin and all breast parenchyma

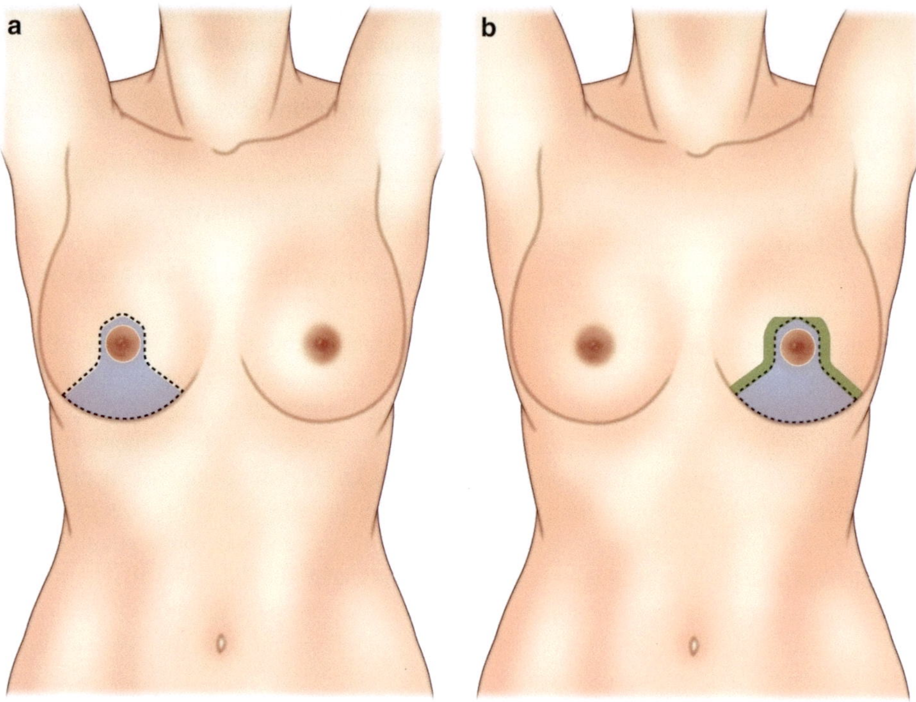

Fig. 15.2 (**a**) Reduction mammoplasty incision without deepithelialization. The *grey area* of skin is excised with the breast tissue. (**b**) Reduction mammoplasty incision with deepithelialization in the cross-hatched area. The *grey area* of skin is excised with the breast tissue

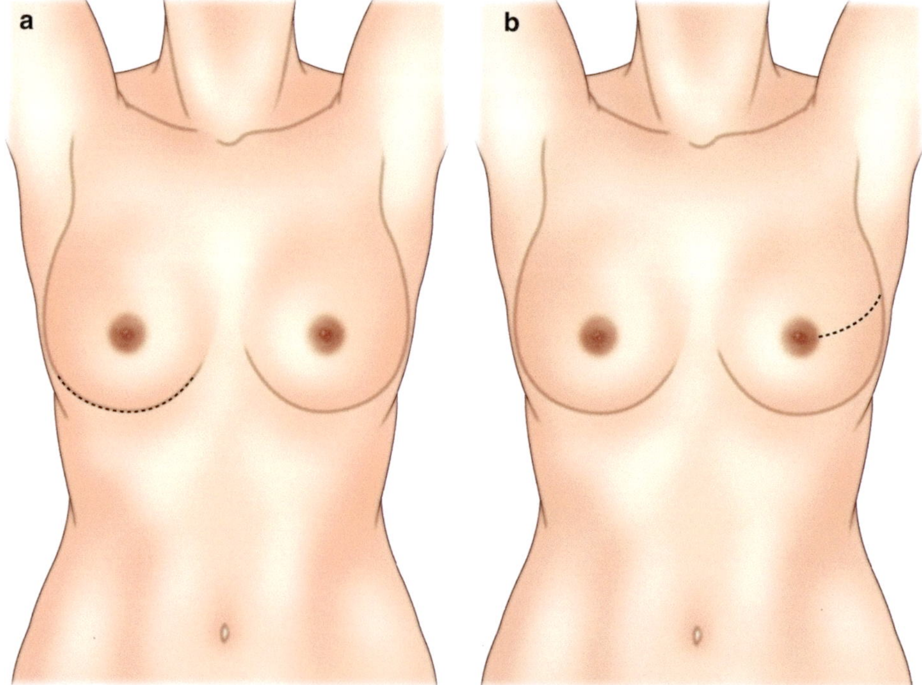

Fig. 15.3 (**a**) Inframammary incision for nipple-sparing TSSM. (**b**) Lateral radial incision for TSSM, which can be extended into the NAC itself if needed

rior part of the breast may be confidently removed in its entirety (Fig. 15.3a). The scar is easily hidden in this natural skin crease postoperatively. The lateral radial incision is similar to the tennis-racquet incision without encirclement of the areola (Fig. 15.3b). This incision can also be extended into the NAC itself if necessary for adequate resection, as long as 30 % of the nipple is spared. The mastopexy incision is another incision similar to a circumareolar incision, but includes only a crescent of skin above the nipple-areolar complex. If more than one third of the areola is needed to perform a mastectomy through this incision, it is recommended to choose another incision as this will compromise nipple-areolar blood supply. However, this incision does create a nipple lift postoperatively which can be desired in a pendulous breast. Contralateral mastopexy on the unaffected breast may be required to achieve symmetry. This is an ideal approach for breasts with larger areolas or smaller lesions. If at any time the patient's breast tissue is unable to be adequately incised or gross tumor is within 1–2 cm of the nipple-areolar complex, enlarge the incision to include the nipple-areolar complex and convert to a skin-sparing mastectomy without nipple preservation.

Sentinel Lymph Node Biopsy

Mastectomies require a sentinel lymph node biopsy. After general anesthesia, inject methylene blue (2 cc diluted with 2 cc saline) intradermally over the area of skin to be excised and massage into upper outer quadrant. Make curvilinear incision in axilla and do sentinel node biopsy, send for frozen section. If the frozen section is positive, then an axillary dissection can be performed prior to starting the reconstruction of choice. It is important to include all nodal tissue below the axillary vein, extending to the latissimus dorsi towards the tissue at the medial aspect of the pectoralis minor.

Creating the Skin Flaps

Create the incision that has been preoperatively determined on the affected breast. Raise skin flaps cephalad and caudad using skin hooks and Richardson retractors to create countertraction while pulling down on the breast tissue with your free hand. Typically scissors, scalpel, or electrocautery can be used to raise flap with long even strokes in parallel with the flap to minimize buttonholes or burns. Continually grasp flap between index and thumb to ensure even flap thickness. The flap should be 5- to 10-mm thick (7–8 mm ideal). Preserve parasternal and infraclavicular perforating vessels if possible, without compromising the oncological element of the procedure, to improve the viability of the skin flaps.

Breast Excision

Remove all fibroglandular tissues within the borders of a simple mastectomy: the clavicle superiorly, inframammary crease inferiorly, latissimus dorsi laterally, and sternum medially. Dissect breast tissue off pectoralis major. The investing fascia of the pectoralis can be preserved if the tumor is small and the muscle is not involved, otherwise, excise the fascia and involved muscle. Separate the axillary tail from the pectoralis major and minor and the serratus anterior while sacrificing the lateral branches of the medial pectoral neurovascular bundle. Divide the breast tissue from the axillary contents with clamp and tie approach. If appropriate, continue to immediate reconstruction.

Potential Pitfalls

Difficulty in performing an adequate mastectomy through a limited incision; thicker flaps have shown increased rates of recurrence

Care must be taken not to thin the flaps to the point of skin perforation (buttonhole) or devascularization

Initial preservation of the nipple-areolar complex with may require removal in a second stage operation if pathologic analysis reveals positive margins

Nipple necrosis secondary to devascularization during tissue mobilization and removal

Descending below the inframammary fold affects the cosmesis of the breast

Reconstruction complications, namely implant loss, wound infection, and myocutaneous or free flap necrosis, depending on the type of reconstruction chosen

Postoperative Care

Postoperatively, the patient should be kept in the hospital overnight for observation. A drain should be placed in the axilla to monitor excessive drainage and collapse any dead space. The patient will require teaching regarding care of the drain. An expanding hematoma at the mastectomy site may require operative evacuation. Hematomas of this nature are often impossible to aspirate at bedside. As for rehabilitation needs, patients are often discharged home with their drains and wound care teaching on postoperative day 1. They can follow-up in the office within 1 week for removal of the drain. They will have pain in the chest and axilla and should likely avoid strenuous activity with that extremity, but can manage the daily activities of living without too much difficulty. Physical therapy may be of assistance, after the initial healing period is complete, for retraining and strengthening surrounding musculature.

Common Complications

Local recurrence (0–3 %)
Surgical skin infections
Hematoma
Seroma

Lymphedema

Injury to the nerves (long thoracic, thoracodorsal, or intercostal brachial)

Flap necrosis

When to Transfer

Performing an SSM with immediate reconstruction requires some additional skills on the part of the general surgeon. Many courses exist for the development of reconstructive techniques, such as the myocutaneous flaps. Free flaps, such as the gluteal, require expertise, likely at the hand of a plastic surgeon with access to microsurgical equipment. Those general surgeons with experience performing mastectomies should find the SSM a relatively straightforward adjustment to their own technique. If the facility supports a plastic surgeon, it is advisable that they assist in the reconstructive portion of the surgery until the general surgeon is confident enough of the remodeling to act alone. If the facility where the surgeon is employed does not have a plastic surgeon, then perhaps assisting in the reconstruction procedure at a nearby facility could be arranged. Other components of reconstruction include nipple tattooing, which may or may not be available in a more rural setting. Another indication for referral might consist of contralateral breast mammoplasty, but again this depends on the comfort and experience of the surgeon performing the original SSM. There are relatively few emergencies in an SSM procedure that would require urgent transfer to another facility for specialized care, but if the patient desires a reconstructive procedure that is not within the realm of the surgeon's skill base, then transferring the patient with all of their preoperative evaluation, scans, consultations, and oncologic details, such as pathology, is acceptable.

Suggested Reading

Agrawal A, Sibbering DM, Courtney CA. Skin sparing mastectomy and immediate breast reconstruction: a review. Eur J Surg Oncol. 2013;39(4):320–8.

Carlson GW, Styblo TM, Lyles RH, Bostwick J, Murray DR, Staley CA, Wood WC. Local recurrence after skin-sparing mastectomy: tumor biology or surgical conservatism? Ann Surg Oncol. 2003;10(2):108–12.

Fortunato L, Loreti A, Andrich R, Costarelli L, Amini M, Farina M, Santini E, Vitelli CE. When mastectomy is needed: is the nipple-sparing procedure a new standard with very few contraindications? J Surg Oncol. 2013;108(4):207–12.

Garwood ER, Moore D, Ewing C, Hwang ES, Alvarado M, Foster RD, Esserman LJ. Total skin-sparing mastectomy: complications and local recurrence rates in 2 cohorts of patients. Ann Surg. 2006; 249:26–32.

Romics Jr L, Chew BK, Weiler-Mithoff E, Doughty JC, Brown IM, Stallard S, Wilson CR, Mallon EA, George WD. Ten-year follow-up of skin-sparing mastectomy followed by immediate breast reconstruction. Br J Surg. 2012;99(6):799–806.

Tokin C, Weiss A, Wang-Rodriguez J, Blair SL. Oncologic safety of skin-sparing and nipple-sparing mastectomy: a discussion and review of the literature. Int J Surg Oncol. 2012;2012:921821.

Guy J. Petruzzelli and Emily A. Norris

Indications

Epistaxis occurs commonly and the vast majority of cases are self-limited. It represents 0.5 % (or approximately 500,000 cases) of all visits to emergency rooms yearly in the United States. Emergency department visits are more common in the winter and are related to desiccation of the nasal mucosa by dry heat. Hospitalization for epistaxis is rare (approximately 30,000 admissions/year) and it is associated with trauma (17 % of cases) or an exacerbation of an underlying comorbidity (see below). Emergency room visits for epistaxis are most common in patients 70–80 years old and are likely related to the prevalence of hypertension and the use of anticoagulants in this population. The second most common incidences in patients 10 years old or less is related to trauma. Deaths directly due to epistaxis are rare and are most often reported in elderly patients with several comorbidities. The management of patients with epistaxis remains highly variable and while general treatment guidelines are in place no large prospective studies exist to direct therapy.

In addition to assisting with managing patients with epistaxis in the Emergency Department the rural surgeon may be asked by hospitalists to urgently evaluate and treat patients with nasal bleeding admitted with other diagnoses. Severe epistaxis can develop from either local disease or trauma to the nose, nasal cavity, or paranasal sinuses. Local causes of severe epistaxis include craniofacial trauma, benign or malignant sinonasal deformities or neoplasms, prior surgery, or intranasal pharmaceuticals (prescribed or illicit). Systemic causes of severe epistaxis include autoimmune or vascular diseases, disorders of coagulation (either acquired or congenital), anticoagulation or antiplatelet therapy (see Table 16.1). Correction of underlying coagulopathy may be necessary for definitive control of nasal hemorrhage in some patients.

Preoperative Preparation

Traditionally nasal hemorrhage has been divided into anterior and poster epistaxis based on the site of the bleeding. The nasal septum and lateral nasal wall have a rich vascular supply based on an anastomosing network of the internal and external carotid circulations. The external carotid artery blood supply to the nasal septum is derived from the septal branches of the superior labial division of the facial artery and the greater palatine artery; posteriorly the septum is supplied by the dorsal septal branches of the sphenopalatine artery. Superiorly the nasal septum is supplied by the anterior and posterior ethmoidal branches of the ophthalmic division of the internal carotid artery. The most frequent site of epistaxis is the dense vascular plexus overlying the anterior cartilaginous septum or Kesselbach's plexus, formed by the anterior ethmoidal and anterior septal arteries. The blood supply to the lateral nasal wall is derived from terminal divisions of the sphenopalatine artery with smaller contributions anteriorly from the anterior ethmoid and superiorly from the posterior ethmoid arteries. The most common site of posterior epistaxis is the posterior lateral nasal wall at the terminal divisions of sphenopalatine artery at the base of the middle turbinate.

The treatment of the patient with epistaxis can be significantly streamlined and frustration for the managing providers reduced by assembling all the proper equipment prior to manipulating the nasal cavity. The patient needs to be examined in the sitting position. Examining patients supine will direct blood posteriorly into the pharynx and larynx precipitating coughing and making epistaxis control significantly more challenging. Necessary equipment includes a headlight,

G.J. Petruzzelli, M.D., Ph.D., F.A.C.S. (✉)
Department of Surgery, Mercer University School of Medicine—
Savannah Campus, 4700 Waters Avenue, Savannah,
GA 31404, USA
e-mail: guypetruzzelli@memorialhealth.com

E.A. Norris, M.D.
General Surgery, Naval Medical Center Portsmouth,
Portsmouth, VA 23708, USA

A.L. Halverson, D.C. Borgstrom (eds.), *Advanced Surgical Techniques for Rural Surgeons*,
DOI 10.1007/978-1-4939-1495-1_16, © Springer Science+Business Media New York 2015

Table 16.1 Etiology of epistaxis

Trauma
Craniofacial trauma
Nasal/nasoseptal fracture
Digital trauma (nose picking)
Foreign body
Nasal instrumentation (Nasogastric tubes, nasal intubation)
Barotrauma
Postsurgical trauma
Structural
Nasal septal deviation
Septal spur
Septal perforation
Necrosis of septum—intranasal illicit drugs
Neoplasms (local or systemic)
Juvenile angiofibroma
Nasal polyposis
Inverted papilloma
Hemangio (glomangio)-pericytoma
Malignant neoplasm of the nasal cavity or paranasal sinus
Infections, inflammatory or autoimmune
Rhinosinusitis
Nasal diphtheria
Wegner's granulomatosis
Disorders of coagulation
Acquired
Antiplatelet therapy
Anticoagulation
Thrombolytics
Cirrhosis (alcohol or infectious)
Uremia
Systemic
Leukemia
Hemophilia
Von Willebrand or other inherited clotting disorder
Sickle cell disease
Vascular
Hypertension
Hereditary hemorrhagic telangiectasia

Table 16.2 Equipment for epistaxis management

Personal protective equipment
Gowns, gloves, mask, protective eye wear
Suction
Yankauer or tonsil and Frazier (nasal) suction tips
Headlight
Kidney basin
Ice water
Equipment
Nasal speculum, bayonet forceps
Topical anesthetics and vasoconstrictors
4 % plain lidocaine
Epinephrine 1:10,00 topical
Oxymetazoline
Cotton balls or neurosurgical 1×3 neurosurgical pledgets
Topical hemostatic agents
Silver nitrate, Gelfoam sheet, Surgical sheet
Vaseline impregnated gauze 0.5×72 in.
Nonabsorbable tamponade sponges
Anterior–posterior balloon packing device
Foley catheter 20 cc balloon

Table 16.3 Treatment of epistaxis (escalation of invasive techniques)

Level 1 (site-directed therapy)
Digital pressure and topic oxymetazoline
Topical hemostatic agents
Oxidized cellulose
Microfibrillar collagen
compressed gelatin
Electrocautery
Level 2
Nonabsorbable nasal packing
Polyvinyl acetal (PVA) sponge
Petrolatum gauze
Balloon packing
Level 3
Vascular control
Endoscopic sphenopalatine and/or anterior ethmoid artery ligation
Trans-antral sphenopalatine artery ligation
Ligation of anterior ethmoid artery (medial canthotomy)
External carotid artery ligation (extremely rare)
Trans-catheter angiography and embolization

nasal speculum, suction, personal protective equipment, topical vasoconstrictors, absorbable hemostatic material, and nonabsorbable packing or tamponade devices (Table 16.2).

Management Strategy

Control of nasal hemorrhage should proceed in a systematic fashion from these least to most invasive methods (Table 16.3). The provider should assure durable hemostasis and not discharge the patient until after a minimum of 2 h of observation and no further bleeding is identified. Persistent poor control of anterior bleeding, need for multiple packing, bleeding through packing, or bleeding posteriorly into the pharynx indicate inadequate hemostasis and are indications for anterior–posterior packing, vascular intervention, and likely transfer.

When the rural surgeon is called to assist in managing an individual with epistaxis it is likely that the patient will have failed previous attempts at hemostasis and the hemorrhage will have become severe. Initial assessment and management should include the basic life support algorithm of establishing a secure airway, maintaining unobstructed spontaneous breathing, and confirming appropriate intravascular volume to maintain adequate circulation. The past medical history should be obtained with attention to a history of illicit drug use, systemic anticoagulation or antiplatelet therapy, bleeding diathesis, current medications, and ischemic heart disease. The patients should be examined sitting upright and leaning forward to direct blood anteriorly away from the pharynx with digital pressure pinching the naris alternating sides. This maneuver will help elucidate the side of the bleeding and whether the bleeding is anterior or posterior. The severity of the hemorrhage should be approximated by reviewing the history of duration of bleeding, estimated blood loss present in suction canisters, towels etc., and clinical indications of hypoxemia such as hypotension, tachycardia, and reduced oxygen saturation. Intravenous access, fluid resuscitation, supplemental oxygen or rarely transfusion of blood or blood products may be acutely necessary. Based on the severity of the bleeding, the patient's comorbidities and hemodynamic status blood should be drawn for baseline hemoglobin and hematocrit levels, serum biochemistry studies, and type and cross match in the event of continued bleeding requiring transfusion of packed red blood cells, or platelets. Prothrombin time (PT), partial thromboplastin time (PTT), the internal normalized ratio (INR), and thromboelastogram (TEG) can also be obtained based on a history of the use of anticoagulation or antiplatelet medications or illicit substance abuse or an anticipated need to administer coagulation factors.

On rare occasions patients will present with uncontrolled severe epistaxis with blood literally pouring unabated from the nose and mouth. In this situation initial management is to place a Foley catheter into the nasopharynx, inflating the balloon with saline, placing gentle anterior traction on the catheter and seating the balloon in the nasopharynx by palpating the soft palate (Fig. 16.1). The surgeon can then proceed to bilateral anterior packing with vasoconstrictors as described below. Massive uncontrolled hemodynamically significant nasal bleeding, particular with oxygen desaturation or evidence of myocardial ischemia may require urgent orotracheal intubation to secure the airway and prevent continued aspiration of blood.

Once the initial resuscitation is complete the nasal cavity should be racked bilaterally with vasoconstrictor impregnated cotton balls or neurosurgical cotton pledgets. Packs are first placed along the nasal floor and layered superiorly. Effective topical vasoconstrictors include 0.5 % phenylephrine, epinephrine diluted 1:10,000, or 0.05 % oxymetazoline all of which can be mixed directly with 4 % plain (topical) lidocaine to achieve both intranasal hemostasis and anesthesia (Fig. 16.2). Historically, 4 % topical cocaine has been used to achieve intranasal hemostasis and anesthesia but it is more likely associated with hypertension, tachyarrhythmias, and agitation and has been replaced by these other agents.

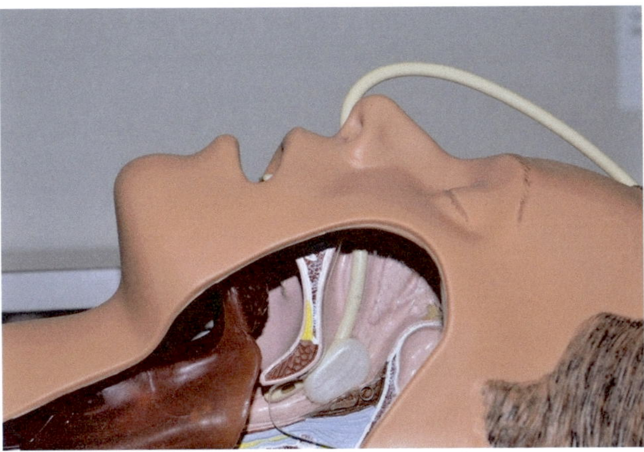

Fig. 16.1 Acute balloon tamponade of the posterior nasal cavity with Foley catheter

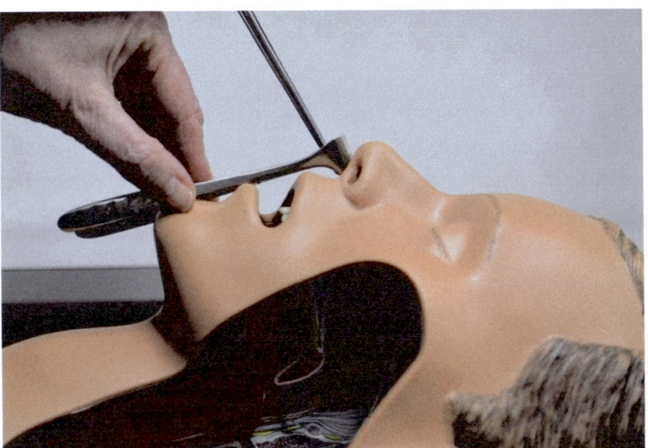

Fig. 16.2 Approach for instrumenting the anterior nose

With acute bleeding under control the lateral nasal wall and septum can be clearly inspected to identify potential bleeding sites. Headlight, nasal speculum, or an otoscope with the largest adult ear speculum, and suction will help clear blood from the nasal cavity and facilitate identification of the bleeding site(s). Optimum examination of the nasal cavity is performed with a 4 mm diameter 0° nasal endoscope.

Operative Techniques

Site-specific hemostasis can be performed with chemical or thermal cautery and supplemented with dissolvable hemostatic material. The nasal mucosal should be topically anesthetized as described above prior to any manipulation. Additional intranasal anesthesia can be accomplished anteriorly by injecting 1 % plain lidocaine into the lateral nasal wall anterior to the root of the middle turbinate. If more posterior anesthesia is needed a sphenopalatine nerve block is needed. This be performed by injecting 1 % plain lidocaine at the posterior aspect of the middle turbinate and directing it superiorly and laterally into the sphenopalatine foramen. If nasal bleeding precludes safe visualization of the lateral nasal wall, the sphenopalatine nerve can be anesthetized via an intraoral greater palatine nerve block. This is performed by first injecting lidocaine 1 % 1:100,000 with epinephrine into the mucosa of the hard palate 1 cm medial to the second molar tooth using a 25-gauge needle bent 60 % 2 cm from the tip. The needle is then advanced superiorly into the greater palatine canal and injecting 1.5–2 cc of local anesthetic resulting in anesthesia of the greater palatine and sphenopalatine nerves and subsequently the posterior lateral nasal wall.

Chemical cautery is most effective for localized bleeding from the nasal septum and is most commonly performed with commercially available 75 % silver nitrate – 25 % potassium nitrate applicators. While site-specific hemostasis is the ultimate objective, chemical cautery is challenging in the face of active bleeding. Therefore hemostasis can be achieved by first lightly cauterizing the mucosa circumferentially around the bleeding site, thereby reducing the severity of the active hemorrhage and allowing for eventual control of the principal bleeding site by direct contact. Care must be exercised in the use of the silver nitrate applicators. Excessive cautery of the anterior septum can lead to full thickness avascular necrosis of the septal cartilage and eventual perforation. Therefore, simultaneous bilateral silver nitrate cautery of the anterior nasal septum should not be performed. Undirected cautery of the septum and lateral nasal wall may lead to scar and synechiae formation. Finally, silver nitrate cautery leads to black staining of the nasal mucosa which can result in a permanent black tattoo.

Thermal cautery can be performed with disposable battery-powered cautery pens. It is more precise than chemical cautery in controlling epistaxis and can be used in the setting of active bleeding. With this technique suction is used to remove the active bleeding and facilitate identification of the bleeding source (Fig. 16.3). The cautery device is then activated and hemostasis is achieved. The use of an integrated suction cautery for posterior epistaxis is effective but requires a more specialized equipment and familiarity with intranasal anatomy.

Nasal packing can either be used as an adjunct to site directed hemostasis or as primary treatment of more sever epistaxis when site directed treatment cannot be performed. Nasal packing can either be nonabsorbable (balloons, tampons, or gauze strips), absorbable hemostatic material, or newer devices which are combinations of the previous two.

A wide variety if topical hemostatic products are available and are classified based on the mechanism of enhancing coagulation. An understanding of the nature of the intranasal hemorrhage and any potential underlying disorders of hemostasis due to either medications, hematologic diseases, or

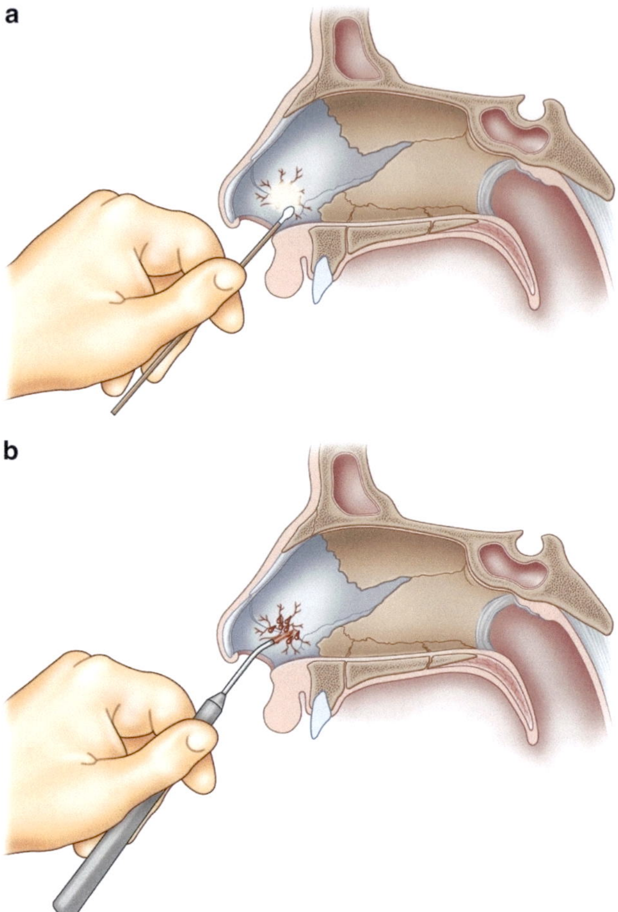

Fig. 16.3 Control of anterior epistaxis with either chemical (**a**) or electrocautery (**b**). From Eibling DE, Epistaxis in Operative Otolaryngology Head and Neck Surgery, First edition., Myers EN (ed) p 7., WB Saunders, Philadelphia

inborn errors of the coagulation cascade are important in determining the correct topical hemostatic agent to use. Mechanical hemostatic agents are matrices which provide a surface which facilitates platelet aggregation and promote a clot to form. The effectiveness of mechanical hemostatic agents is dependent on the patient having acceptable production and function of coagulation factors and normal platelet function. Examples of mechanical hemostatic agents are oxidized regenerated cellulose (Surgical, Oxycel), porcine gelatin sponge or foam (Gelfoam), bovine microfibrillar collagen (Avitene), and carboxymethyl cellulose. These are often used to enhance the efficacy of site directed intranasal hemostasis. Topical thrombin preparations are a form of active hemostatic agents which facilitate the conversion of fibrinogen to fibrin. Topical thrombin is available as either bovine, pooled human plasma, or recombinant thrombin and each carry risk of possible infection or allergic complications. These agents are rarely effective intranasally because they are washed away by active bleeding and are rarely used. A third type of absorbable

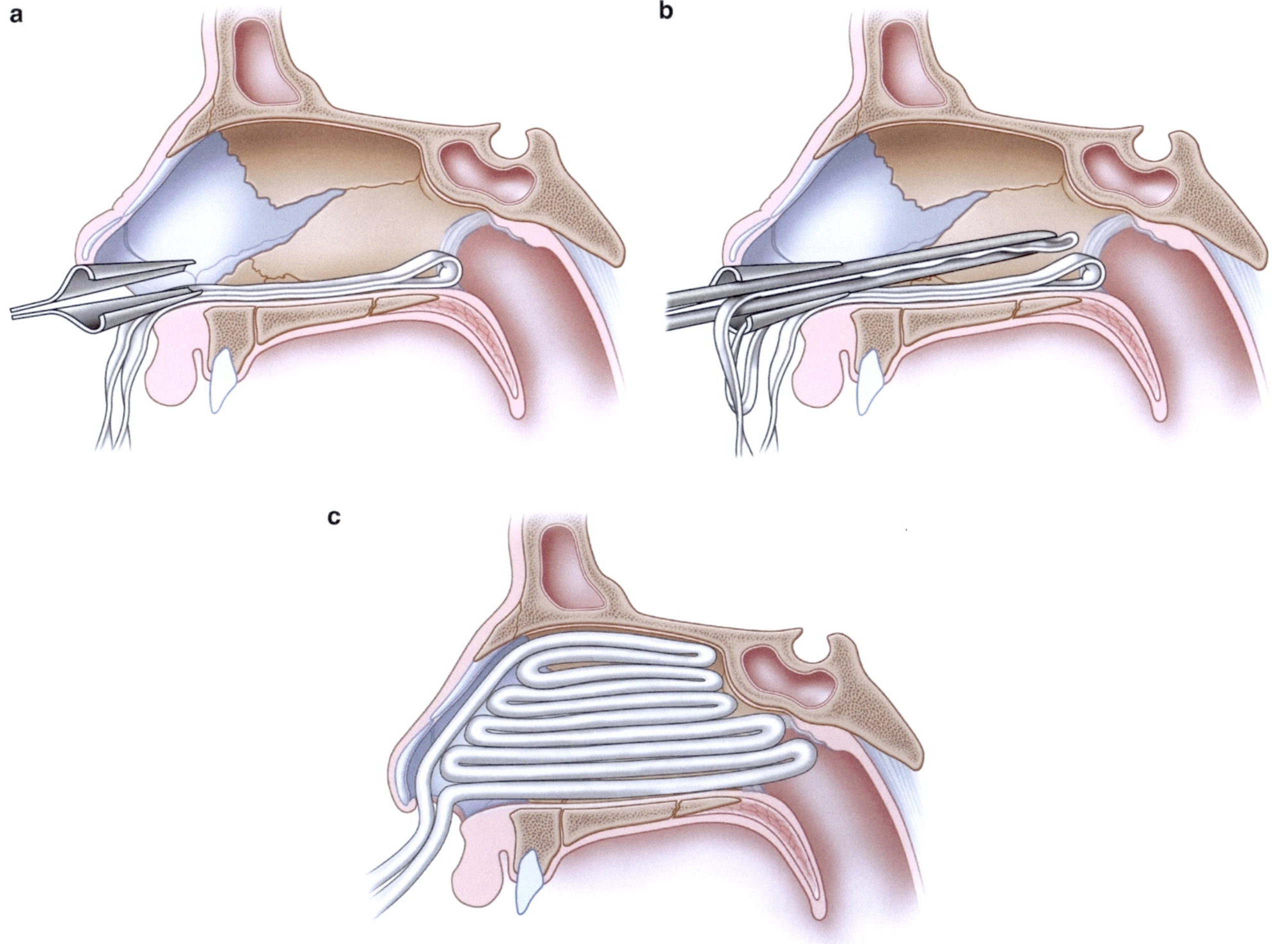

Fig. 16.4 Sequence of ribbon gauze nasal packing beginning on the floor of the nose and layering the packing superiorly until the nasal cavity is filled and the bleeding is controlled. (**a**) Anterior nasal packing with ribbon gauze begins by placing a loop of gauze along the floor of the nose. (**b**) Subsequent layers of ribbon gauze are placed in an inferior to superior fashion. The nasal speculum is used to stabilize the existing packing while additional gauze is layered superiorly. (**c**) Completed packing of the nasal cavity with antibiotic impregnated ribbon gauze extending from the nasal floor to the roof of the ethmoid

hemostatic material is the flowable compounds. These are hybrid products composed of either cross-linked bovine gelatin granules and pooled human thrombin (Flo-seal) or porcine gelatin granules used with either bovine, recombinant, or pooled human plasma thrombin. The common mechanism of these agents is that thrombin and gelatin work to mechanically reduce bleeding and facilitate conversion of fibrinogen to fibrin. These agents are effective in the management of nasal bleeding and are being used with increasing frequency. Other types of topical hemostatic agents or sealants used for other surgical procedures such as fibrin sealants, polyethylene-glycol (PEG) polymers, albumin–glutaraldehyde, and cyanoacrylate adhesives have little or no application in the management of epistaxis.

Traditionally, nasal nonabsorbable packing was performed with a 36 in. length of ½″ to ¾″ wide petroleum or antibiotic impregnated ribbon gauze. Using a bayonet forceps and nasal speculum the packing is inserted flat along the floor of the nose. Subsequent layers of packing are placed inferior to superior using the nasal speculum to hold the layered packing in place while additional gauze is introduced into the nasal cavity until the packing fills the superior nasal vault and hemostasis is achieved (Fig. 16.4). This method is poorly tolerated by patients and contributed to the development of a variety of highly pure, biocompatible, porous polyvinyl alcohol expandable foam intranasal tampons. These devices are produced by several companies and are available in a wide range of sizes and configurations. The benefits that these devices include are less trauma during insertion, they conform to the size of the nasal cavity, and are less likely to be colonized by *Staphylococcus aureus* or other nasal pathogens. Prior to insertion, the tampons are coated with a topical

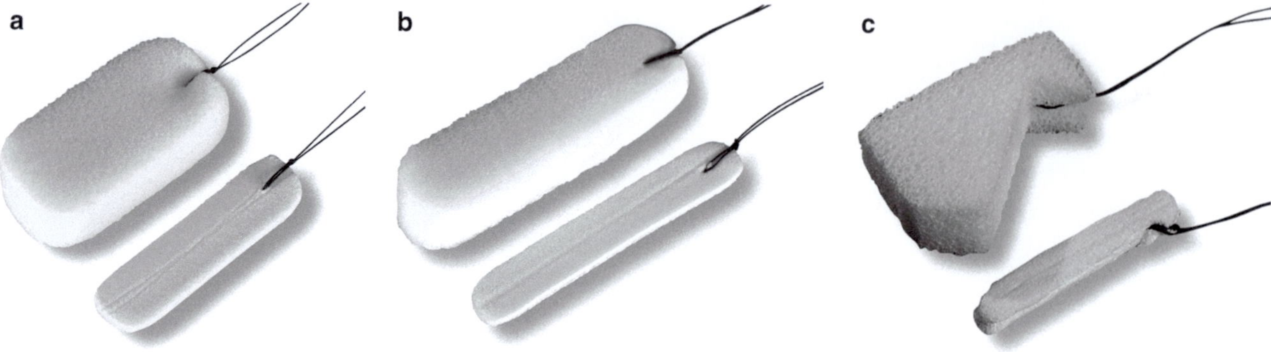

Fig. 16.5 Merocel intranasal tampons. Photos courtesy of Medtronic, Inc.®

antibiotic ointment (bacitracin or mupirocin) then placed into the nasal cavity along the floor of the nose. Ten milliliters of normal saline injected into the device expanding the tampon to fill the nasal cavity and tamponade the bleeding. Depending on the location of the hemorrhage (anterior or posterior) varying sizes and lengths of the devices are available to extend posteriorly into the nasopharynx if necessary (Fig. 16.5).

In cases of posterior epistaxis or if the expandable sponges are ineffective or unavailable, silicon balloon catheters can be used. These devices consist of two balloons a long broad anterior balloon and a smaller rounder posterior balloon with separate inflation ports. Like the expandable sponges, this device is placed along the floor of the nose until the anterior balloon is completely within the nasal cavity. The anterior balloon is the inflated and the oropharynx inspected for continued posterior bleeding. If posterior bleeding persists then the posterior balloon is inflated to tamponade the sphenopalatine artery (Fig. 16.6).

Recently a hybrid device has been developed which leverages the tamponade pressure generated by a nonabsorbable balloon with an absorbable hemostatic agent. The Rapid Rhino Epistaxis Device (ArthroCare Corporation, Austin, TX) is composed of a balloon catheter covered by a hydrophilic absorbable carboxymethylcellulose fabric designed to promote platelet aggregation and facilitate hemostasis. Application of this device begins by hydrating the carboxymethylcellulose fabric thus converting it to a gel which provides a more acceptable insertion and removal without compromising hemostasis. The device is passed into the nasal cavity along the nasal floor and the balloon is inflated with air and pilot balloon is included to prevent over inflation (Fig. 16.7).

Anterior–Posterior Packing

In the face of profuse nasal hemorrhage a formal anterior–posterior packing may be necessary to achieve hemostasis. Historically posterior nasal (nasopharyngeal) packs were constructed from gauze or large tonsillectomy sponges

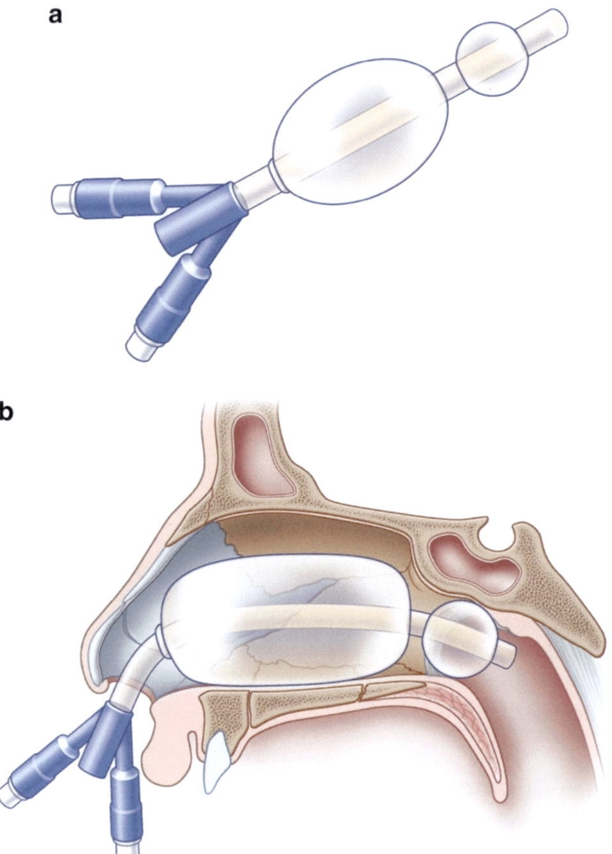

Fig. 16.6 Balloon epistaxis catheters. (**a**) Commercially available double-balloon epistaxis catheters for severe anterior or anterior–posterior epistaxis. (**b**) Schematic representation of correct placement of catheter in the nasal cavity

attached to umbilical tapes or heave silk sutures placed into the nasopharynx through the mouth. The entire nasal cavity was then packed with ribbon gauze against the posterior pack which was secured anteriorly with a clamp or rolled gauze bolster. Currently, we use a Foley catheter with a 10 cc balloon filled with saline secured over the anterior pack with an umbilical clamp (Fig. 16.8).

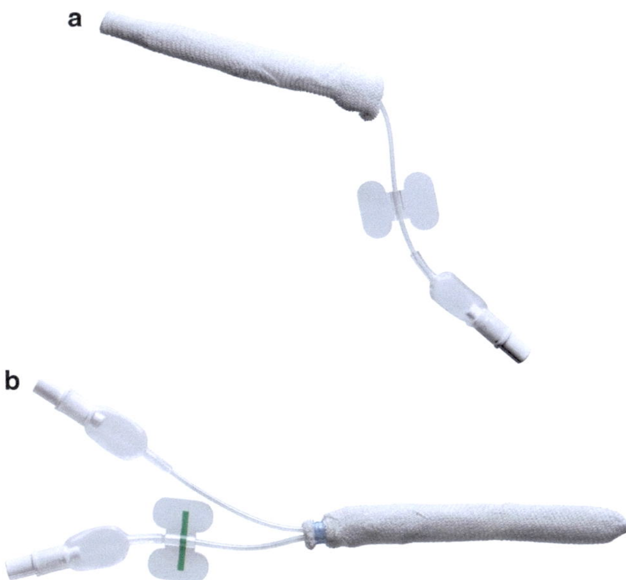

Fig. 16.7 Rapid Rhino devices. (**a**) Rapid Rhino® 751 Epistaxis Device—single-balloon anterior pack, and (**b**) Rapid Rhino® 900 Epistaxis Device—double-balloon anterior–posterior pack. Rapid Rhino® is a registered trademark of ArthroCare, Corp.

Following the placement of any type of nasal packing the oropharynx should be carefully examined to insure there is satisfactory hemostasis and there is no blood draining posteriorly. Patients should be observed in the emergency department for 2 h to insure hemostasis prior to discharge. Nonabsorbable nasal packing should remain in place for at least 24 h. Patients treated with small amounts of dissolvable packing or unilateral anterior nonabsorbable anterior nasal packing can be discharged home with otolaryngology follow-up. Patients with posterior or anterior–posterior nasal packing should be admitted to the hospital, administered humidified supplemental oxygen, and monitored with pulse oximetry due to the propensity to develop hypoxemia, exacerbation of underlying sleep apnea, and cardiac arrhythmias. Other complications from posterior packing are listed below in the Common Complications section.

The open surgical management of intractable epistaxis evolved from external carotid artery ligation to serial ligation of external carotid artery branches to ligation of the internal maxillary artery posterior to the maxillary sinus (trans-antral internal maxillary artery ligation) to the current practice of

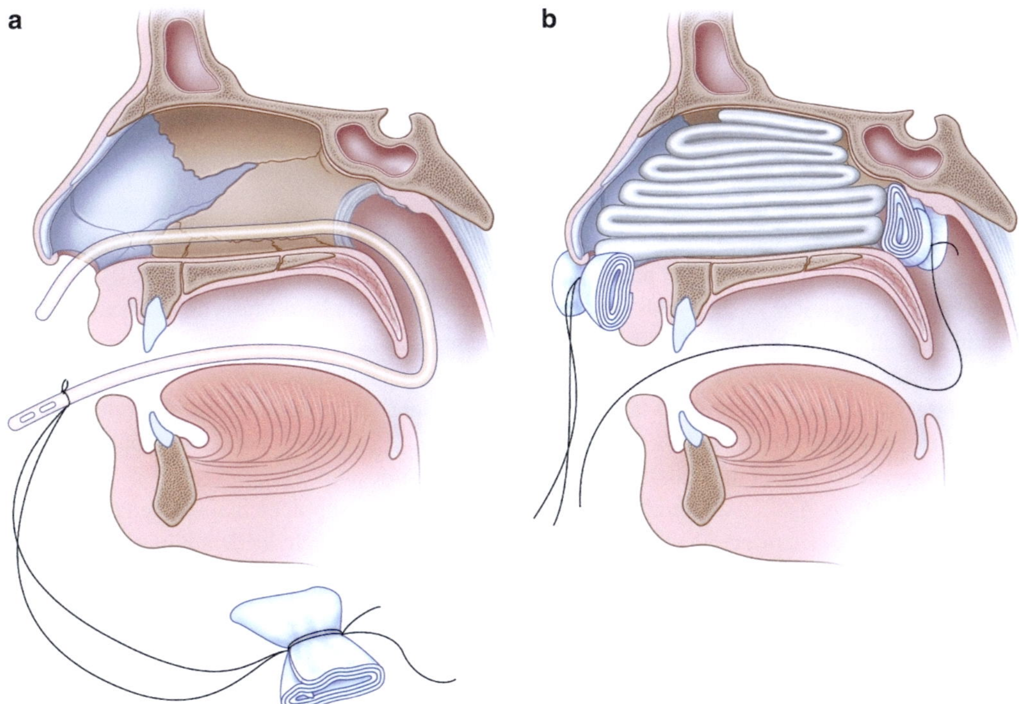

Fig. 16.8 Placement of the anterior–posterior nasal packing. (**a**) A flexible catheter is placed through the nose and nasopharynx, brought out through the mouth. A gauze roll or tonsil sponge is secured to the catheter and as the catheter is withdrawn, the gauze is seated into the nasopharynx. (**b**) The gauze roll is manually seated in the nasopharynx to serve as a buttress for layered gauze packing placed anteriorly to control bleeding

selective endoscopic (trans-nasal) sphenopalatine ligation or trans-femoral catheter embolization of the sphenopalatine artery. Ligation of the external carotid artery or its branches is infective due the multiple anastomoses between the branches of the external carotid artery and the potential for internal–external carotid anastomoses as well. Due to the lack of efficacy at managing the collateral circulation and the potential for vagus and hypoglossal nerve injuries this practice has largely been abandoned. Direct ligation of the internal maxillary artery through the maxillary sinus is effective but can be complicated by permanent or temporary numbness of the ipsilateral face, palate, and upper gum. Additional complications of palatal necrosis, oroantral fistula, and nasolacrimal duct injury have also been reported. Trans-femoral selective arteriography embolization of the sphenopalatine artery has been shown to be effective but requires endovascular expertise and specialized equipment. Several recent comparative studies have demonstrated that is cases of sever posterior epistaxis endoscopic trans-nasal sphenopalatine artery ligation or cautery is safer, more effective, and results in a significant cost saving compared to endovascular techniques.

Endoscopic sphenopalatine artery ligation or cautery is performed under general anesthesia using a 4 mm 30° rigid endoscope. After the induction of anesthesia previously placed nasal packs are removed and replaced with cotton pledgets soaked in 0.05 % oxymetazoline. A generous middle meatus antrostomy is needed to perform the procedure therefore the surgeon should be prepared to perform a nasal septoplasty, anterior ethmoidectomy, resection of the uncinate process or a portion of the middle turbinate as needed to obtain clear visualization. The middle meatus antrostomy should be extended inferiorly to the lateral attachment of the inferior turbinate, superiorly to 5 mm below the plane of the orbital floor and posteriorly until it is flushed with the posterior wall of the maxillary antrum. The mucosa is then gently elevated from the posterior aspect of the lateral nasal wall and the sphenopalatine artery is identified as it exists in the foramen just inferior to the posterior attachment of the middle turbinate at the supero-medial corner of the maxillary sinus.

The sphenopalatine artery is dissected laterally into the pterygomaxillary space to provide correct identification and allow for satisfactory clip placement. A 1–2 mm Kerrison rongeur is used to precisely remove the bone overlying the artery and expose it laterally. The artery is then gently circumferentially mobilized with a blunt hook or other atraumatic dissector and stabilized while clips or bipolar ere are applied to ligate the vessel (Fig. 16.9a–e). Five milliters of dissolvable flowable nasal packing can be placed on the artery. If a septoplasty was performed or other mucosal disruptions occurred silastic nasal splints are needed to prevent synechiae between the septum and lateral nasal wall. Coughing and straining on extubation are to be avoided and the patients can be discharged within 24 h.

The anterior ethmoid artery is fortunately a much less common source of intractable nasal bleeding and is more frequently associated with surgical or other traumatic injury to the upper craniofacial skeleton. The anterior ethmoid artery arises from the ophthalmic branch of the internal carotid artery. Endovascular manipulation of the ophthalmic artery risks thrombotic complications and blindness and is therefore contraindicated in all but the most usual settings. Open or endoscopic ligation of the anterior ethmoid arteries has been described but only by experienced sinus, head and neck, and orbital surgeons and is beyond the scope of this chapter.

Potential Pitfalls

Underestimating the hemodynamic consequences of prolonged nasal bleeding

Failing to obtain baseline laboratory studies, particularly in elderly patients with serious comorbidities

Not carefully examining the posterior oropharynx and missing posterior nasalhemorrhage

Neglecting screening neurological and cranial nerve examinations and failing to order imaging studies on patients with traumatic epistaxis and missing an intracranial injury

Premature discharge of patients without observation to assure satisfactory hemostasis

Discharging patients with anterior-posterior nasal packing

Failing to stress the need for otolaryngology follow-up

Postoperative Care

Insure complete hemostasis and effectiveness of packing

Administer prophylactic antibiotics to patients with nonabsorbable nasal packing

For patients requiring anterior–posterior nasal packing
    Admit patients for continuous pulse oximetry and EKG monitoring
    Administer supplemental oxygen by face mask
    Administer prophylactic antibiotics
    Obtain otolaryngology and other consultations as needed

Common Complications

Failure to obtain hemostasis from initial site directed cautery

Failure to obtain hemostasis from poorly placed nasal packs or dressings

Nasal septal perforation from overaggressive or bilateral chemical or thermal cautery of the mucosal overlying the cartilaginous nasal septum anteriorly

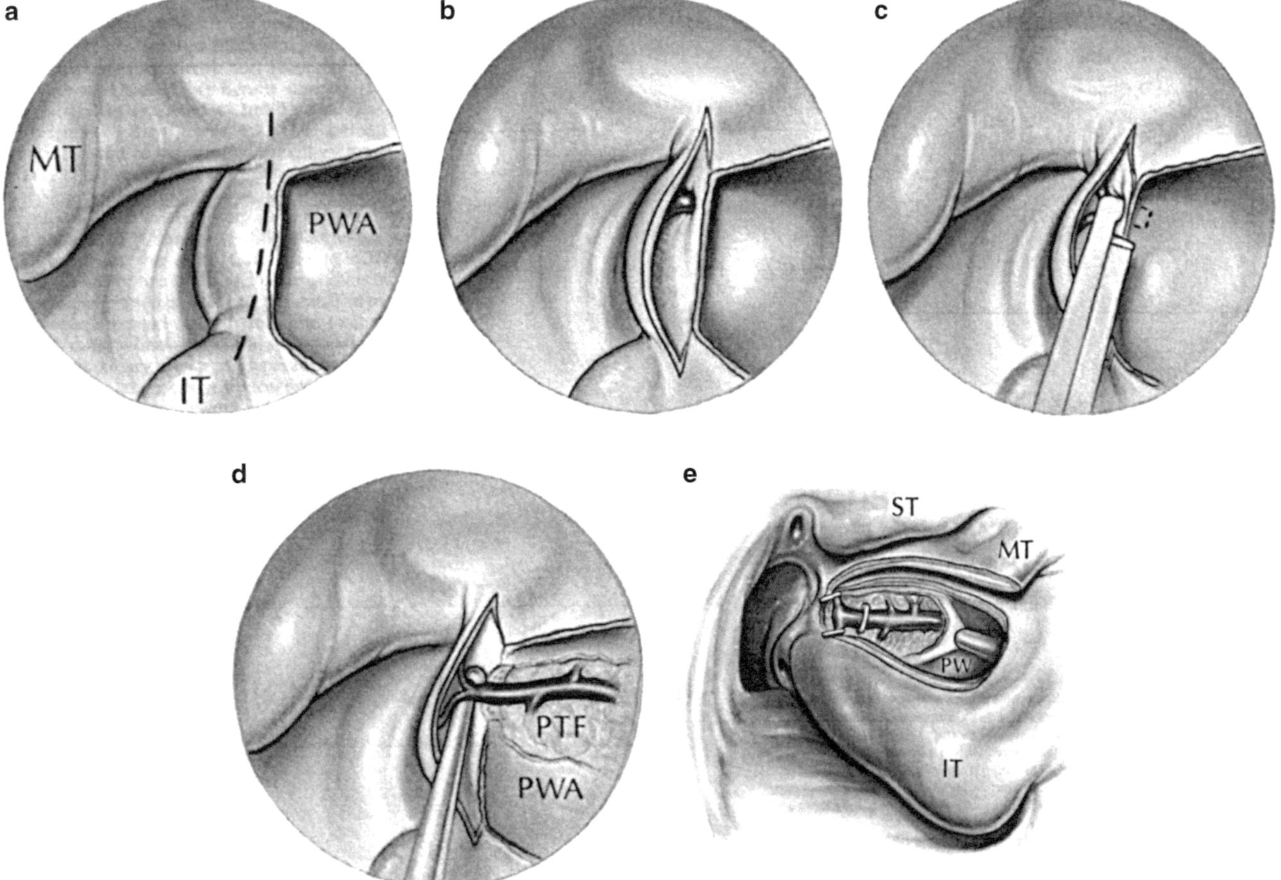

Fig. 16.9 Endoscopic sphenopalatine artery ligation. (**a**) Creation of wide middle meatus antrostomy, the area of submucosal elevation identified by *dotted line*. (**b**) Identification of sphenopalatine artery at the superior medial aspect of the antrostomy. (**c**) A 1 mm rongeur engages the medial aspect of the sphenopalatine foramen and precisely removes the overlying bone in a medial to lateral direction. (**d**) Mobilization of the sphenopalatine artery laterally into the pterygopalatine fossa fossa. (**e**) Clip placement on the sphenopalatine artery and the distal branches. *Abbreviations*: *IT* inferior turbinate, *MT* middle turbinate, *PTF* pterygopalatine fossa, *PWA* posterior wall of maxillary antrum, *ST* superior turbinate. From Snyderman CH, Carrau RL, Endoscopic ligation of the sphenopalatine artery for epistaxis, Operative Tech in Otolaryngol-Head Neck Surg 8 (1997:85–89)

Intranasal synechia and scarring from excessive mucosal trauma

Hypoxemia and oxygen desaturation from bilateral anterior nasal or anterior–posterior nasal packing.

Necrosis of the nasal skin from overinflated packing

Posterior or anterior–posterior packing can result in:

   Hypoxemia and/or exacerbation of sleep apnea and secondary cardiac arrhythmia

   Necrosis of the nasal skin, philtrum, nasal ala, and palate

   Displacement and aspiration of the packing with airway obstruction

   Post-obstructive sinusitis and toxic shock syndrome from colonization with *Staphylococcus aureus* and endotoxin production

When to Transfer

Indications for transfer of patients with epistaxis are directly related to the availability of otolaryngology support for definitive management at the primary facility. As a general principle patients with anterior epistaxis in whom the bleeding has been successfully controlled should be observed for 2 h or so to confirm satisfactory hemostasis and then discharged. Patients with unilateral anterior epistaxis that have been controlled using intranasal vasoconstriction with topical oxymetazoline, digital pressure, and local chemical or thermal cautery can be discharged with otolaryngology follow-up as needed. Patients with anterior epistaxis controlled with unilateral nasal packing can also be discharged, however, otolaryngology follow-up should be arranged to remove the nasal packing and perform office nasal endoscopy. Patients with craniofacial trauma and sever epistaxis should be imaged with contrast CT and/or CT angiography and transferred to an appropriate trauma facility. Any patient suspected to have an intranasal mass should have a prompt evaluation by an otolaryngologist – head and neck surgeon. Patients with anterior–posterior nasal pack should be admitted to the hospital for airway monitoring. Finally, we should stress that the major causes of morbidity and mortality in patients with non-traumatic epistaxis are in elderly individuals and are related to exacerbations of underlying comorbidities exacerbated either by the bleeding itself (hypotension, shock, tissue ischemia) or the interventions (packing, anesthesia, embolization, imaging contrast load, transfusion, etc.) needed to control the bleeding.

Suggested Reading

Barnes ML, Spielmann PM, White PS. Epistaxis: a contemporary evidence based approach. Otolaryngol Clin North Am. 2012;45:1005–17.

Cullen MM, Tami TA. Comparison of internal maxillary artery ligation versus embolization for refractory posterior epistaxis. J Otolaryngol Head Neck Surg. 1998;118(5):636–42.

Dedhia RC, Desai SS, Smith KJ, Lee S, Schaitkin BM, Snyderman CH, et al. Cost-effectiveness of endoscopic sphenopalatine artery ligation versus nasal packing as first-line treatment for posterior epistaxis. Int Forum Allergy Rhinol. 2013;3(7):563–6.

Eibling DE. Epistaxis. In: Myers EN, editor. Operative otolaryngology—head and neck surgery. Philadelphia: WB Saunders Co; 1997. p. 2–20.

Douglas R, Wormald P-J. Update on epistaxis. Curr Opin Otolaryngol Head Neck Surg. 2007;15:180–3.

Goddard JC, Reiter ER. Inpatient management of epistaxis: outcomes and cost. Otolaryngol Head Neck Surg. 2005;132(5):707–12.

Kasperek ZA, Pollock GF. Epistaxis: an overview. Emerg Med Clin North Am. 2013;31:443–54.

Loughran S, Hilmi O, McGarry GW. Endoscopic sphenopalatine artery ligation—when, why and how to do it. An on-line video tutorial. Clin Otolaryngol. 2005;30:539–43.

Nikoyan L, Matthews S. Epistaxis and hemostatic devices. Oral Maxillofac Surg Clin North Am. 2012;24:219–28.

Pallin DJ, Chng Y-M, McKay MP, Emond JA, Pelletier AJ, Camargo Jr CA. Epidemiology of epistaxis in US emergency departments, 1992 to 2001. Ann Emerg Med. 2005;46(1):77–81.

Shargorodsky J, Bleier BS, Holbrook EH, Cohen JM, Busuba N, Metson R, et al. Outcomes analysis in epistaxis management: development of a therapeutic algorithm. J Otolaryngol Head Neck Surg. 2013;149(3):390–8.

Singer AJ, Blanda M, Cronin K, LoGiudice-Khwaja M, Gulla J, Bradshaw J, et al. Comparison of nasal tampons for the treatment of epistaxis in the emergency department: a randomized controlled trial. J Ann Emerg Med. 2005;45(2):134–9.

Snyderman CH, Carrau RL. Endoscopic ligation of the sphenopalatine artery for epistaxis. Operat Tech Otolaryngol Head Neck Surg. 1997;8(2):85–9.

Speilmann PM, Barnes ML, White PS. Controversies in the specialist management of adult epistaxis: an evidence-based review. Clin Otolaryngol. 2012;37:382–9.

Villwock JA, Jones K. Recent trends in epistaxis management in the United States 2008-2010. JAMA Otolaryngol Head Neck Surg. 2013;6. http://www.jamaotolaryngology.com. Accessed 10 Aug 2013.

Von Buchwald C, Tranum-Jensen J. Endoscopic sphenopalatine artery ligation or diathermy. Operat Tech Otolaryngol. 2006;17(1):28–30.

Willems PWA, Farb RI, Agid R. Endovascular treatment of epistaxis. AJNR Am J Neuroradiol. 2009;30:1637–45.

Thyroid Surgery

David R. Schmidt and Wallace F. Martin

Introduction

Surgeons have performed thyroid surgery safely since the changes developed and instituted by Theodore Kocher in the late nineteenth century for which he was awarded the Nobel Prize in 1909. Thyroid diseases can be treated with minimal risk of complication by experienced high volume surgeons as well as the excellent and careful rural surgeon who may not perform as many thyroidectomies in their practice. Understanding the indications of the procedure; knowing the anatomy of the thyroid gland, recurrent laryngeal and superior laryngeal nerve and parathyroid glands; performing the procedure meticulously; and avoiding the complications can lead to a successful outcome in these sometimes challenging patients.

Indications

Thyroid surgery is indicated for the treatment of thyroid diseases that can be classified into malignant disease, thyroid nodular disease including symptomatic or increased risk of cancer development, or hyperthyroid disease states. The clearest indication is for thyroid malignancy that has been determined with preoperative fine needle aspiration. Papillary cancer can often be diagnosed on FNA, but follicular carcinoma commonly requires removal of the nodule with histological determination of capsule invasion for follicular cancer to be diagnosed. Hurthle cells can also be seen, which are a type of follicular cells with an increased risk of malignancy. Thyroid nodules can also be classified as atypical or indeterminate on the cytological evaluation of the FNA specimen with surgery being a viable plan of care as well as

D.R. Schmidt, M.D., F.A.C.S. (✉) • W.F. Martin, M.D., F.A.C.S.
General Surgery, Gwinnett Surgical Associates,
Lawrenceville, GA 30046, USA
e-mail: schmidt31@comcast.net

observation or repeat biopsy. Nodules which have increased in size, are larger than 4 cm, are "cold" on nuclear scan, or occur in patients with a strong family history or exposure to radiation all have an increased risk of developing malignancy. A complex cyst may be indicative of a degenerating tumor and does not convey the sense of benign disease seen with other cysts seen throughout the body. Thyroidectomy is indicated if a large cyst recurs or persists after aspiration. In addition to malignant or potentially malignant disease, thyroidectomy may be indicated in patients with symptomatic thyroid enlargement becoming symptomatic goiters as they interfere with swallowing and eventually airway obstruction. A toxic thyroid adenoma is a clear indication for thyroid lobectomy with an excellent cure rate of these patients' hyperthyroidism. Thyroidectomy, thyroid medications, and/or I 131 therapy can treat Graves disease or hyperthyroidism. Near total or total thyroidectomy provides an excellent cure rate, avoids the risk associated with radioactive iodine therapy, achieves its result quickly immediately after surgery, and avoids the risk of malignancy developing in a nodule exposed to radioactive therapy in the future.

Operative Technique

Patient is placed under a general anesthetic and in the semi-fowler (beach chair) position with the neck extended gently. A standard Kocher incision is made approximately 2 fingerbreadths above the sternal notch in or along the direction of a skin crease. The thin platysma muscle is divided in the same direction as the skin incision. Subplatysmal flaps are then raised with electrocautery in the avascular plane below the muscle while elevating the muscle with several Allis clamps. The dissection is carried superior to the thyroid cartilage and inferiorly to the sternal notch. The next layer, the investing fascia of the strap muscles, is opened in the midline from sternal notch to thyroid cartilage staying between the muscles and blood vessels and above and on top of the thyroid isthmus. Next the strap muscles are freed from the thyroid gland in another avascular plane. As this plane is developed, the strap muscles are elevated and retracted laterally exposing the surface of the thyroid gland. The middle thyroid vein is then divided as the gland is rotated medially between right angle clamps and ligated with silk suture. As the strap muscles are retracted laterally with retractors, the gland is mobilized medially after division of the middle thyroid vein. The superior pole is then dissected free with a right angle clamp and divided between 2- silk suture ties or right angles. This can be a potential site of bleeding postoperatively and secure ligation is imperative. A newer technique using a harmonic scalpel or blood vessel coagulating device can be used, but we prefer to at least ligate the superior thyroid artery to prevent bleeding. Above the superior aspect of the gland lies the external branch of the superior laryngeal nerve, which should be looked for to prevent injury during the superior dissection and take down of the superior pole. After take down of the superior pole the gland is rotated medially and inferiorly. The recurrent laryngeal nerve is next identified in the tracheal esophageal groove. The gold standard is to identify the nerve and trace it up to the thyroid cartilage as the thyroid gland is dissected away. The nerve is identified with blunt dissection and classically has a blood vessel traveling along its superior surface, the so-called racing stripe. The use of a nerve monitor may assist in identifying the nerve but it has not replaced the visualization of the nerve as a means to prevent injury. We do not routinely use a nerve monitor, having found that it is not needed to locate the nerve in our cases and requires some experience and training for the monitoring device and endotracheal tube to become useful. After careful dissection of the gland away from the nerve, identification of the superior and inferior parathyroid glands is necessary. The superior glands are commonly located along the back and side of the gland superior to the nerve. The inferior glands are more variable and often found within a centimeter of the recurrent laryngeal nerve. They are identified by their characteristic brown pigmentation and are small with a tenuous blood supply, which needs to be preserved and handled delicately. Multiple branches of the inferior thyroid artery are divided as they enter the gland. Commonly we dissect the gland away from the recurrent laryngeal nerve and divide the vessels as they enter along the inferior aspect of the gland. As the gland is mobilized away from the nerve, it is retracted medially and superiorly and off of the trachea as Berry's ligament is divided. The pyramidal lobe extends superiorly above the isthmus and is removed with the gland. The isthmus may be divided and the lobe removed. In a total thyroidectomy we often leave the isthmus intact and place the gland on top of the skin as we operate on the opposite lobe. A total thyroidectomy should remove the entire gland. A near total thyroidectomy may leave a small portion of the gland near the nerve and parathyroid glands to lessen the likelihood of injury. A subtotal thyroidectomy can leave a rim of normal thyroid tissue along the trachea and near the recurrent laryngeal nerve. Although leaving a moderate amount of tissue may decrease the likelihood of the need for thyroid replacement, this needs to be weighed against the chance of enlargement and growth in the future resulting in recurrent hyperthyroidism in patients with Graves disease. As the thyroid gland can be vascular, especially in the Graves disease patient, care is taken to carefully dissect the gland without entering its capsule with the result of brisk bleeding. When performing a subtotal procedure, we will over sew the remaining parenchyma prior to division with interrupted 3-0 silk sutures. After completion of the resection, the neck is irrigated and inspected carefully for hemostasis with any bleeding sites suture ligated to prevent a postoperative bleed or hematoma. We do not use drains even in enormous gland resections, and drains should not be relied upon to prevent a postoperative hematoma if hemostasis is not adequate. Rarely will we use Surgicel if oozing occurs, but will not close the neck if any bleeding or oozing is seen. The neck is then closed with interrupted 3-0 silk sutures in the investing fascia, which was opened in the midline. The platysma muscle is reapproximated with interrupted 3-0 Vicryl sutures. The skin is closed with a running 4-0 Vicryl subcuticular suture. The scrub nurse maintains her sterile instruments and field until the patient is extubated and the airway is proven to be adequate. A bilateral recurrent laryngeal nerve injury will leave the vocal cords paralyzed rendering the airway inadequate requiring an emergency tracheostomy. A rapidly developing hematoma may obstruct the airway and require immediate evacuation to relieve an airway obstruction. We do not routinely have the anesthesiologist examine the cords on extubation. We have a sterile trach tray accompany the patient in the recovery room and surgical floor as a postop hematoma bleed can obstruct the airway rapidly.

Potential Pitfalls

The performance of a thyroidectomy relies on a thorough understanding of the anatomy, a delicate and meticulous technique, and is best performed in the hands of an experienced surgeon performing several thyroidectomies a month. The potential pitfalls of this procedure are related to injury to the recurrent laryngeal nerve, external branch of the superior laryngeal nerve, and removal of or damage to the parathyroid glands. Care must be taken in mobilizing and dividing the superior thyroid artery as losing control of this vessel can lead to intraoperative difficulties as well as a postoperative hematoma. The proper visualization and identification of the recurrent laryngeal nerve must be established to avoid a traction injury with resultant voice loss and a dreaded bilateral nerve injury resulting in airway obstruction and a tracheostomy. The parathyroid glands are small, variable in location, and may be intimately related and attached to the thyroid gland and a careful search for these small brown-pigmented glands is necessary to avoid postoperative hypocalcemia.

Postoperative Care

Patients are usually monitored in the PACU and short stay hospital beds for airway management. A postoperative hematoma can develop rapidly and cause airway obstruction acutely. We have a trach tray at the bedside while the patient is in the hospital. Pain is controlled with po or IV narcotics, and swallowing can be uncomfortable but patients are usually able to tolerate a normal soft diet. Patients can be monitored for postoperative hypocalcemia either clinically or with calcium levels. Our practice is to have a serum calcium level drawn the afternoon of surgery and in the following morning. Thyroid hormone replacement is usually begun as an outpatient. Our patients are routinely discharged on an oral pain medication, thyroid replacement hormone (usually synthroid 0.125 μg), and oral calcium supplements. Our preference is to have patients remain for a 24-h observation stay, but routine lobectomies in a reliable patient with strong family support have been discharged the same afternoon in selected cases.

Common Complications

Complications are unusual in thyroid surgery and the three complications unique to thyroid surgery include recurrent laryngeal nerve injury, postoperative hypocalcemia, and postoperative neck hematoma. The most severe would be a recurrent laryngeal nerve injury. Most are thought to be a traction injury where the nerve does not function after being stretched or manipulated during the performance of the thyroidectomy. The nerve must be identified and handled with meticulous dissection and extreme care. Avoidance of the use of electrocautery and thermal spread from ligation devices in the area near the nerve is advised to prevent a thermal injury to the nerve. Mild postoperative hypocalcemia can be asymptomatic and easily tolerated by the patient, but more severe hypocalcaemia can become symptomatic and dangerous if left untreated. Initial symptoms include paresthesias around the mouth and lips and of the hands and feet. Chvotek's sign should be checked for by tapping the facial nerve in front of the ear, which if positive elicits a twitching of the mouth or eyes. Trousseau's sign occurs when carpel spasm is elicited when the blood pressure cuff is inflated. Hypocalcemia is usually treated with oral calcium carbonate, but may require rocalcitol in increasing doses to assist in calcium absorption. In severe hypocalcemia (symptomatic patients with calcium levels less than 7.5) a calcium drip may be required. Patients with persistent hypocalcemia should also have their magne-

sium levels checked as hypomagnesaemia may make their hypocalcemia refractory to treatment. A postoperative hematoma can expand rapidly and lead to stridor and airway compromise. A relatively small amount of bleeding into the operative space and neck can lead to a feeling of fullness and pressure. If bleeding continues it can compress the trachea and the airway can be lost suddenly. Bleeding can occur from the superior laryngeal artery or a branch of the inferior thyroid arteries and care should be taken when ligating these structures. The development of stridor or the inability to phonate indicates airway loss is imminent and treatment must be rendered immediately. The opening of the wound and subcutaneous layer through the investing fascia is required to alleviate the obstruction. This can be performed in the control surroundings of the operating room with anesthesia involved, but if airway loss is imminent or occurring, this can and must be performed at the bedside. The best treatment is prevention and therefore ligation of these vessels should be performed with care and skill, and the neck should not be closed until pristine hemostasis is achieved. The development of hypothyroidism after total thyroidectomy is not considered a complication, but is the result of surgery. Patients should be advised preoperatively that there might be a need for lifelong thyroid hormone replacements after their surgery. There is also the possibility of further surgery if a malignancy is identified in the final pathology of a patient who underwent a thyroid lobectomy. Thyroid storm is a rare and potentially life-threatening complication that may be precipitated by the stress of surgery, anesthesia, and the manipulation of the hyperthyroid gland during thyroidectomy. It is of extreme importance that we render our hyperthyroid patients as close to euthyroid as possible with antithyroid drugs prior to surgery.

When to Transfer

Studies indicate that the outcomes of patients undergoing thyroid surgery are improved when performed by well-trained, experienced, and high volume surgeons. Data from one study showed that complications were less when performed by a surgeon completing more than 30 cases a year than someone performing fewer. Surgeons operating on more than 100 patients a year were even better regarding outcomes and complication rates. The decision to transfer a patient would be best done prior to performing a surgery that could lead to a devastating complication. Patients who may be transferred to a high volume experienced surgeon include patients who have had a previous thyroid procedure, or have a massively enlarged gland causing tracheal deviation or narrowing, or have a large substernal goiter. Patients with a large cancer with extensive lymph node involvement or possible tracheal involvement would also require extensive surgery that would best be performed in experienced hands.

Suggested Reading

Richmond BK, Eads K, Flaherty S, Belcher M, Runyon D. Complications of thyroidectomy and parathyroidectomy in the rural community hospital setting. Am Surg. 2007;73(4):332–6.

Sosa JA, Bowman HM, Tielsch JM, Powe NR, Gordon TA, Udelsman R. The importance of surgeon experience for clinical and economic outcomes from thyroidectomy. Ann Surg. 1998;228: 320–30.

Edwin Kaplan, MD. Surgery of the thyroid gland. In: Thyroid disease manager. Department of Surgery, The University of Chicago, Chicago, IL.

Cooper DS, Doherty GM, Hangen BR, et al. Revised American Thyroid Association management guidelines for patients with thyroid nodules and differentiated thyroid cancer. Thyroid. 2009;19: 1167–214.

Parathyroidectomy

William F. Nowlin

Developments in Laboratory Diagnosis

The development of the immunoassay for the measurement of parathyroid hormone and other peptides by Berson and Yalow in 1936 was a seminal discovery that earned them the Nobel Prize. The introduction of the serum chemical autoanalyzer improved serum calcium determinations and a better understanding of calcium diseases. This dramatically increased the number of patients diagnosed with primary hyperparathyroidism [1].

Signs and symptoms of hyperparathyroidism have changed dramatically in recent years largely due to the introduction of serum channel autoanalyzers. Precipitous increase in the number of cases that are asymptomatic, asignomatic, or both occurred with parallel reduction in kidney stones and bone disease.

The current recommendation of the National Institutes of Health Consensus Development Conference for surgical intervention in patients with asymptomatic primary hyperthyroidism is as follows: (1) markedly elevated serum calcium (greater than 1 mg/dL above normal); (2) history of episode of life-threatening hypercalcium; (3) reduced creatinine clearance; (4) presence of one or more kidney stones detected by abdominal radiography; (5) markedly elevated 24-h urinary calcium excretion; and (6) substantially reduced bone mass as determined by direct measurement (dual energy X-ray absorptiometry 5-score less than 2.5).

Even though a National Institutes of Health (NIH) consensus conference was conducted and another workshop was held in 2002 on the management of asymptomatic primary HPT, there is still no consensus among endocrinologists and endocrine surgeons about whether to administer nonoperative medical therapy and monitor patients or to refer them for early parathyroidectomy.

W.F. Nowlin, M.D., F.A.S.C.R.S. (✉)
Porter Regional Hospital, Valparaiso, ID 46383, USA
e-mail: nowlinp@aol.com

History

At the Annual Churchill Lecture of the American College of Surgeons in April of 1998, Dr. Claude H. Organ described the history of parathyroid surgery [2]. This was presented at the American College of Surgeons Spring meeting in Baltimore, Maryland. He described the history of parathyroid surgery as parallel to the development of modern surgery in both Europe and the United States.

The ravages of hyperparathyroidism are all too well known including renal manifestations, bony manifestations, gastrointestinal complaints, and depression.

The pitfalls of the loss of parathyroid glands were well documented by the world's leading surgeon, William Halsted. "It seems hardly creditable that the loss of bodies so tiny as the parathyroid should be followed by a result so disastrous." Jacob Erdheim from the University of Vienna was the first to associate bone disease with parathyroid glands. Professor Frederick von Recklinghausen, of Strausburg, described seven patients with bone disease and at least one had osteitis fibrosis cystica. Issac Y. Olch, MD, an attending surgeon at Barnes Hospital performed the first successful parathyroidectomy in the United States on August 1, 1928 [2].

Presenting Signs and Symptoms

The presenting signs and symptoms of HPT have dramatically changed since the introduction of the serum channel autoanalyzers. A dramatic increase in the number of asymptomatic patients with hypercalcemia, kidney stones, and bone disease has been noted.

The National Institute of Health consensus group concluded that medical monitoring was permissible in patients with moderate hypercalcemia and no renal disease, bone disease, or life-threatening conditions. No consensus on specific laboratory monitoring or predictive factors was identified to alert clinicians.

A.L. Halverson and D.C. Borgstrom (eds.), *Advanced Surgical Techniques for Rural Surgeons*, DOI 10.1007/978-1-4939-1495-1_18, © Springer Science+Business Media New York 2015

Surgical Approach

The surgical approach that is recommended for surgeons in low volume centers is a standard bilateral neck exploration. In high volume centers, pre-op scanning and intra-op PTH testing allows focused parathyroidectomy with outcomes comparable to bilateral neck exploration [3].

A preoperative localization with technetium 99m sestamibi is the technique of choice.

Most community hospitals offer this procedure and it is sufficiently sensitive and cost effective.

The sestamibi scan does not diagnose multiglandular disease; however accurately localizes parathyroid adenomas. Bilateral neck exploration for hyperparathyroidism is 95 % effective for localization and removal by examining all four parathyroid glands.

Intraoperative PTH assays should be performed before incision and at 5 and 10 min after excision. Care must be taken to avoid massaging the thyroid and doing any dissection while waiting for the results of the PTH assay test.

Nuclear Medicine Parathyroid Scans

Patient #1: History of Hypercalcemia

Following the administration of 25 mCi technetium 99m sestamibi, delayed images are obtained. Delayed images are obtained for clearance of the radionuclide from the thyroid. Increased uptake in the lower aspect of the thyroid at 2-h is consistent with parathyroid adenoma (Fig. 18.1).

Patient #2: History of High Calcium

Following the administration of 24 mCi of Tc99m sestamibi injected intravenously, immediate and delayed imaging of the head, neck, and upper chest were obtained in the anterior projection.

The impression of abnormal sestamibi scan demonstrated persistent activity in the projection of the inferior right thyroid. A prior ultrasound demonstrated a hypoechoic nodule in the right inferior thyroid lobe (Fig. 18.2).

Operative Procedure

A 5–6 cm low collar incision is made two finger-breadths above the suprasternal notch and deepened through the cervical fascia and platysma. The strap muscles are carefully separated in the midline and care is taken to avoid injury to the anterior jugular veins (Figs. 18.3 and 18.4).

After separating the strap muscles in the midline, the soft tissues around the thyroid are gently dissected using a stroking motion. The middle thyroid veins are double clipped and divided. The thyroid gland is grasped gently and elevated. The recurrent laryngeal nerve is found in the tracheoesophageal groove and the middle thyroid artery is noted and may be superficial or deep to the recurrent laryngeal nerve.

The superior parathyroid is present adjacent to the gland 80 % of the time. It is much more reliable in its position on the superior aspect of the thyroid gland.

The inferior parathyroid, however, is more variable with some reports noting up to 42 % variation in the location of the inferior glands. A careful inspection on the surface is done and if not found then a careful dissection inferiorly of the tissue beneath the thyroid dissecting down to the thymus and into the anterior mediastinum may be done.

In gently massaging an area suspected of containing the inferior gland and then obtaining a rapid PTH assay is one technique for localization of the gland. Most parathyroid surgeons have carried out many thyroid operations and understand the need for a meticulous and purposeful dissection. The anatomy on the left side proves to be much easier to find the recurrent laryngeal nerve in the tracheal esophageal groove than the right side. A focused dissection of the parathyroid gland is done based upon the preoperative sestamibi scan (Fig. 18.5).

The right side, however, is localized in much the same manner by dividing the middle thyroid veins and gently dissecting the thyroid gland toward the midline. Careful Kittner dissection to expose the recurrent laryngeal nerve traveling vertically and the horizontal thyroid artery is done (Fig. 18.6). Occasionally it is necessary to dissect the thymus and expose the surface of that gland in order to identify the mediastinal parathyroid.

The actual removal of the adenoma should be done with direct vision by dividing the artery on the proximal side of the adenoma. Careful exposure of the recurrent laryngeal nerve and its relationship to the middle thyroid artery is mandatory to avoid injury.

Although the upper parathyroids on the left and right are more predictable in their location, occasionally one of these may be hidden in the carotid sheath. The carotid sheath can be easily opened with hemostat dissection and superior lateral retraction. This dissection can be carried upward toward the pharynx.

The adenoma is identified as a dark brown, smoothly rounded structure. The lower parathyroid glands migrate with the thymus. The unusual parathyroid gland may be

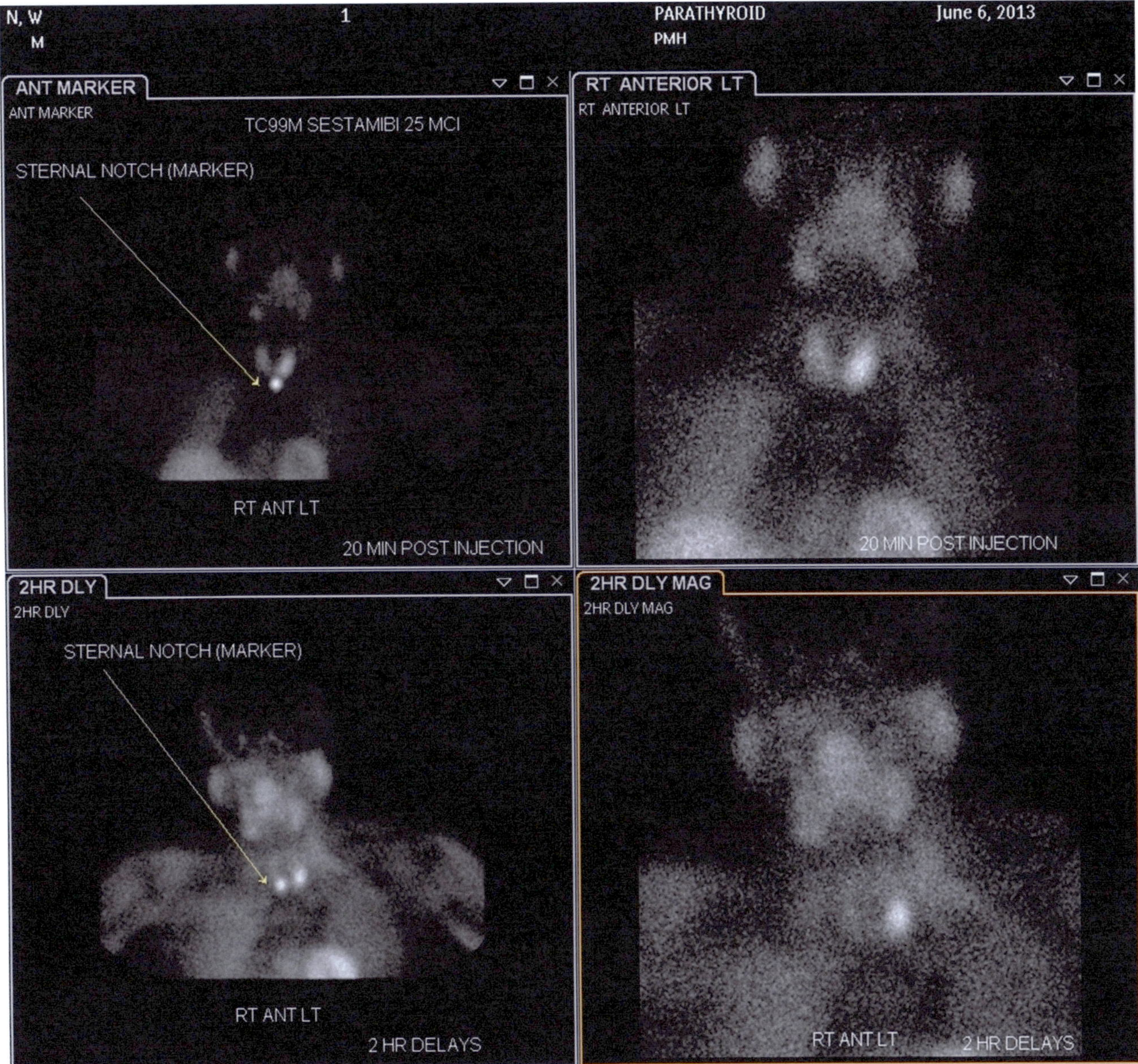

Fig. 18.1 Increased uptake lower left thyroid consistent with parathyroid adenoma

intrathyroidal and may require resection of the thyroid lobe to identify and remove this parathyroid adenoma (Fig. 18.7).

In summary, the upper gland is likely to be in its anticipated position in the majority of patients; however occasionally in the carotid sheath. The lower gland is more variable and may be inferior to the thyroid and may require dissection down to the thymus gland.

For good exposure of the thymus, a retractor should be used to elevate the sternum and provide good exposure of the thymus gland. The adenoma may be found on the surface of the thymus gland and should be removed with resection of that portion of the thymus.

Parathyroid hyperplasia may be identified during bilateral neck dissection. All four glands are diffusely enlarged, dark brown, and with uneven surfaces and appear cystic. The microscopic appearance is typical of clear cell hyperplasia.

The recommended treatment for patients with four gland enlargement is removal of 3½ parathyroid glands.

The use of intraoperative rapid parathyroid hormone assay is very helpful and one must wait 5–10 min after

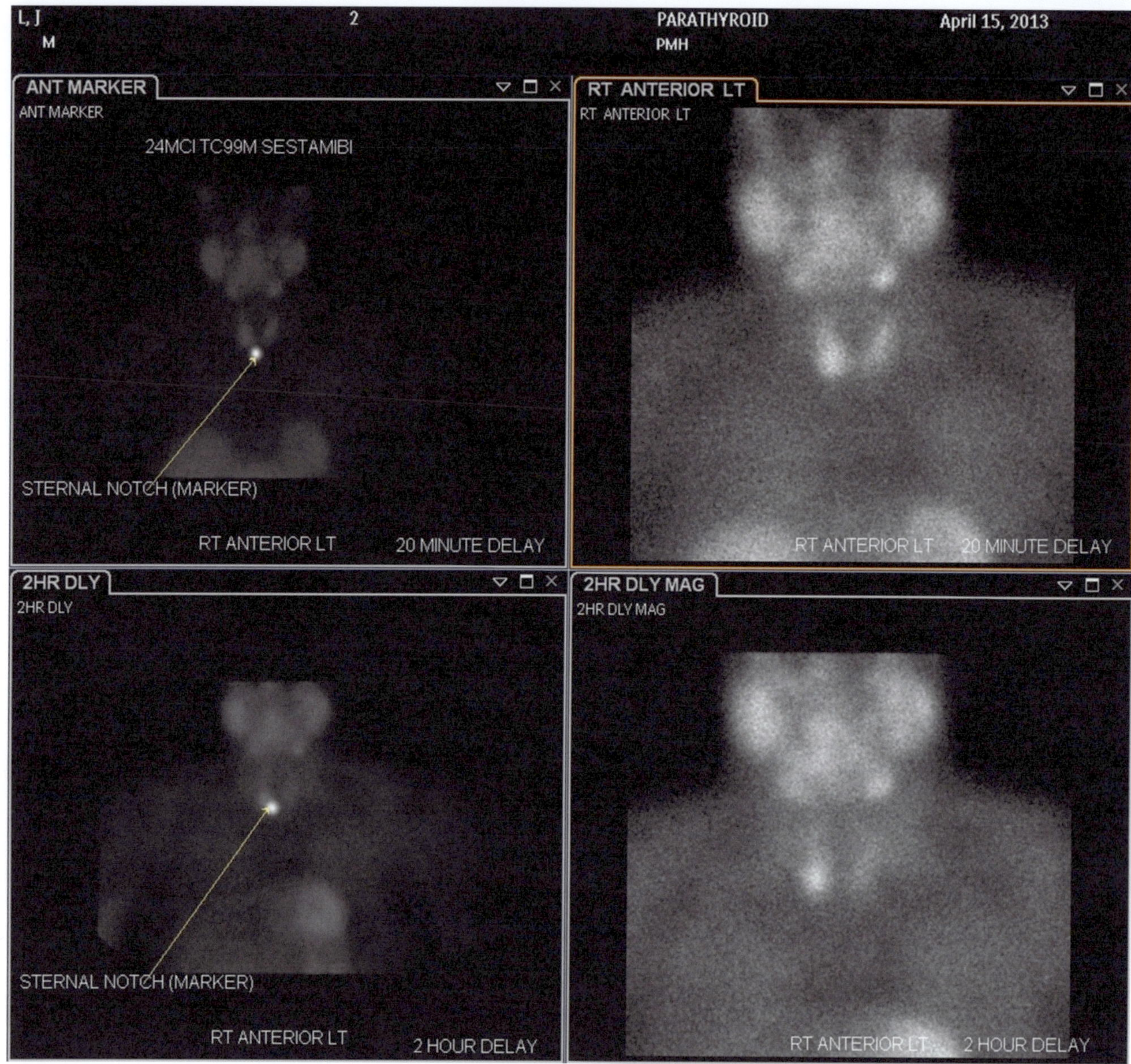

Fig. 18.2 Increased uptake lower right thyroid consistent with parathyroid adenoma

excision of the adenoma to demonstrate a decrease of at least 50 % in the level of parathyroid hormone.

The intraoperative PTH is most reliable with a single adenoma and least reliable with parathyroidectomy for hyperplasia.

Surgical Pathology

Microscopic appearance of normal parathyroid shows a mixture of chief cells and oxyphil cells (Figs. 18.8, 18.9 and 18.10).

The typical parathyroid adenoma on the other hand shows numerous chief cells and oxyphil cells (Figs. 18.11, 18.12, 18.13 and 18.14).

Conclusion

In summary, the National Institute of Health held a consensus conference in 1990 advising surgeons about the appropriate indications for parathyroidectomy.

The established criteria being >1 to 1.4 mg/dL above normal; typical age less than 50; calcium renal calculi; urinary

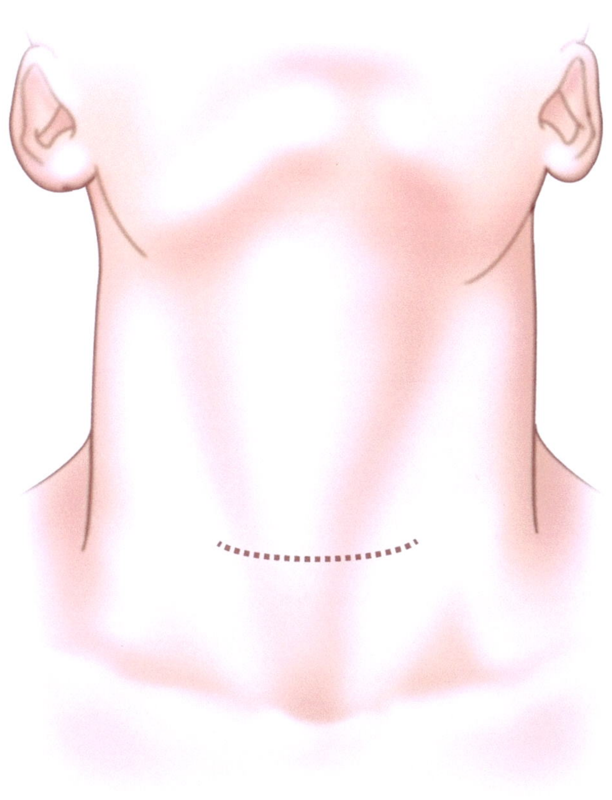

Fig. 18.3 The incision is 5–6 cm in length and two finger-breadths above the suprasternal notch

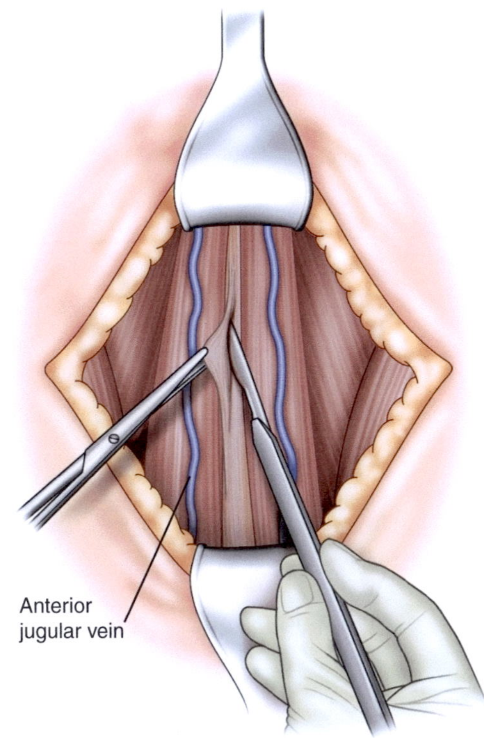

Fig. 18.4 The strap muscles are gently separated taking care not to injure the anterior jugular vein

calcium >400 mg per 24 h; bone density >2 standard deviations from normal; reduced renal function or co-existing disease that would make observation inappropriate.

Now 23 years since those recommendations were made with the increasing accuracy of measuring bone densities and improving quality and outcomes of parathyroidectomy, it is clear that other indications exist for patients with elevated serum calcium levels including patients with diabetes mellitus and hypercalcemia.

Can biochemical abnormalities predict symptomatology? This question was addressed by Anna Bargren, M.D., et al., at the University of Wisconsin in the September 2011 issue of the Journal of the American College of Surgeons.

Their conclusion was that the degree of parathyroid hormone elevation and the presence of Vitamin-D deficiency do not correlate well with the presence of symptoms in patients. Significant hypercalcemia was associated with nephrolithiasis, but interestingly, milder hypercalcemia had significantly more depression, bone or joint pain, and constipation, suggesting that these symptoms are mediated in a different manner [4].

In conclusion, bilateral neck exploration for hyperparathyroidism is recommended for lower volume settings. In high volume settings, focused unilateral parathyroidectomy with intraoperative rapid PTH assays is quite feasible. Rapid PTH has a margin of error and cost is a consideration.

Parathyroid hormone elevation alone does not establish the diagnosis of hyperparathyroidism but with simultaneous elevation of the serum calcium level, the finding is virtually diagnostic.

Caution to Surgeons

Remember the limitation of histological diagnosis of hyperplasia.

Carefully avoid injury to the recurrent laryngeal nerve.

Wait 5–10 min before excision of a hyperfunctioning gland and not disturb the surgical field while waiting for intraoperative PTH assay.

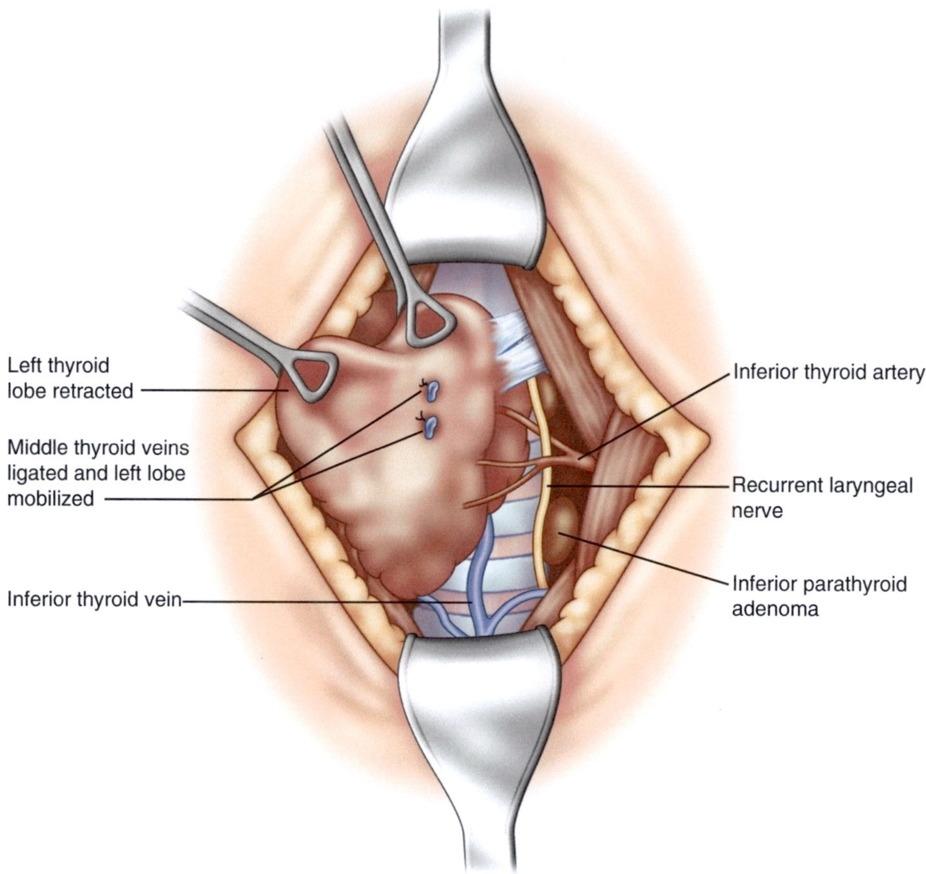

Fig. 18.5 (*Left*) The soft tissues around the thyroid are dissected and the middle thyroid veins are clipped and divided. The thyroid is grasped, elevated, and retracted to the midline to expose the tracheoesophageal groove

In hard to find adenomas, look for the inferior gland from the tracheoesophageal groove down to the thymus. Mediastinotomy is indicated in only 1 % of patients and should be delayed to allow confirmation of surgical findings and repeat of imaging [5].

For the hard to find superior gland, look in the carotid sheath.

Remember that sestamibi scans are not always accurate. False positive and false negative readings do occur.

Postoperative monitoring of calcium levels is exceedingly important in parathyroidectomy surgery and the administration of supplementary calcium during the postoperative period is wise and recommended.

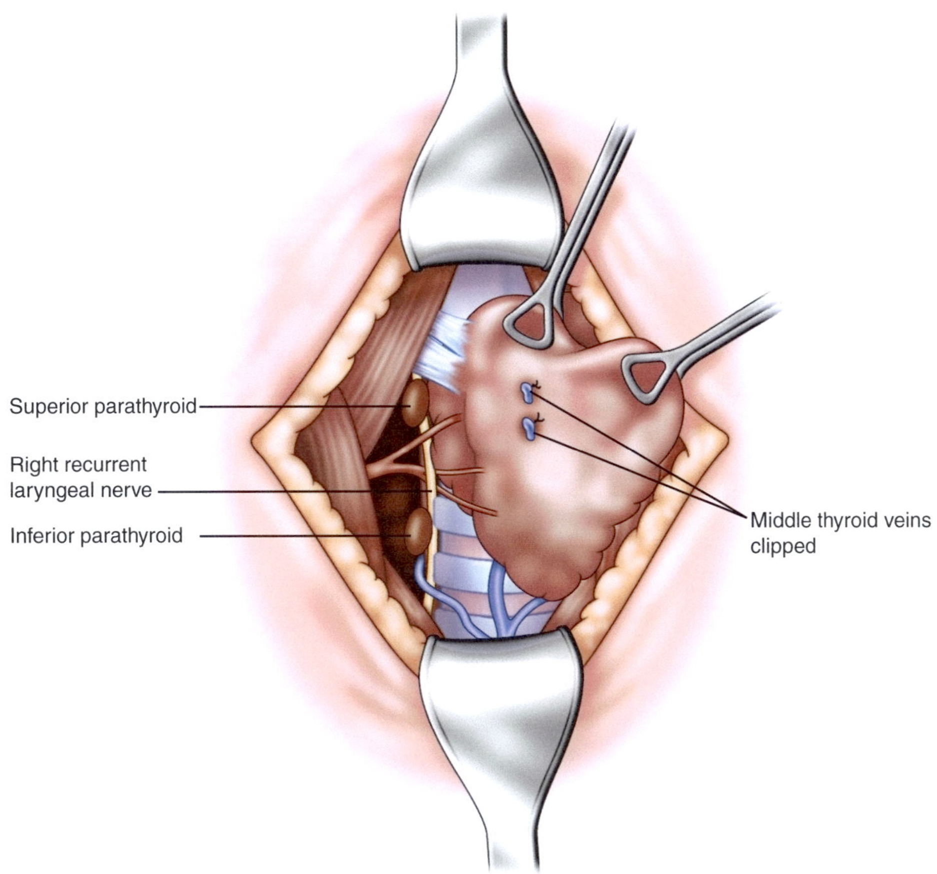

Fig. 18.6 (*Right*) Retract the right thyroid lobe to expose and ligate the middle thyroid veins. The right recurrent laryngeal nerve usually ascends in a groove between the esophagus and larynx

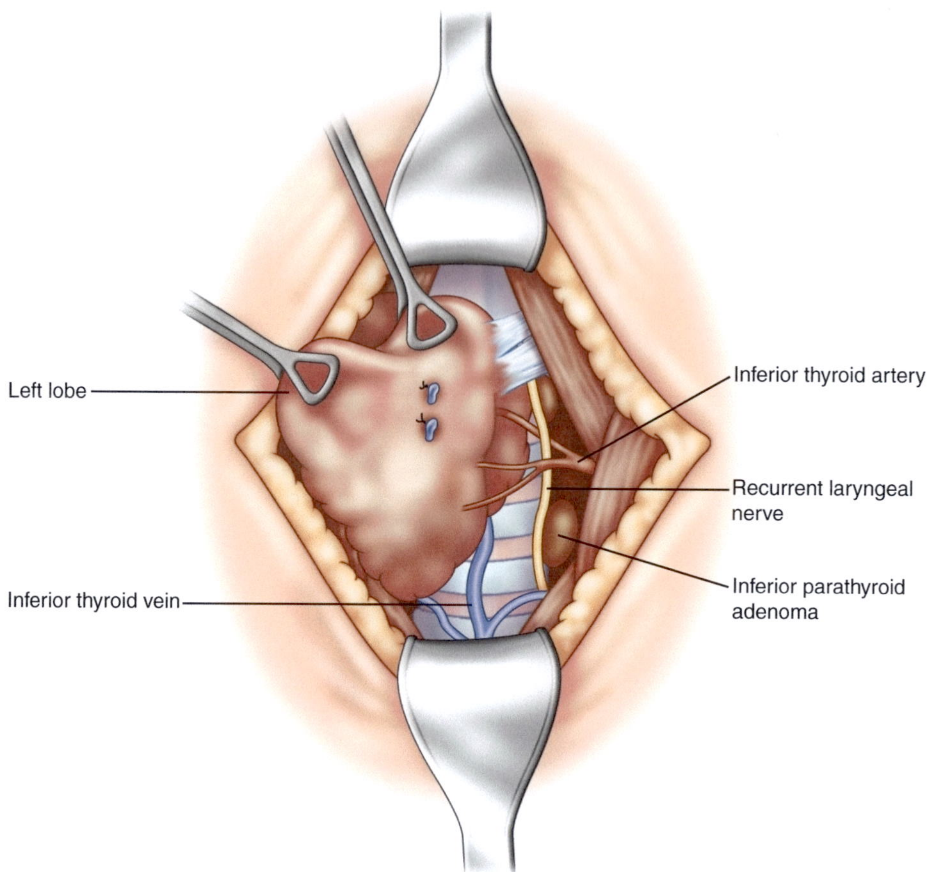

Fig. 18.7 (*Left side*) The inferior thyroid artery and the recurrent laryngeal nerve are identified. The artery may cross over or under the nerve. The dark brown parathyroid adenoma is located according to the results of the sestamibi scan

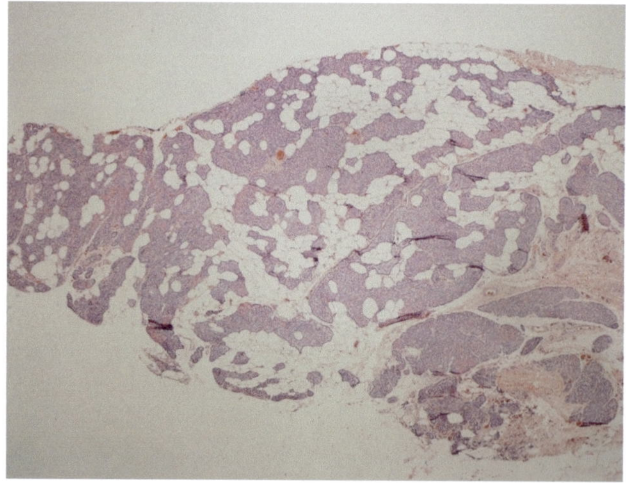

Fig. 18.8 Normal parathyroid low power

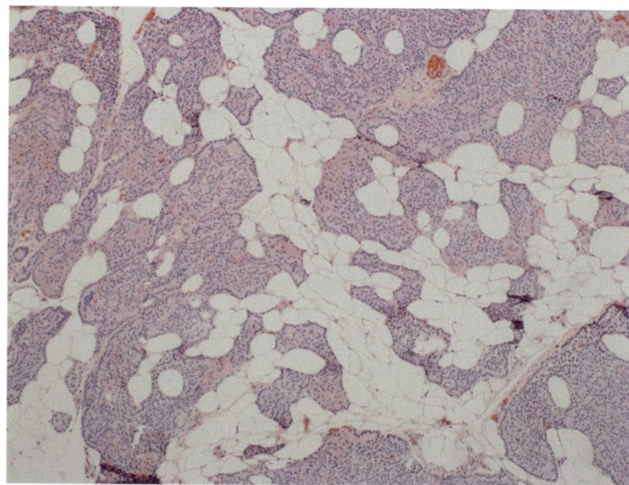

Fig. 18.9 Normal parathyroid medium power

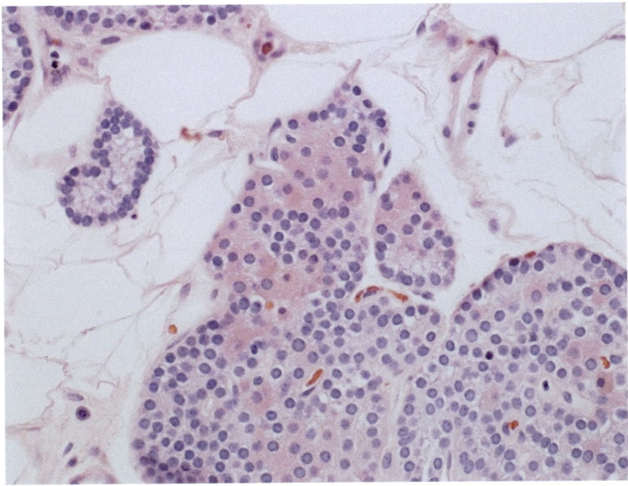

Fig. 18.10 Normal parathyroid high power. Mixture of chief and oxyphil cells

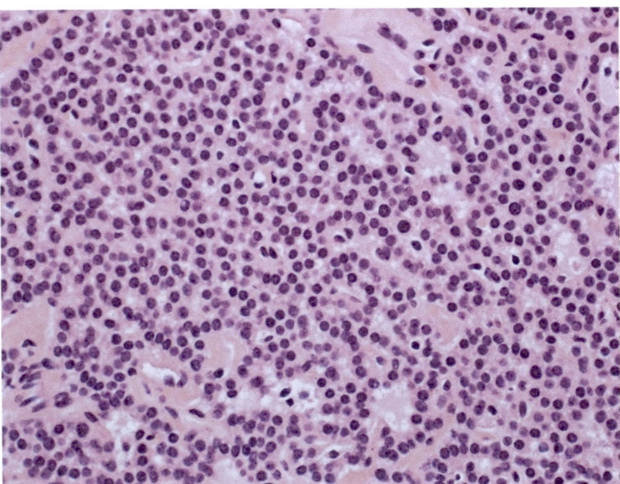

Fig. 18.13 Parathyroid adenoma high power. Numerous chief cells

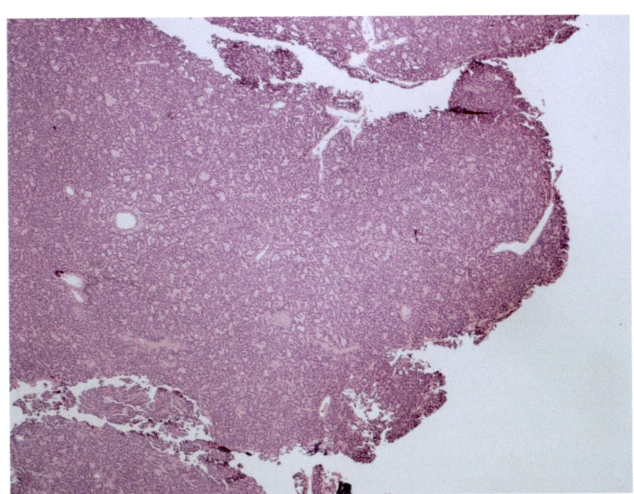

Fig. 18.11 Parathyroid adenoma low power

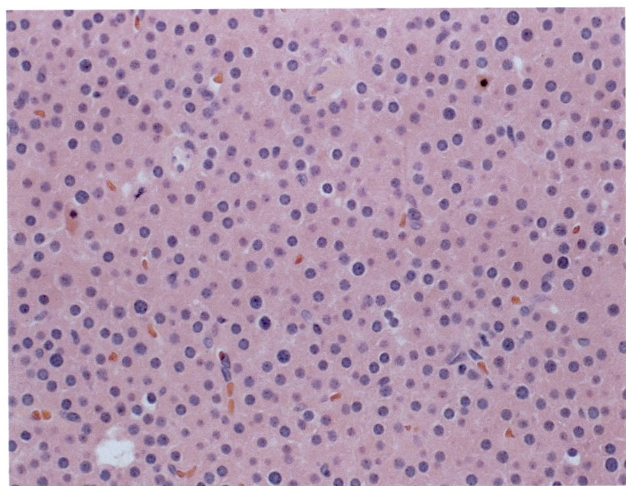

Fig. 18.14 Parathyroid adenoma high power. Numerous oxyphil cells

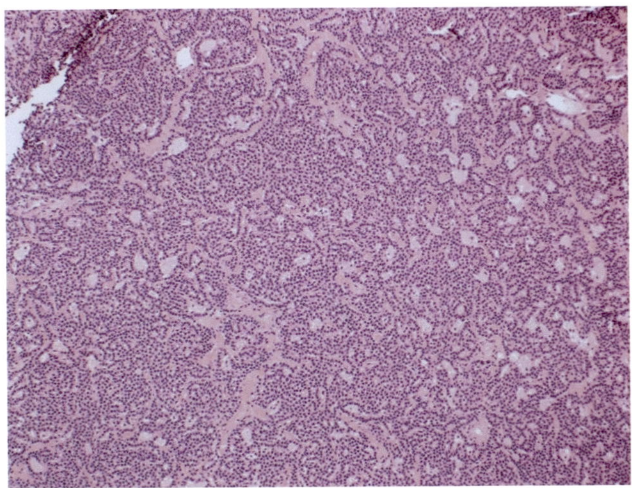

Fig. 18.12 Parathyroid adenoma medium power

References

1. Berson SA, Yalow RS, Aurbach GD, Potts JR. Immunoassay of bovine and human parathyroid hormone. Proc Natl Acad Sci U S A. 1963;49:613–7.
2. Organ CH. The history of parathyroid surgery, 1850-1996; the Excelsior Surgical Society 1998 Edward D Churchill Lecture. J Am Coll Surg. 2000;191:284–99.
3. Numann P. Endocrine surgery. J Am Coll Surg. 2000;190:129–33.
4. Bargren A, Repplinger D, Chen H, Sippel R. Can biochemical abnormalities predict symptomatology in patients with primary hyperparathyrodism? J Am Coll Surg. 2011;213(3):410–4.
5. Doherty GM, Moley JE. Conventional exploration for hyperparathyroidism. In: Udelsman R, van Heerden J, editors. Operative techniques in general surgery, vol. 1. Philadelphia: W.B. Saunders; 1999. p. 4–17.

Part V

Vascular

Central Venous Access for Rural Surgeons

Ervin B. Brown

Introduction

Over a 30-year career at University of Texas M.D. Anderson Cancer Center, I have placed over 7,000 implanted ports. Virtually all have been done with real-time ultrasound guidance for the initial venous access. In this chapter I will illustrate the value of ultrasound guidance in central venous access. I will then describe the evolution of my technique in implanted port insertion, and offer practical suggestions that have helped to maintain consistent results in our patients. I will then present some unusual cases that have arisen, the consideration of which may help the practicing surgeon.

Indications

Long-term venous access for medication administration or parenteral nutrition

Intravenous access for individuals with limited peripheral venous access

Preoperative Preparation

All patients are evaluated in our Port Clinic prior to surgery. Our port team includes dedicated physician assistants, nurses from our Infusion Therapy Clinic, and schedulers. At the preoperative assessment, a complete history and physical examination is done. Important aspects of the patient's history include a history of current or prior venous thromboembolism, and anticoagulation or antiplatelet therapy. The patient's prior central venous catheter history is reviewed, including types of catheters, date of insertion and removal,

E.B. Brown, M.D., F.A.C.S. (✉)
Department of Surgical Oncology, University of Texas
M.D. Anderson Cancer Center, Houston, TX 77030, USA
e-mail: ebbrown@mdanderson.org

and associated catheter related complications. Prior surgery or injury of the chest, neck and axilla, and prior radiation therapy are noted. The patient's chest is evaluated for skin lesions including rashes and wounds, and venous collaterals. Recent chest CT scans or MRIs are evaluated to assess the veins for potential access. If necessary, an upper extremity venous Doppler may be ordered preoperatively, or the patient may be evaluated in the Port Clinic with ultrasound. Patients with pacemakers or defibrillators have their devices interrogated prior to the procedure.

Patients on warfarin are usually bridged with low-molecular weight heparin. Plavix is typically stopped 5 days prior to the scheduled procedure. Aspirin is held the morning of surgery. If a patient has a drug-eluting cardiac stent, aspirin is not held. Antibiotic prophylaxis is given preoperatively. Cefazolin is used if patients do not have penicillin or cephalosporin allergies. Vancomycin or clindamycin are used for penicillin allergic patients. Vancomycin is used for patients with a history of MRSA infection, or for carriers. We routinely prep the patients with ChloraPrep. We use Betadine for patients who are allergic to chlorhexidine. We prefer the patient's absolute neutrophil count to be 1.0×10^3/cu mm or greater, and the platelet count to be at least 50×10^3/cu mm. If the patient's ANC is low because of a nadir from recent chemotherapy, the procedure is postponed until the counts recover, either spontaneously or with supportive treatment.

Operative Strategy

Central venous access can be divided into two types of access; (1) tunneled catheters with implanted ports, including chest ports and arm ports, and (2) non-implanted central venous catheters, including PICC lines, subclavian catheters, and tunneled catheters without implanted subcutaneous ports. Most commonly, central venous access is achieved via the internal jugular vein or subclavian vein, or via upper limb veins for PICC lines and arm ports. Femoral veins are seldom used, but may become necessary in selected situations.

A.L. Halverson and D.C. Borgstrom (eds.), *Advanced Surgical Techniques for Rural Surgeons*,
DOI 10.1007/978-1-4939-1495-1_19, © Springer Science+Business Media New York 2015

The choice of access and the type of catheter depends upon multiple factors, including the reasons for central venous access, the anticipated duration of access, the venous sites available, and the operator's judgment. The history of vascular access has been chronicled by Dudrick [1].

Central Venous Access by Anatomic Landmarks vs. Ultrasound-Guided Central Venous Access

Multiple government agencies and societies advocate routine ultrasound guidance for central venous access [2]:
AHRQ-Agency for Healthcare Research and Quality
NICE-National Institute for Health and Clinical Excellence
CDC-Centers for Disease Control and Prevention
American College of Surgeons
American College of Emergency Physicians
American College of Chest Physicians
American Board of Internal Medicine
American Society of Anesthesiologists
Association for Vascular Access

Central venous access can be performed with the anatomic landmark technique or with ultrasound guidance. Techniques for central venous access insertion are well known by all surgeons. Complications of insertion of central venous catheters include pneumothorax, vascular injury, and nerve injury. Indwelling complications include infection and thrombosis. Kusminsky provided an excellent review of complications of central venous complications [3]. Real-time ultrasound guidance can reduce the risk of injuries from central venous access. Ultrasound allows one to determine the adequacy of the vein for access. Is the size adequate? Is the vein compressible? Is there evidence of thrombosis? Is the vein absent? One is able to follow the needle into the vein. Keys to success include maintaining a low rate of complications, which include pneumothorax, vascular injury, nerve injury, thrombosis, infection, and malposition. It is important to be consistent with the technique of insertion, port location, and catheter tip location. Strict attention should be given to sterile technique, gentle tissue handling, meticulous hemostasis, and accurate wound closure.

The decision to place a subclavian or internal jugular port is determined by factors which include operator's preference, patient's anatomy, and patient's preference. The subclavian vein is used by most surgeons, while the internal jugular vein is used by most interventional radiologists. The femoral vein is useful if there is no route to access the superior vena cava. There are advantages to using the internal jugular vein rather than the subclavian vein. The internal jugular vein has a lower reported incidence of symptomatic venous thrombosis than does the subclavian vein. Araujo et al., in 2008, reported in 1,231 ports a 5 %

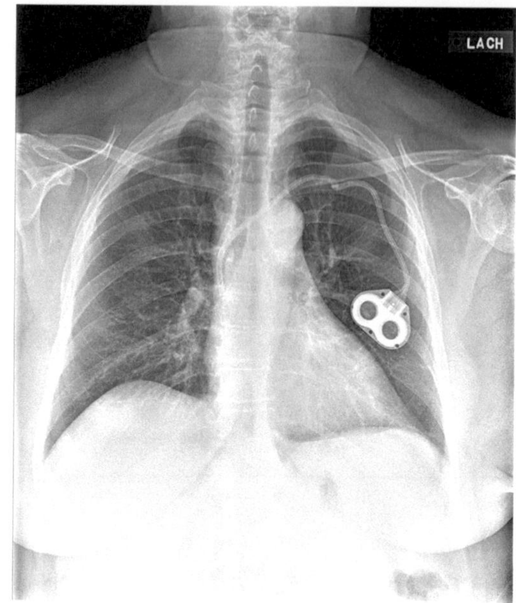

Fig. 19.1 CXR. Left subclavian dual lumen implanted port with pinch-off and kinking of catheter with catheter malfunction

thrombosis rate with subclavian catheters, and a 1.5 % with jugular catheters [4].

Another advantage of internal jugular ports is that there is no risk of catheter pinch-off. Catheter pinch-off is a potential complication of subclavian catheters. As the subclavian vein passes over the first rib and beneath the clavicle, a subclavian catheter is at risk of being repeatedly compressed between the clavicle and first rib. This risk is increased with more medial access of the subclavian vein. The risk may be decreased with ultrasound-guided subclavian access, as the entrance in the vein is more lateral, allowing for some movement of the catheter within the vein. There is no risk of pinch-off with internal jugular ports, as the catheter goes over the clavicle and not between the clavicle and first rib. Pinch-off can result in malfunction of the catheter, due to kinking of the catheter (Fig. 19.1). It may result in fracture of the catheter, with risk of extravasation, or complete transection of the catheter, with embolization of the distal catheter fragment (Figs. 19.2 and 19.3).

Once the vein for access has been chosen, one needs to decide which type of port is to be used. Since there is a high likelihood that our patients will need contrast injection for either CT scans or MRIs, most of our patients will get implanted ports that are rated for pressure injection. Generally, I choose the size of the port proportional to the size of the patient. I use full sized ports for most morbidly obese patients. It is also my preference to use a full sized port for patients who are receiving multi-day infusions, as it seems to provide a more stable platform for access. If the patient is more slender and needs multi-day infusion, an intermediate size port is used. Small, low profile ports are useful for extremely thin patients. If a patient is extremely thin, the pocket for the port may be created deep to the pectoralis fascia for a little more tissue coverage. The size of the catheter is another consideration. In general, smaller sized catheters are preferred. We currently use 6-French and 8-French single lumen catheters. Dual ports are not frequently requested at our institution, but are available with various sized ports and catheters.

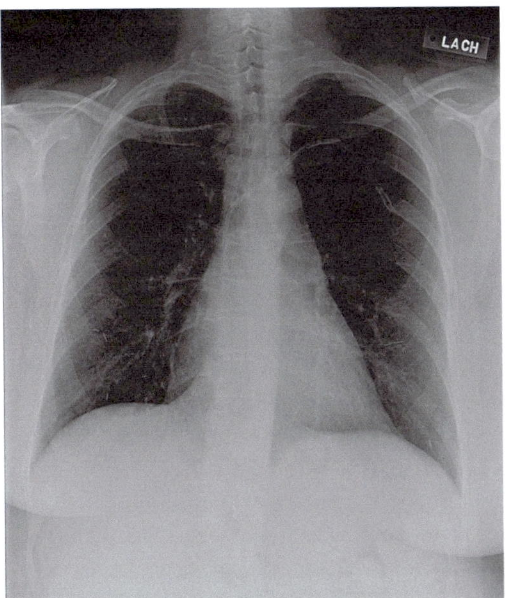

Fig. 19.2 Patient with left subclavian implanted port

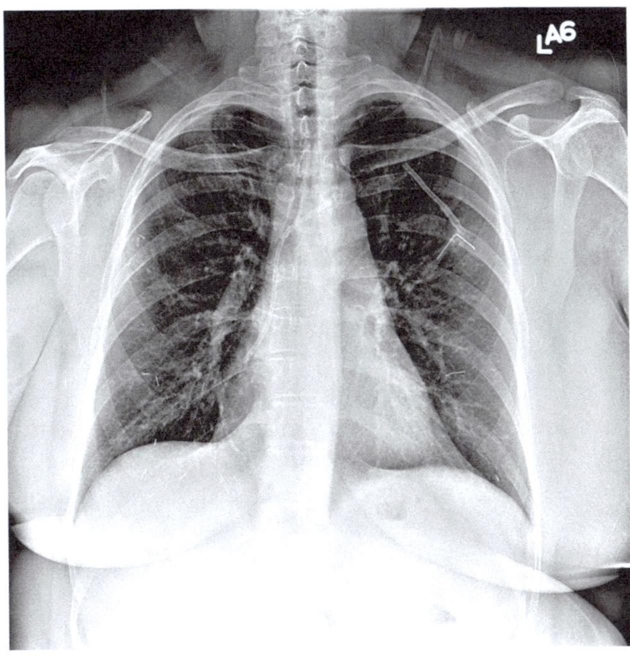

Fig. 19.3 Transection of subclavian catheter in patient in Fig. 19.15

Operative Technique

I use an ultrasound probe with an attachable needle guide (Site-Rite) (Fig. 19.4). The needle guide attaches on the side of the ultrasound probe, so that the targeted vein is visualized in cross section. The angle of the needle guide determines the depth at which the needle tip will cross the ultrasound beam. For internal jugular vein access the probe is stabilized by resting it on the clavicle below, lateral to the sternal notch (Fig. 19.5). The appropriate needle guide is used so that the needle crosses the ultrasound beam at the depth of the lumen of the vein. After appropriate local anesthesia, the 21-gauge needle is slowly advanced through the guide (Fig. 19.6). The tissue can be seen moving anterior to the vein. The needle can usually be seen entering the vein, and is imaged within the lumen of the vein. The needle is released from the needle guide and the 0.018″ wire is inserted through the needle and

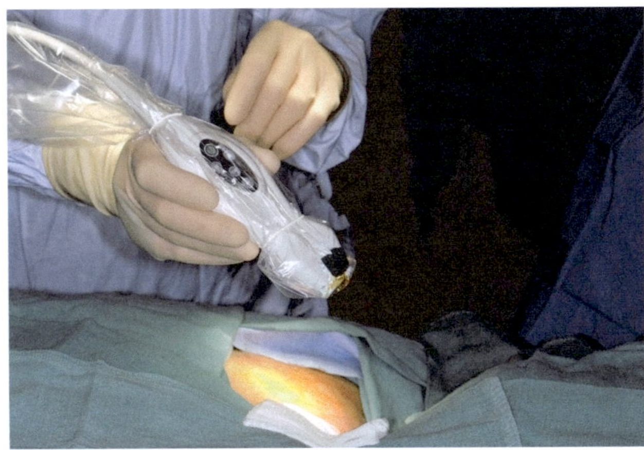

Fig. 19.4 Ultrasound probe with an attachable needle guide (site-rite)

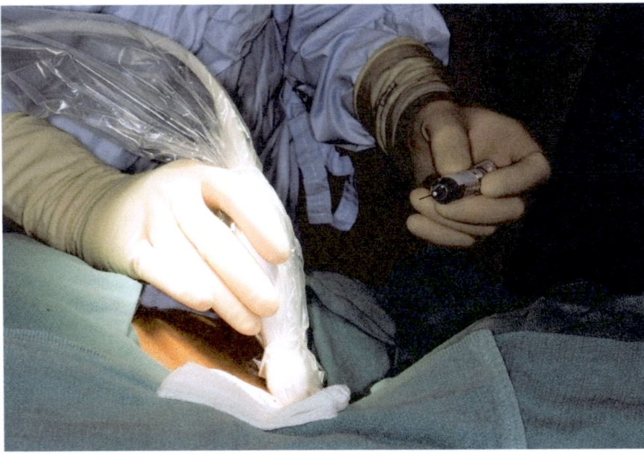

Fig. 19.5 Internal jugular vein access: Ultrasound probe stabilized by resting it on the clavicle below, lateral to the sternal notch

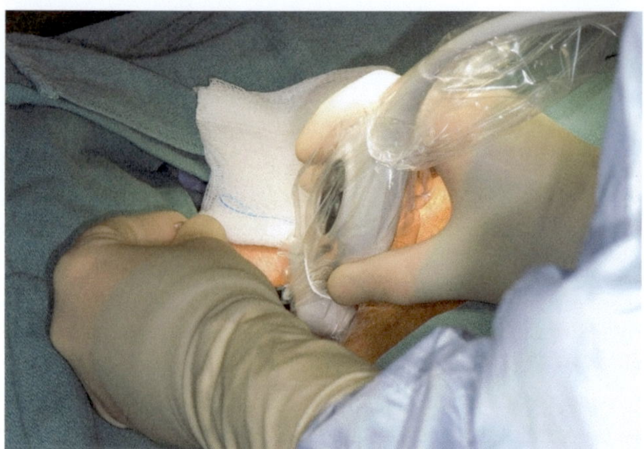

Fig. 19.6 21-gauge needle advanced through needle guide

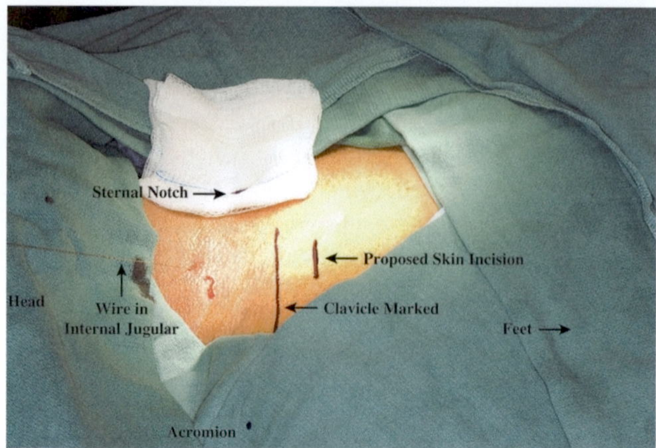

Fig. 19.7 Location of proposed skin incision marked parallel and inferior to clavicle

advanced into the superior vena cava. For subclavian vein access, the subclavian vein is also visualized in cross section. The needle guide is directed towards the patient's feet. After local anesthesia, the 21-gauge needle is slowly advanced through the guide. The tissue anterior to the vein can be seen moving prior to the needle entering the vein. The 0.018″ wire is threaded through the needle into the vein. The vein may also be accessed freehand without the use of a needle guide. Care must be taken to avoid passing the needle too deep, to avoid the underlying lung.

Techniques for Insertion of Implanted Ports

For over 20 years the subclavian vein was my preferred vein for central venous access. The subclavian vein was accessed using the anatomic landmark technique. In order to help to avoid catheter retraction and malposition, I routinely tape the female patient's ipsilateral breast inferiorly. I also tape the male chest wall inferiorly if there is considerable laxity in the tissues or significant gynecomastia. This is especially important for morbidly obese patients. The needle entrance site is half way between the sternal notch and acromion, where the clavicle bends posteriorly. After infiltration of local anesthesia, an 18-gauge needle is advanced beneath the clavicle, keeping the needle parallel to the ground, and directing it one fingerbreadth above the sternal notch, while aspirating with the syringe. When venous blood return is obtained, a 0.035″ J-wire is inserted through the needle. The skin incision for the pocket is marked centered upon the wire and parallel to the clavicle. The incision is deepened to the pectoralis fascia and the pocket made inferiorly. An introducer is passed over the J-wire. The catheter is threaded through the introducer, which is then removed. The catheter is positioned so that the tip of the catheter is in the region of the cavoatrial junction. The catheter is trimmed to the

appropriate length and attached to the port. The port is positioned within the pocket and sutured to the pectoralis fascia.

With real-time ultrasound guidance, the subclavian vein is accessed with a micro-introducer kit. The ultrasound probe is placed inferior to the clavicle approximately midway between the sternal notch and the acromion. The subclavian vein is accessed with a 21-gauge needle and a 0.018″ wire threaded through the needle. The incision is made centered upon the wire parallel to the clavicle. The pocket is created inferiorly at the level of the pectoralis fascia. A 4-French introducer is passed over the 0.18″ wire, which is exchanged for a 0.035 J-wire. An introducer is passed over the J-wire. The catheter is threaded through the introducer, which is removed. The catheter is positioned so that the tip of catheter is in the region of the cavoatrial junction. The catheter is trimmed to the appropriate length and attached to the port. The port is positioned within the pocket and sutured to the pectoralis fascia.

When I place a jugular port, I access the internal jugular vein low in the neck, supporting the ultrasound probe on the clavicle inferiorly. The internal jugular vein is accessed using real-time ultrasound guidance using a 21-gauge needle, and a 0.018″ wire is threaded through the needle. The wire position is confirmed with fluoroscopy. The proposed infraclavicular skin incision is marked parallel to the clavicle, and centered upon a point midway between the sternal notch and acromion (in a location similar to my subclavian ports) (Fig. 19.7). The proposed subcutaneous tunnel is marked between the infraclavicular incision and the wire entrance site (Fig. 19.8). Additional local anesthesia is used in the infraclavicular fossa and along the proposed subcutaneous tunnel between the pocket and the wire entrance site. The infraclavicular pocket is created (Figs. 19.9, 19.10, and 19.11). The 0.018″ wire is exchanged for a 0.035″ J-wire (Figs. 19.12 and 19.13). The introducer is passed over the

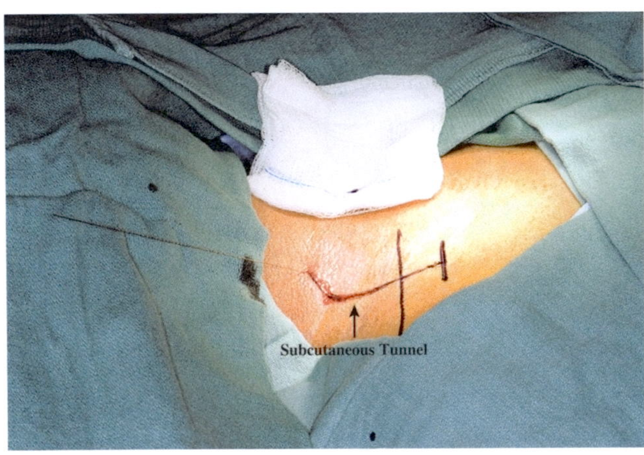

Fig. 19.8 Location of proposed subcutaneous tunnel marked between infraclavicular incision and wire entering internal jugular vein

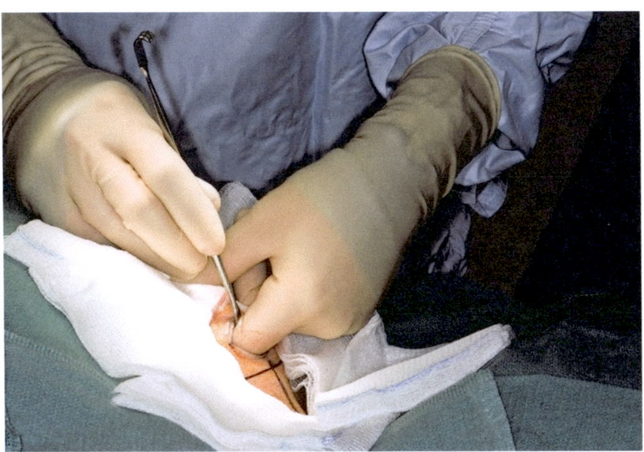

Fig. 19.11 Pocket created inferiorly at the level of pectoralis fascia

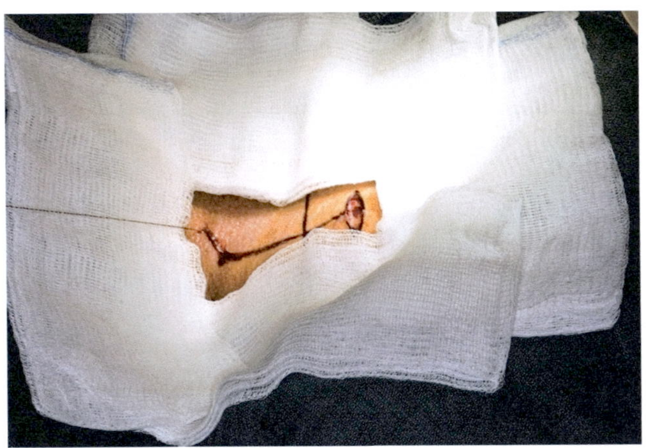

Fig. 19.9 Infraclavicular incision

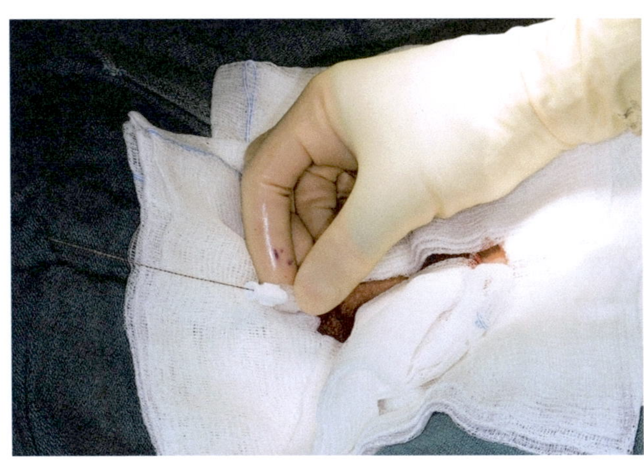

Fig. 19.12 4-French introducer advanced over 0.018″ wire

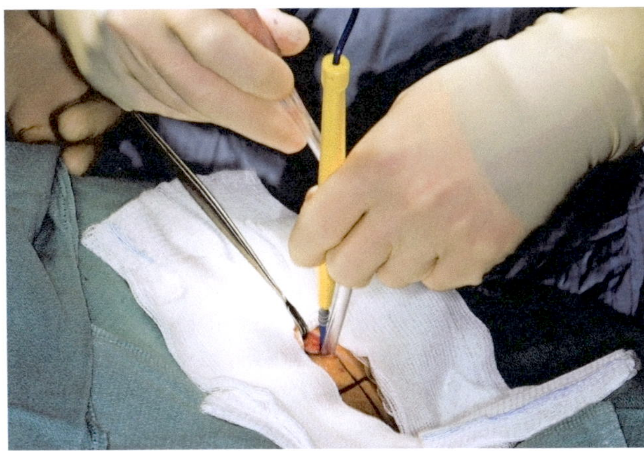

Fig. 19.10 Infraclavicular incision deepened to pectoralis fascia

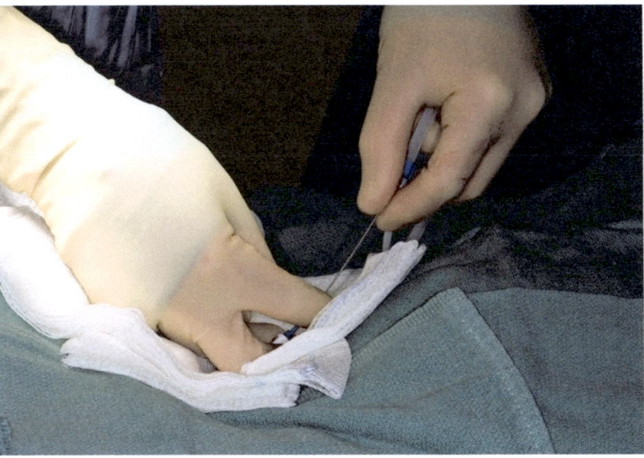

Fig. 19.13 J-wire passed through 4-French introducer

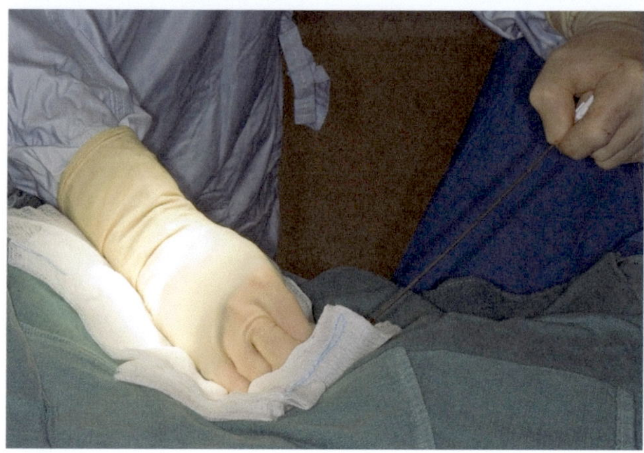

Fig. 19.14 Introducer passed over J-wire

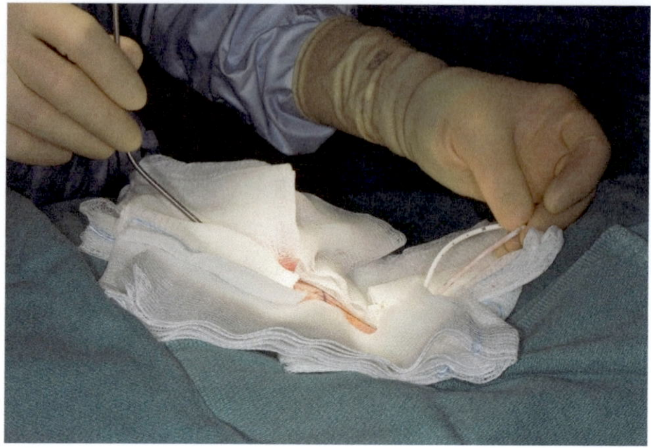

Fig. 19.16 Catheter attached to tunneler. Tunneler drawn through subcutaneous tunnel down to pocket bringing catheter down to pocket

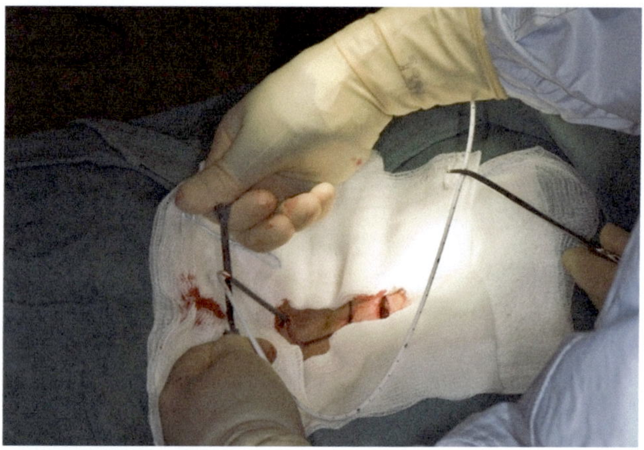

Fig. 19.15 Catheter threaded through introducer. Introducer peeled away

J-wire (Fig. 19.14). The catheter is threaded through the introducer, which is removed (Fig. 19.15). The tunneler is passed from the infraclavicular incision to the cervical incision. The catheter is attached to the tunneler and brought down to the pocket (Fig. 19.16). The catheter tip is positioned in the region of the cavoatrial junction. The catheter is trimmed to the appropriate length and connected to the port with the locking device. The port is positioned within the pocket and sutured to the pectoralis fascia. As can be seen in the operative photographs, I try to isolate the incision(s) with Ray-Tec® sponges, to avoid as much as possible my touching the skin, and to avoid either the catheter or port touching the skin. After hemostasis has been assured, and the port sutured within the pocket, the incision(s) are meticulously closed. I suture the deep subcutaneous tissue with running absorbable suture (4-0 Vicryl), and the dermis with interrupted 4-0 Vicryl deep dermal sutures, followed by subcuticular absorbable monofilament suture (4-0 Monocryl). Further illustration of my technique for insertion of implanted ports has been previously published [5].

Venous Access in the Morbidly Obese Patient

In my 7,000 implanted ports there have been over 400 morbidly obese patients (BMI $\geq$ 40), including 39 patients with BMI 50–60 and 13 patients with BMI > 60. The highest BMI in one of my port patients was 78. That patient underwent successful insertion of a right internal jugular implanted port. The right internal jugular vein was easily accessed with ultrasound guidance. The vein was accessed using a 2 cm needle guide. The center of the right internal jugular vein was at 2 cm depth. Accessing the subclavian vein for this patient using the anatomic landmark technique would certainly have been a challenge. The patient's port is still in use over 2½ years post insertion. It is extremely important to tape the female breast down on the side of port insertion. In morbidly obese male patients the chest wall is also taped inferiorly. This is done in order to place the tissues in a position similar to that when the patient is in the upright position. Following venous access with ultrasound it is helpful to elevate the patient's back prior to marking the proposed port site incision in the infraclavicular fossa, and the subcutaneous catheter tract. The patient's back is also elevated during creation of the port pocket. The patient is returned to flat or slight Trendelenberg position for insertion of the catheter. The back is then elevated for tunneling the catheter and for the remainder of the procedure.

Potential Pitfalls

Pneumothorax
Malpositioned Catheter tip
Central-line-associated blood stream infection
Arrythmia

Malpositioned Catheter Tip

The ideal location of the catheter tip is in the distal superior vena cava, near the junction of the superior vena cava and the right atrium. Catheters with tips that extend deep into the right atrium may cause cardiac arrhythmias and have increased thrombosis rate. Catheters with tips in the proximal superior vena cava and inlet vessels (brachiocephalic veins) and subclavian veins also have higher thrombosis rates. Caers, in a retrospective review of catheter tip position and thrombosis in 437 patients showed that the lowest thrombosis rate (1.5 %) occurred if the catheter tip was in the distal SVC. Those with tips in the proximal SVC had a 19 % thrombosis rate. Those in the brachiocephalic vein had a 45 % thrombosis rate [6]. Cadman, et.al, in a retrospective review of 428 central venous catheters in 334 patients, reviewed CXRs, cathetergrams, venograms, and Doppler ultrasounds. A single radiologist assigned catheter tip locations. They concluded "the position of the tip of tunneled CVC on the post-insertion radiographs was the only significant factor that could be used to predict venous thrombosis." Catheters with the tips in the proximal SVC or higher inlet vessels were 16 times more likely to develop venous thrombosis than those with the tips in the lower third of the SVC and below [7]. Nakazawa published a helpful review of catheter tip location in the Journal of the Association for Vascular Access [8]. Catheters that are clearly malpositioned include those with the tip in the subclavian vein, internal jugular vein, brachiocephalic vein, and at or near the junction of the brachiocephalic veins.

Organizations' Positions on Catheter Tip Location

2006—Infusion Nursing Society Standards of Practice: Central vascular access devices shall have the distal tip dwelling in the lower one third of superior vena cava to the junction of the superior vena cava and the right atrium [8].

2010—Society of Cardiovascular and Interventional Radiology (SCVIR): "Image-guided percutaneous central venous access is defined as the placement of a catheter with its tip in the cavoatrial region or right atrium with the assistance of real-time imaging. The cavoatrial junction has been defined as two vertebral body units below the carina" [9]. Successful placement of a catheter is where the tip is in the desired location and the catheter functions for its intended use [10].

In a review of central venous catheter tip position Vesely noted the significant changes in the position of the catheter tip when the patient changes position [11]. This occurs with PICC lines as well as with subclavian and internal jugular catheters. Catheters are placed when the patient is in the supine position. When the patient sits or stands, the abdominal contents and mediastinal structures shift, and the tip of the catheter is pulled upward. This change in catheter tip position is also affected by downward movement of the female breast, or adipose tissue in the morbidly obese patient. What appears to have been an appropriately positioned catheter at the time of insertion may become malpositioned with the catheter tip withdrawing into the proximal superior vena cava or the brachiocephalic vein. My technique of placing the port in the infraclavicular fossa, taping down female breasts and redundant chest wall tissue in the morbidly obese, and elevating the head of the bed at the time of creating the pocket in morbidly obese patients seems to decrease the subsequent catheter movement.

Catheter lengths for my right subclavian ports are typically between 17 and 20 cm. Catheter lengths for my left subclavian ports are typically between 20 and 24 cm. The catheter length for my right internal jugular implanted ports is typically between 21 and 23 cm. Optimal catheter length is more constant on the right due to the relatively straight course of the right internal jugular vein down to the superior vena cava. The patient's height is the main variable, with taller patients requiring longer catheters. The catheter length for left internal jugular implanted ports is more variable; lengths typically range from 23 to 26 cm. The girth of the patient's chest is also a factor, with a barrel chested patient needing a longer catheter. The angle at which the left brachiocephalic vein crosses the midline is an additional factor. Patients in whom the vein crosses in a more horizontal manner need longer catheters, while those with the brachiocephalic vein being more vertical need shorter catheters. The patient's BMI is also important. The appropriate length for the individual patient is that which allows the tip of the catheter to be positioned in the distal superior vena cava near the cavoatrial junction.

Some central venous catheters are malpositioned because they are too short. I have had patients referred who had subclavian implanted ports whose catheters were 12 and 13 cm long (Fig. 19.17). Other catheters are too long. For example, one patient had a left internal jugular port with a catheter length of 36 cm. The catheter extended deep into the right atrium (Fig. 19.18). Another patient had a right subclavian implanted port with a catheter length of 40 cm (Fig. 19.19). The catheter tip was in the right ventricle just below the outflow tract. This patient had arrhythmias.

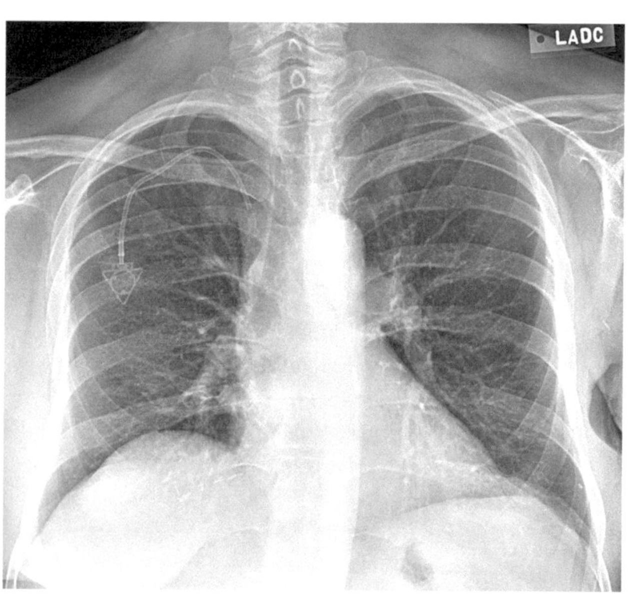

Fig. 19.17 CXR. Right subclavian implanted port. Tip right brachiocephalic vein. Catheter length 12.2 cm

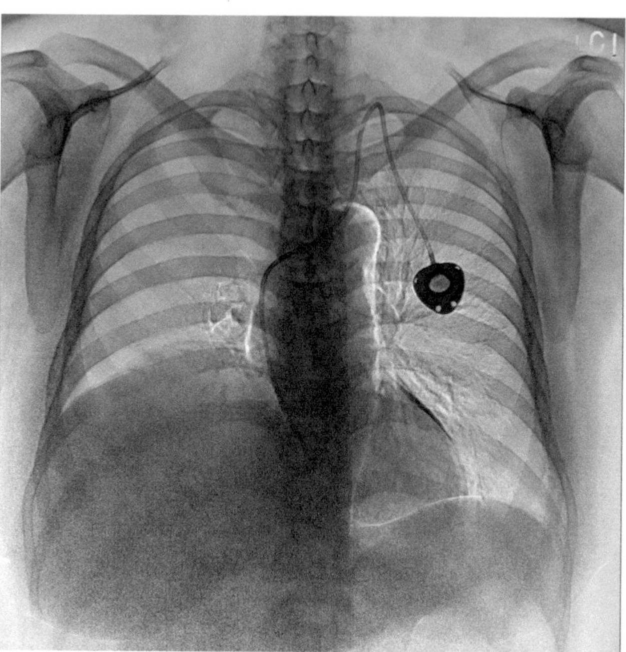

Fig. 19.18 CXR. Left internal jugular implanted port. Catheter tip deep in right atrium. Catheter length 36 cm

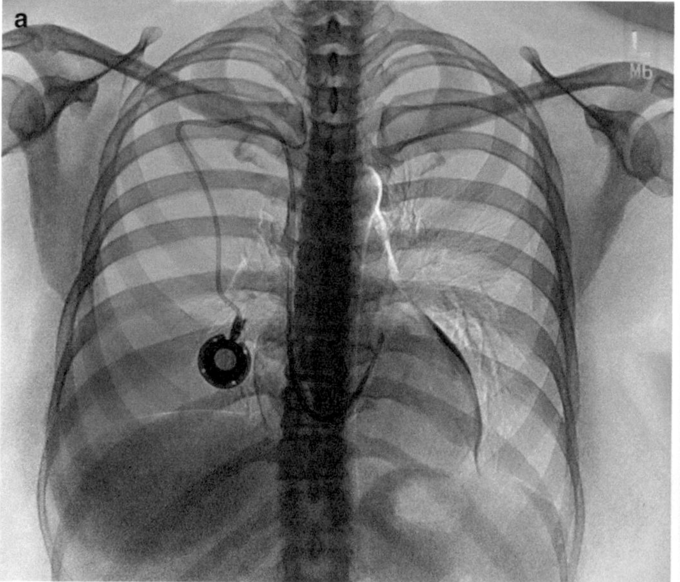

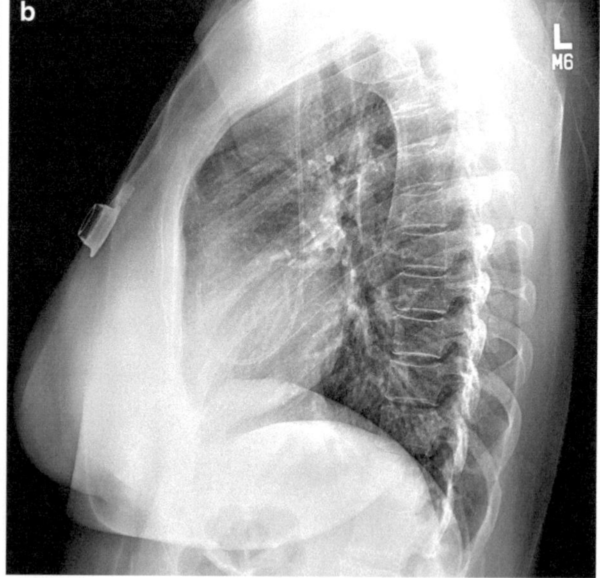

Fig. 19.19 CXR. Right subclavian implanted port. (**a**) Catheter tip in right ventricle below outflow tract. Patient had arrhythmias. Catheter length 40 cm. (**b**) Lateral CX

References

1. Dudrick SJ. History of vascular access. JPEN J Parenter Enteral Nutr. 2006;30:S47.
2. Sonosite.com/ultrasound-evidence/iatrogenic-pneumothorax-central-line-safety.
3. Kusminsky RE. Complications of central venous catheterization. J Am Coll Surg. 2007;204(4):681–96.
4. Araujo C, Silva JP, Antunes P, Fernandes JM, Dias C, Pereira H, Dias T, Fougo JL. A comparative study between two central veins for the insertion of totally implantable venous access devices in 1201 cancer patients. Eur J Surg Oncol. 2008;34(2):222–6.
5. Spencer A, Brown EB. Central venous access in breast oncology patients. In: Kuerer HM, editor. Kuerer's breast surgical oncology. New York: McGraw-Hill; 2010. p. 745–51.
6. Caers J, Fontaine C, Vinh-Hung V, De Mey J, Ponnet G, Oost C, Lamote J, De Greve J, Van Camp B, Lacor P, et al. Catheter tip position as a risk factor for thrombosis associated with the use of subcutaneous ports. Support Care Cancer. 2005;13(5):325–31.
7. Cadman A, Lawrance JA, Fitzsimmons L, Spencer-Shaw A, Swindell R. To clot or not to clot? That is the question in central venous catheters. Clin Radiol. 2004;59(4):349–55.
8. Nakazawa N. Challenges in the accurate identification of the ideal catheter tip location. JAVA. 2010;15(4):196–201.
9. Baskin KM, Jimenez RM, Cahill AM, Jawad AF, Towbin RB. Cavoatrial junction and central venous anatomy: implications for central venous access tip position. J Vasc Interv Radiol. 2008;19(3):359–65.
10. Dariushnia SR, Wallace MJ, Siddiqi NH, Towbin RB, Wojak JC, Kundu S, Cardella JF. Quality improvement guidelines for central venous access. J Vasc Interv Radiol. 2010;21(7):976–81.
11. Vesely TM. Central venous catheter tip position: a continuing controversy. J Vasc Interv Radiol. 2003;14(5):527–34.

Suggested Reading

Seldinger SI. Catheter replacement of the needle in percutaneous arteriography; a new technique. Acta Radiol. 1953;39(5):368–76.

Niederhuber JE, Ensminger W, Gyves JW, Liepman M, Doan K, Cozzi E. Totally implanted venous and arterial access system to replace external catheter in cancer treatment. Surgery. 1982;92(4):706–12.

Irwin RB, Greaves M, Schmitt M. Left superior vena cava: revisited. Eur Heart J Cardiovasc Imaging. 2012;13(4):284–91.

Goyal SK, Punnam SR, Verma G, Ruberg FL. Persistent left superior vena cava: a case report and review of literature. Cardiovasc Ultrasound. 2008;6:50.

Povoski SP, Khabiri H. Persistent left superior vena cava: review of the literature, clinical implications, and relevance of alterations in thoracic central venous anatomy as pertaining to the general principles of central venous access device placement and venography in cancer patients. World J Surg Oncol. 2011;9:173.

Pacemakers

20

Gene B. Duremdes

Indications

A pacemaker is an electronic device designed to provide an electrical impulse to the heart at a programmed rate in order to maintain adequate cardiac function. A pacemaker is inserted for the following indications: severe bradycardia, i.e., HR 20–30s, sick sinus syndrome, complete heart block, brady-tachy syndrome. A single chamber pacemaker is indicated in those patients with atrial fibrillation. Otherwise, most patients will benefit from a dual chamber pacemaker which would provide additional atrial stroke volume ("atrial kick").

Preoperative Preparation

Rule out metabolic causes of the bradycardia, i.e., hypothyroidism, electrolyte imbalance

Rule out iatrogenic causes of the bradycardia, i.e., patient on B-blockers

Obtain chest X-ray

Determine if a single or dual chamber pacemaker is required

Hold any anticoagulants, i.e., Coumadin, Heparin, Pradaxa, etc.

Ensure that protime and prothrombin time are within normal values. If not, normalize with appropriate therapies such as Vitamin K, FFP

Administer appropriate systemic antibiotics

May utilize external pacemaker as a temporizing measure

Notify in a timely manner the pacemaker technician who will be assisting in the determination of proper lead placement via electrophysiologic parameters.

G.B. Duremdes, M.D., M.B.A., F.A.C.S. (⊠)
Princeton Surgical Group, Inc., Princeton, WV 24740, USA
e-mail: maryandgene@hotmail.com

Pitfalls and Danger Points

Pneumothorax/hemothorax from subclavian venipuncture
Cardiac arrhythmia from atrial or ventricular stimulation
Cardiac tamponade from atrial or ventricular perforation
Dislodgement of atrial or ventricular lead

Operative Strategy

The initial key step in pacemaker insertion is to gain access into the central venous system by way of the subclavian, internal jugular, or cephalic veins. The subclavian approach utilizing the modified Seldinger technique is typically the preferred route of access; however, the internal jugular vein can be accessed via percutaneous puncture and the cephalic vein may be entered via open cutdown approach.

Approaching this insertion from the left side allows for a technically easier insertion of the lead(s) because of the C-shaped course needed to gain entry into the atrial/ventricular chambers. A right-sided approach may be utilized; however, the S-shaped course needed to successfully manipulate the lead(s) into the cardiac chambers is technically more difficult.

Fluoroscopy C-arm is utilized to visualize proper placement of the atrial/ventricular leads. The ventricular lead is typically inserted first and once confirmation of proper placement, the atrial lead (if indicated) is subsequently inserted.

The lead(s) are then secured to the pectoralis muscle fascia with nonabsorbable sutures, taking care not to dislodge the lead(s). The lead(s) are then attached to the pacemaker pulse generator which is then secured in the subcutaneous pocket located on the anterior chest wall.

A.L. Halverson and D.C. Borgstrom (eds.), *Advanced Surgical Techniques for Rural Surgeons*,
DOI 10.1007/978-1-4939-1495-1_20, © Springer Science+Business Media New York 2015

Operative Technique

Incision

Make a transverse skin incision on the anterior chest wall just inferior to the clavicle from its midpoint to the deltopectoral groove. Using electrocautery, continue the dissection down to the pectoral fascia and then make a subcutaneous pocket inferiorly and superiorly toward the clavicle. The inferior pocket should be large enough to accommodate the pacemaker pulse generator. Choosing the left side of the chest for placement of the pacemaker will allow for the lead(s) to follow a C-shaped course into the atrial/ventricular chambers, which may technically be easier to insert compared to the S-shaped course that the lead(s) may travel if coming from a right-sided approach. A self-retaining retractor may aid in exposing the pocket and infraclavicular area in preparation for gaining venous access (Fig. 20.1).

Venous Access

The patient is placed in a slight Trendelenburg position and using the modified Seldinger technique, the subclavian vein, which is the preferred route, may be accessed (Figs. 20.2 and 20.3). Alternatively, the venous access may be obtained via an internal jugular approach or even a venous cutdown onto the cephalic vein in the deltopectoral groove. Once the guidewire is inserted into the vein, fluoroscopy is used to confirm proper positioning of the guidewire in the area of the superior vena cava–right atrial junction.

Lead Placement

If the patient is not in chronic atrial fibrillation, then typically, a dual chamber pacemaker utilizing an atrial and ventricular lead is preferred. This allows for a more physiologic stroke volume by providing the additional atrial volume or "atrial kick" that sequential pacing of the atrial and ventricular chambers provides. The ventricular lead introducer and sheath is curved in order to facilitate easier passage toward the right atrial–superior vena cava junction (Fig. 20.4). The introducer and sheath are passed over the guidewire and then while leaving the guidewire in place, the introducer is removed leaving the sheath in place (Fig. 20.5). The ventricular lead, which is an insulated conducting wire, is then inserted into the sheath (Fig. 20.6) and the Teflon-coated "split" sheath catheter is then removed. The lead has an inner guidewire which is curved in a "pigtail" or "hockey stick" configuration in order to be able to manipulate the lead into the ventricular chamber and assist in optimal positioning of

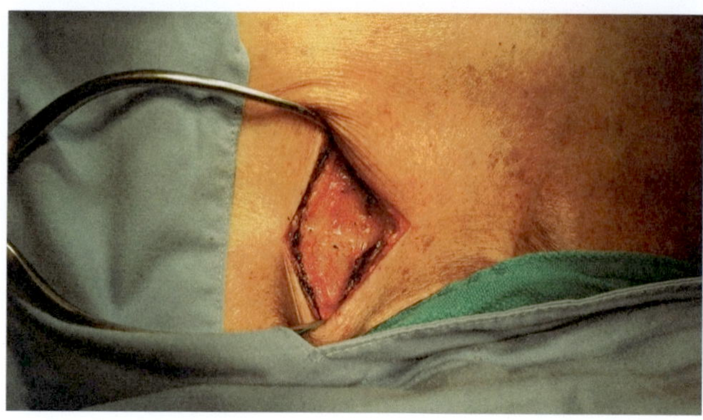

Fig. 20.1 Infraclavicular incision with self-retaining retractor for exposure

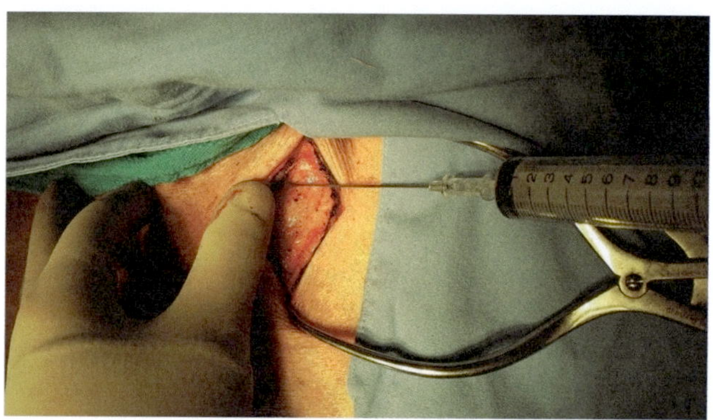

Fig. 20.2 Subclavian vein puncture

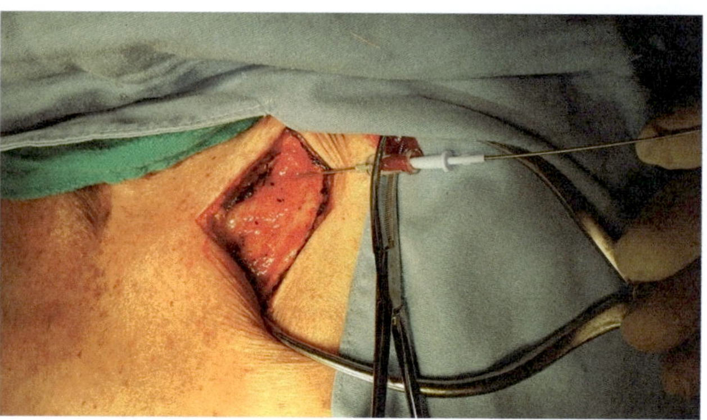

Fig. 20.3 Insertion of guidewire using Seldinger technique

the lead (Fig. 20.7). Under fluoroscopic guidance, the ventricular lead is passed into the atrium through the tricuspid valve and then passed toward the pulmonary outflow tract (Fig. 20.8). The curved guidewire is replaced with a straight guidewire and then under fluoroscopy, the ventricular lead is pulled back into the right ventricle and then directed toward the right ventricular apex. When properly positioned, the ventricular lead has a slightly angled appearance aimed inferiorly and laterally toward the apex of the heart (Fig. 20.9). Once placed, the pacemaker lead is interrogated by attaching

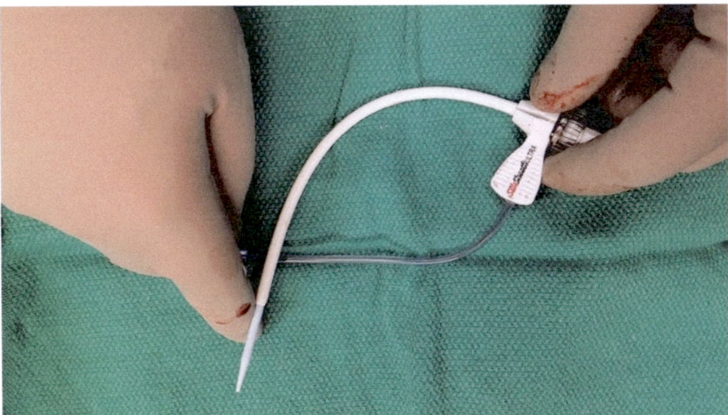

Fig. 20.4 Forming a curved introducer and sheath

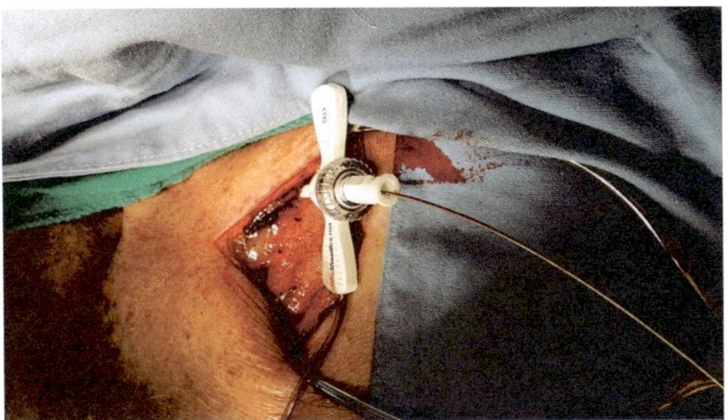

Fig. 20.5 Introducer and sheath with guidewire in place

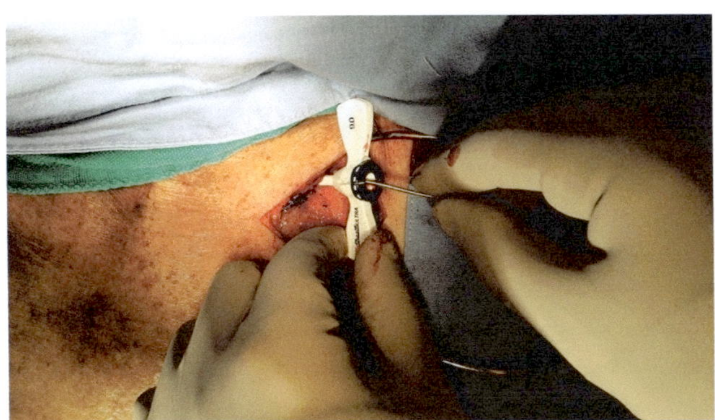

Fig. 20.6 Insertion of ventricular lead through sheath

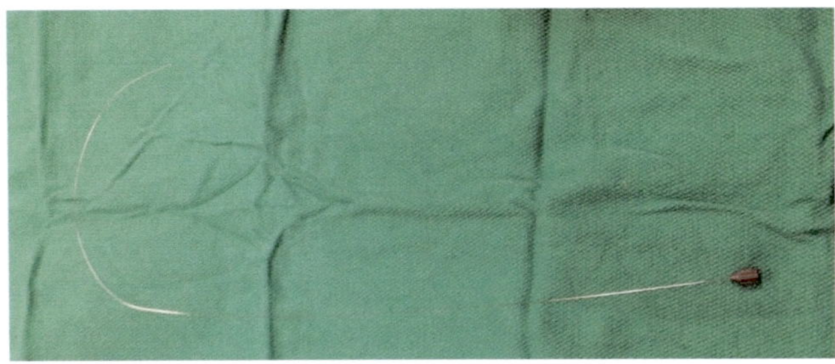

Fig. 20.7 Lead wire curved to form a pigtail conformation

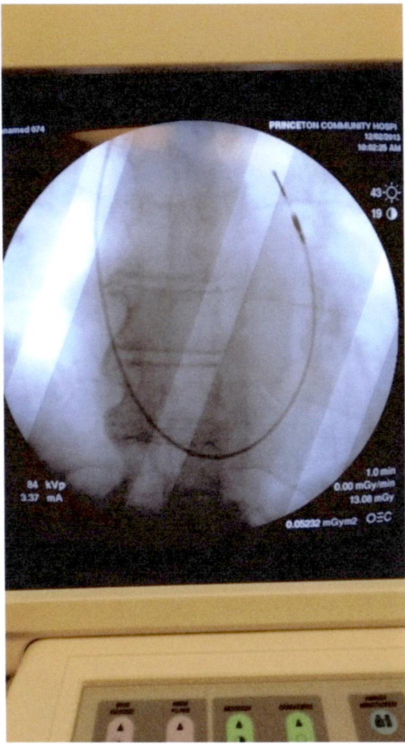

Fig. 20.8 Fluoroscopic view of ventricular lead in pulmonary outflow tract

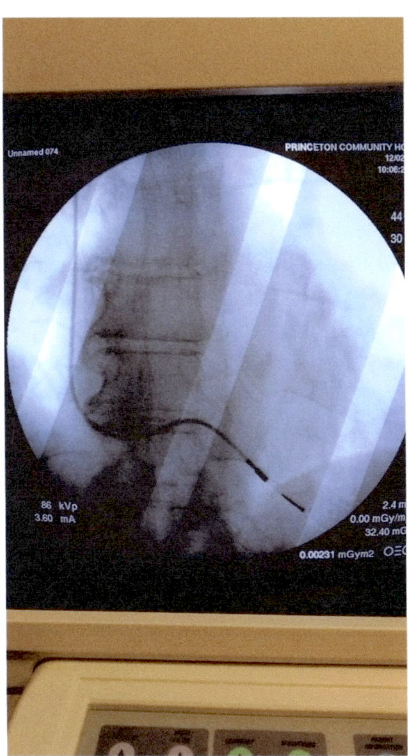

Fig. 20.9 Fluoroscopic view of ventricular lead in the right ventricular apex

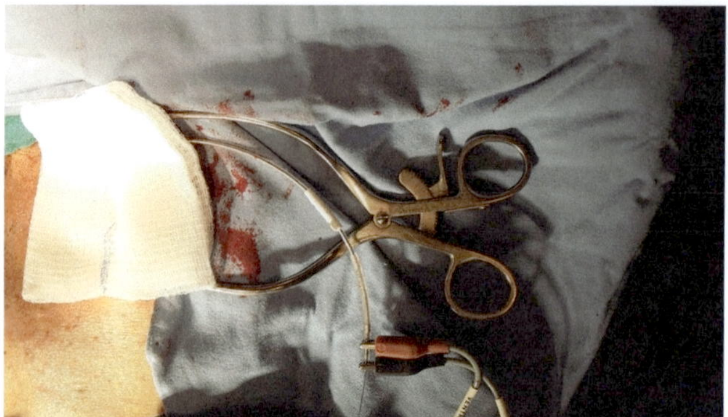

Fig. 20.10 Pacemaker cables attached to lead for pacemaker parameter measurements

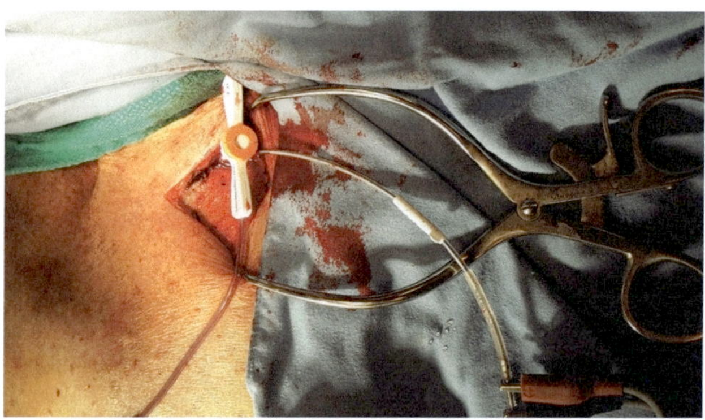

Fig. 20.11 Atrial introducer sheath in place adjacent to ventricular lead

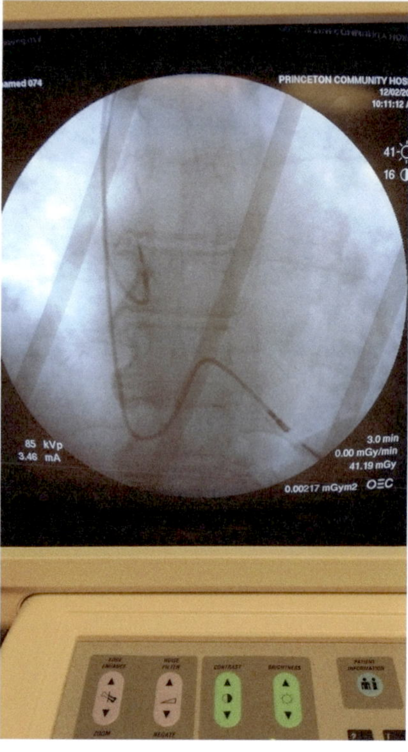

Fig. 20.12 Fluoroscopic view of both atrial and ventricular leads

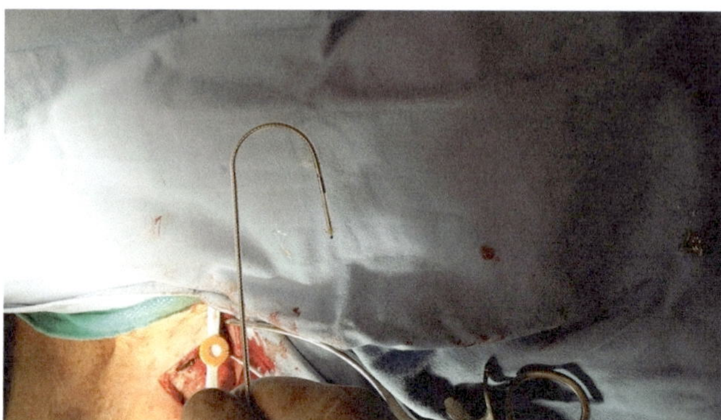

Fig. 20.13 Preformed curve of the atrial lead

the alligator-clipped cables onto the end of the lead in order to obtain and confirm adequate electrophysiologic parameters (Fig. 20.10). This is usually provided with the assistance of the pacemaker technician. Upon obtaining satisfactory cardiac parameters, the ventricular lead is secured in place and the atrial lead (if indicated) is inserted. The atrial introducer and sheath is inserted over the guidewire, which up to this point has been left in the subclavian vein. The guidewire is then removed leaving the introducer–sheath in place because typically the atrial introducer does not have a large enough bore to accommodate both the atrial lead and the guidewire, as was the case with the ventricular lead (Fig. 20.11). The atrial lead, with its guidewire, is inserted into the split sheath introducer. The introducer is removed leaving the lead in place. While visualizing under fluoroscopy, and while insuring that the ventricular lead is not dislodged, the atrial lead is inserted into the region of the right atrium–superior vena cava junction. The atrial lead's guidewire is partially withdrawn to allow the atrial lead to insinuate itself into the right atrial appendage (Fig. 20.12). Most atrial leads have a manufactured J-shaped configuration to allow for easier placement (Fig. 20.13). Once proper position is obtained, interrogation using the pacemaker cables is

performed to confirm that the atrial lead placement is optimal. Upon completion of the lead placement, the guidewires are removed completely from their respective leads and the leads are sutured to the pectoralis muscle fascia using 2-0 Surgidac/Ti-cron (Fig. 20.14).

Pulse Generator Placement

Most pacemakers today are termed "demand" pacemakers in which it will send a stimulating impulse through the wire lead if it senses that the patient's own natural heart rate drops below a certain set limit. They are also "programmable,"

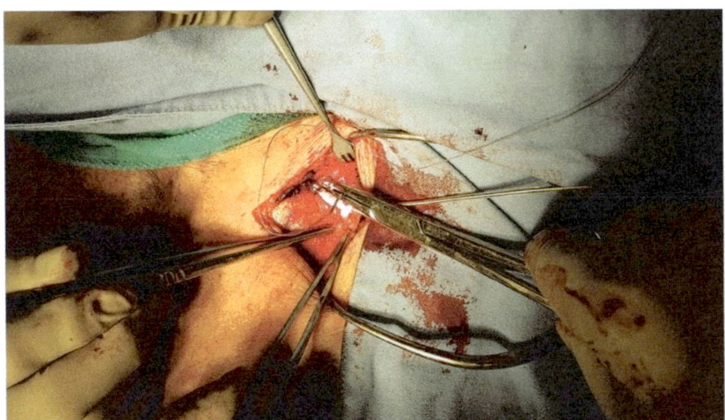

Fig. 20.14 Lead suture fixation to pectoralis fascia

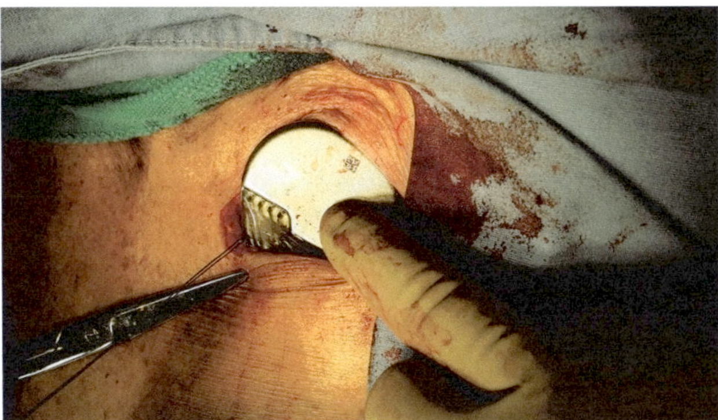

Fig. 20.16 Pulse generator suture fixation to pectoralis fascia

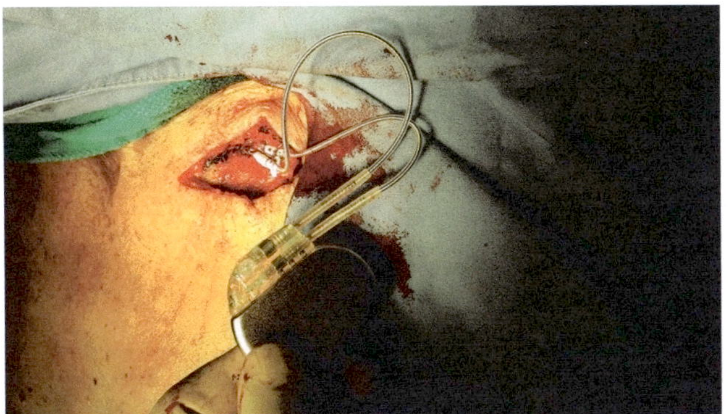

Fig. 20.15 Pulse generator and leads attached

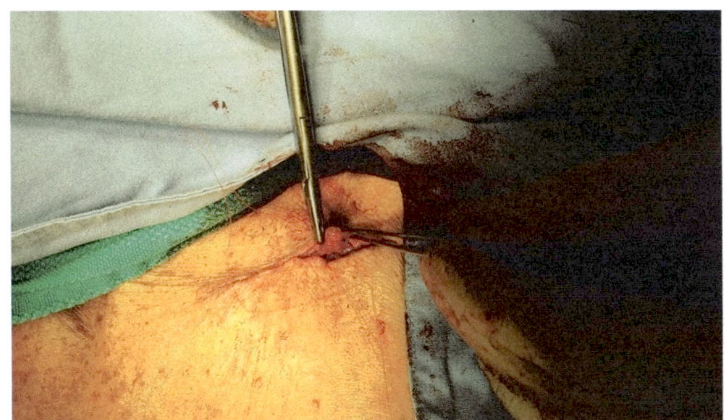

Fig. 20.17 Subcutaneous pocket closure with absorbable suture

where features such as rate, voltage output, sensitivity, and mode of pacing may be adjusted. The pacemaker lead(s) is (are) attached to the pacemaker pulse generator by inserting them into their respective plugs and securing them with the battery screwdriver that comes with the leads (Fig. 20.15). The excess length of pacemaker lead is coiled and placed into the pocket along with the pulse generator. There is a corresponding suture hole on the generator that allows for a 2-0 Surgidac/Ti-cron to be used to suture the generator securely to the pectoral fascia, thereby preventing potential dislodgement of the pacemaker lead(s) (Fig. 20.16). The subcutaneous pocket is then closed with absorbable sutures of 2-0 Polysorb/Vicryl and 5-0 Polysorb/Vicryl for the subcutaneous and subcuticular layers, respectively (Fig. 20.17). Steri-strips are then utilized for completion of the skin closure followed by a gauze dressing.

Potential Pitfalls

- Difficulty gaining venous access
- Difficulty with optimal ventricular lead placement
- Difficulty in properly placing the atrial lead in the atrial appendage. This is especially true if the patient has had open heart surgery and the atrial appendage is distorted or no longer accessible due to the cardiac bypass cannula having been placed through the appendage
- Dislodgement of the lead(s) from their optimal position
- Dislodgement of the pacemaker pulse generator

Postoperative Care

After completion of the procedure and before the patient is placed on a stretcher, a shoulder immobilizer is securely placed to prevent the patient from moving the arm and potentially dislodging the newly placed atrial/ventricular lead(s).

While in the recovery room, the pacemaker technician will perform a postoperative electrophysiologic evaluation on the newly placed pacemaker to ensure proper function.

Additionally, a portable AP chest radiograph is obtained in the recovery room in order to confirm adequate lead and battery positioning.

Once confirmation of both electrophysiologically and radiographically successful placement, the patient may be transferred out of the recovery area and observed on a telemetry unit.

IV antibiotics may be discontinued after 24 h.

Both oral and parenteral narcotics may be used for postoperative pain management.

After 24 h of observation on telemetry without any complications, the patient may be discharged to home.

The shoulder immobilizer may be discontinued after 5 days and switched to a shoulder/arm sling to be worn for 2 weeks. The patient is instructed to avoid lifting the arm above shoulder level during this time period.

Office appointment may be made for 2–3 weeks postoperatively.

Common Complications

- Pneumothorax/hemothorax
- Postoperative wound hematoma
- Dislodgement of pacemaker leads
- Failure of the pacemaker to capture
- Wound infection

When to Transfer

If unsuccessful in obtaining either venous access or proper placement of the pacemaker lead(s), place the patient back on the external pacemaker and seek transfer to a tertiary care facility.

Suggested Reading

1. Aggarwal RK, Connelly DT, Ray SG, Ball J, Charles RG. Early complications of permanent pacemaker implantation: no difference between dual and single chamber systems. Br Heart J. 1995;73(6): 571–5.
2. Armaganijan LV, Toff WD, Nielsen JC, Andersen HR, Connolly SJ, Ellenbogen KA, Healey JS. Are elderly patients at increased risk of complications following pacemaker implantation? A meta-analysis of randomized trials. Pacing Clin Electrophysiol. 2012;35(2):131–4.

The Vein Stripping Ablation and Phlebectomy

Robert Moglia

Indications (Fig. 21.1)

Vein surgery is appropriate for patients manifesting classic venous symptoms of aching leg pain with edema, visible varicose veins, and duplex ultrasound proven superficial venous incompetence.

Preoperative Preparation

A presurgical trial of elastic compression with symptom improvement is predictive of successful surgical results. All patients should have duplex sonographic proof of reflux greater than 0.5 s and saphenous vein diameter >5 mm. Immediately prior to surgery mapping the varicosities with the patient standing facilitates phlebectomy.

Operative Strategy

There are two components to surgery, which may be staged, by surgeons preference
1. Elimination of reflux: endovenous ablation vs. open stripping
2. Phlebectomy of varicosities

Operative Technique (Fig. 21.2)

1. Endovenous ablation using radiofrequency vs. laser energy. Although the hardware required differs somewhat the procedure is similar and entails:
   Ultrasound mapping of the GSV—facilitated by reverse Trendelenburg position.

   Accessing the GSV at the knee and insertion of a sheath to facilitate device insertion. The vein is accessed under ultrasound control using a micro catheter cannulation sheath and then a working sheath of 7F (RFA) or 5F (Laser) is inserted using Seldinger technique. The device is inserted no closer than 2 cm from SaphenoFemoral Junction (SFJ).
   Tumescent anesthesia is infiltrated under ultrasound control by hand or using an infusion pump.
   The patient is positioned in Trendelenburg and the device is activated per manufacturer's protocol.
   Completion ultrasonography to confirm successful treatment and to rule out deep venous thrombosis.
   Sheath removal and compression dressing.
2. Open stripping—Pin vs. Standard (Fig. 21.3)
   GSV at knee and SFJ at groin identified with ultrasound.
   1 cm incision at knee to isolate and control GSV. 2 cm incision at groin crease to isolate SFJ. All branches of SFJ ligated and divided.
   Transverse venotomy in GSV at knee after tying off distally with 3-0 silk ligature.
   Insert and advance internal stripper to groin.
   Flush ligate SFJ and divided GSV at groin and knee.
   Secure proximal end of GSV to stripping device.
   Apply traction to stripping device to remove GSV. The invagination (Pin) technique may be less traumatic in comparison to standard stripping. Incisions are closed with absorbable subcuticular suture.
3. Phlebectomy: With leg elevated for removal of varicosities which were marked preoperatively (Fig. 21.4)
   Small 3–6 mm stab incisions are made with an #11 scalpel.
   The varix is "snagged" with phlebectomy hooks, grasped with hemostats, and gently manipulated free. The placement of incisions is dictated by the length of vein segment removed, on an average every 5–10 cm. A typical case will require 10–15 incisions. All wounds are closed with steri strips and a pressure dressing is applied.

R. Moglia, M.D., F.A.C.S. (✉)
Vascular Surgery, Bassett Hospital, Cooperstown, NY 13326, USA
e-mail: robert.moglia@bassett.org

A.L. Halverson and D.C. Borgstrom (eds.), *Advanced Surgical Techniques for Rural Surgeons*,
DOI 10.1007/978-1-4939-1495-1_21, © Springer Science+Business Media New York 2015

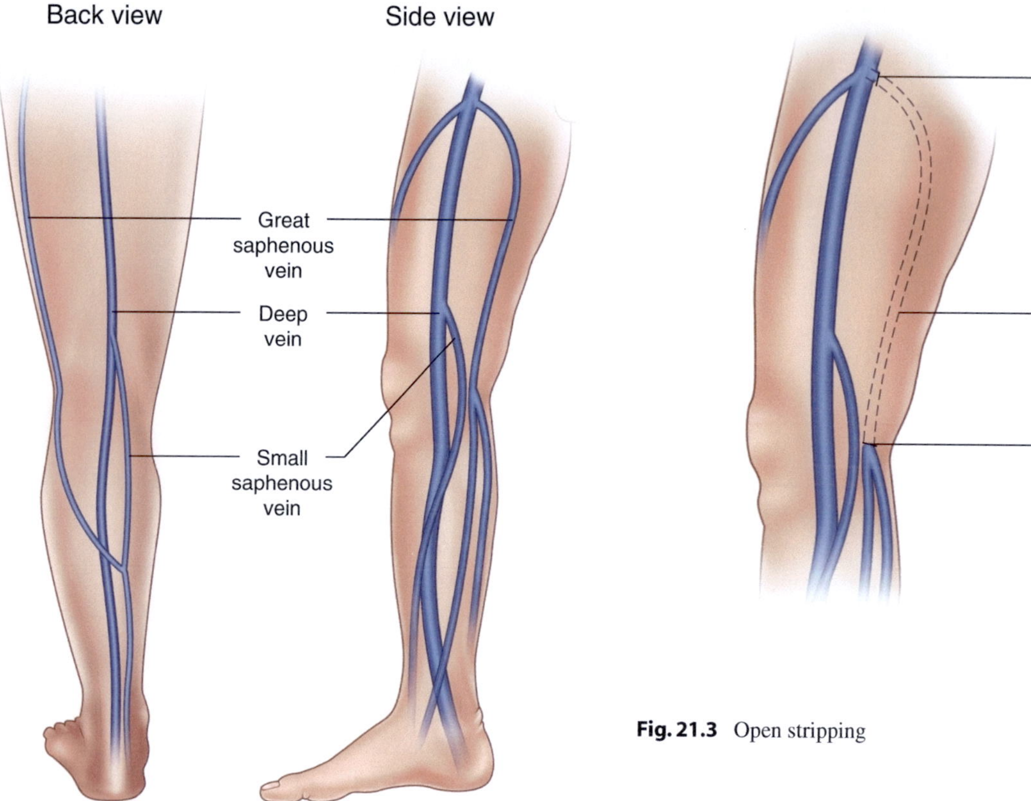

Fig. 21.1 Normal superficial venous anatomy

Fig. 21.3 Open stripping

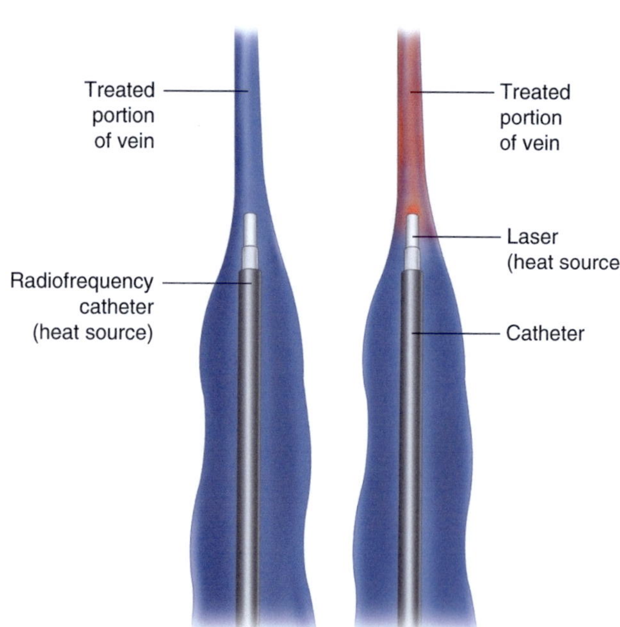

Fig. 21.2 Endovenous catheter mode of action

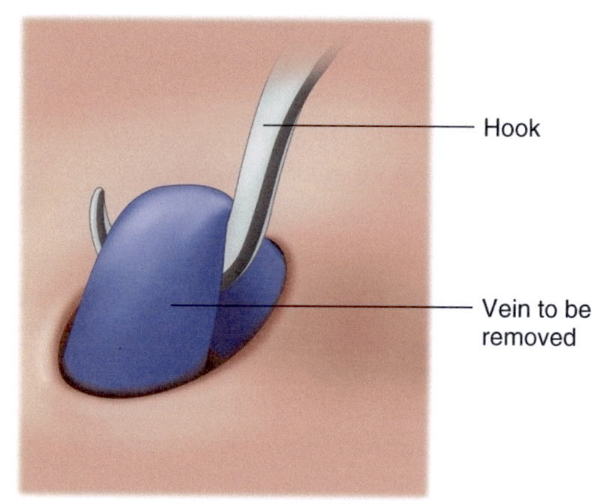

Fig. 21.4 Phlebectomy, magnified view

Postoperative Care

Patient remains in post-op dressing for 48 h. Upon removal a repeat duplex scan is obtained to confirm successful surgery and to rule out DVT. They are then placed in a thigh high compression garment for 2 weeks.

Potential Pitfalls

1. Inability to cannulate GSV at knee. Perform cutdown.
2. Inability to advance device. Insertion over a 0.014 guide-wire may help.
3. Intraoperative bleeding. Minimize with leg elevation.
4. Inability to "hook" veins. Minimize by thorough pre-op mapping.

Common Complications

Minor bruising is expected

Most common complication neuritis due to heat injury or direct trauma

DVT: very rare—anticoagulation

EHIT: endovenous heat induced injury, thrombus at SFJ may require anticoagulation—rare (1)

When to Transfer

Rarely required. If a patient has extensive DVT, postprocedure referral for possible thrombolysis.

Suggested Reading

Bisang U, Meier TO, Enzler M, et al. Results of endovenous closure fast treatment for varicose veins in an outpatient setting. Phlebology. 2012;27:118.

Rosales-Veldorrain A, Gloviczki P, Said SM, et al. Pulmonary embolism after endovenous thermal ablation of the saphenous vein. Semin Vasc Surg. 2013;26:14.

Sadek M, Kabnick LS, Rockman CB, et al. Increasing ablation distance peripheral to the saphenofemoral junction may results in a diminished rate of endothermal heat-induced thrombosis. J Vasc Surg. 2013;3:257.

Spreafico G, Piccioli A, Bernardi E, et al. Six year follow-up of endovenous laser ablation for great saphenous vein incompetence. J Vasc Surg. 2013;1:20.

Part VI

Trauma

Danny R. Robinette and William H. Montano

Indications

Traumatic brain injury (TBI) can be an injury associated with significant mortality and morbidity. Early intervention in surgical candidates can be life saving. Undertaking decompressive craniotomy as a rural surgeon can be extremely intimidating but can be done successfully with appropriate training. Certainly, transfer to a trauma center with neurosurgical capability best serves the brain-injured patient when at all possible. Severe injuries, however, may require early decompression to improve survival and functional capacity. If this procedure is something a rural surgeon plans to undertake, ideally there should be transfer arrangements with your referral center. Collaboration with your neurosurgical consultants is also preferable. Ultimately, the decision to intervene is made when your best judgment is that the delay in institution of treatment will cause harm to your patient. Once a decision has been made to intervene, decompressive craniotomy and control of bleeding is the treatment of choice. Burr holes alone do not generally result in adequate decompression.

The most common surgical approach for TBI is a wide frontotempoparietal craniotomy. Basilar and posterior fossa lesions are technically more demanding and associated with more significant risks of morbidity and mortality. Only surgeons with appropriate training and experience should undertake craniotomy for these lesions.

It is important to inform the patient's family that these are dire circumstances to avoid unrealistic expectations regarding outcomes.

The most common injuries for which decompressive craniotomy are performed are acute epidural hematomas and acute subdural hematomas. Additional lesions, which may require emergent decompression, include intracerebral hematomas, cerebral contusions, depressed skull fractures, and penetrating injuries. Specific indication varies by the type of injury (as do outcomes).

Acute Epidural Hematomas

These injuries often have better outcomes with appropriate and timely intervention, as there is generally less underlying damage to brain tissue.

Indications for decompression of acute epidural hematomas (Fig. 22.1):
Volume of hematoma >30 mL regardless of GCS
Midline shift >5 mm
GCS <9
Thickness of hematoma >15 mm
  Timing of intervention for acute epidural hematomas:
Surgery <2 h after loss of consciousness improves outcomes
Surgery <70 min after clinical signs of brain herniation
  improves outcomes
ASAP for GCS <9 with anisocoria

Acute Subdural Hematomas

These injuries frequently involve more serious damage to underlying brain tissues and often have more disability postinjury for that reason.

Indications for decompression of acute subdural hematomas (Fig. 22.2):
Thickness >10 mm
Midline shift >5 mm
Comatose patient with <10 mm thickness or <5 mm midline shift and either ICP >20 mmHg, pupil abnormalities, or deterioration of 2 or more points in GCS

D.R. Robinette, M.D., F.A.C.S. (✉)
Department of Surgery, University of Washington,
Fairbanks, AK 99701, USA
e-mail: drrobinette@gmail.com

W.H. Montano, M.D., D.D.S., F.A.C.S.
William Montano, MD, Inc., 1919 Lathrop, Suite 204,
Fairbanks, AK 99701, USA

A.L. Halverson and D.C. Borgstrom (eds.), *Advanced Surgical Techniques for Rural Surgeons,*
DOI 10.1007/978-1-4939-1495-1_22, © Springer Science+Business Media New York 2015

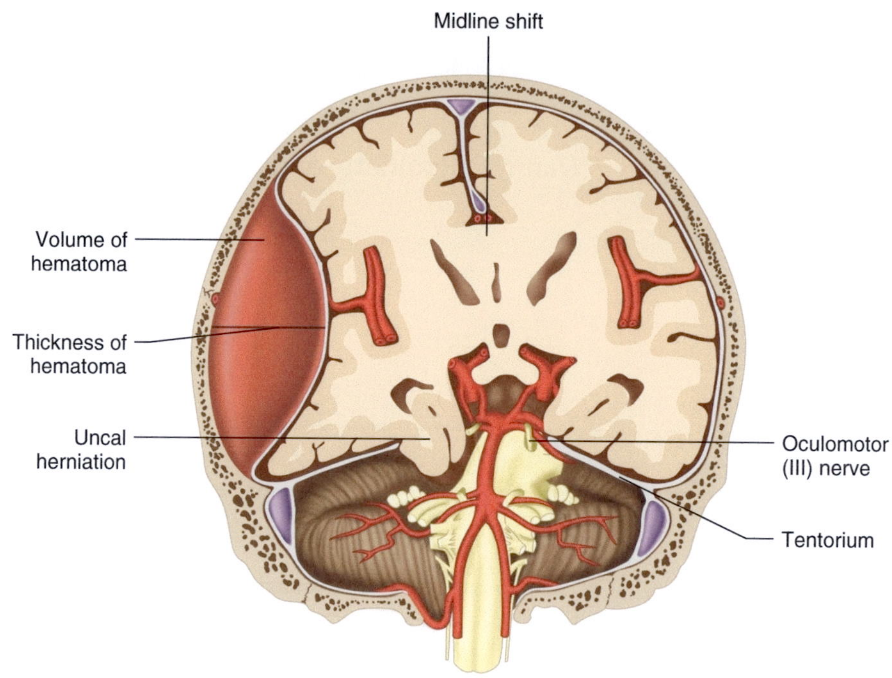

Fig. 22.1 Indications for surgery for acute epidural hematoma

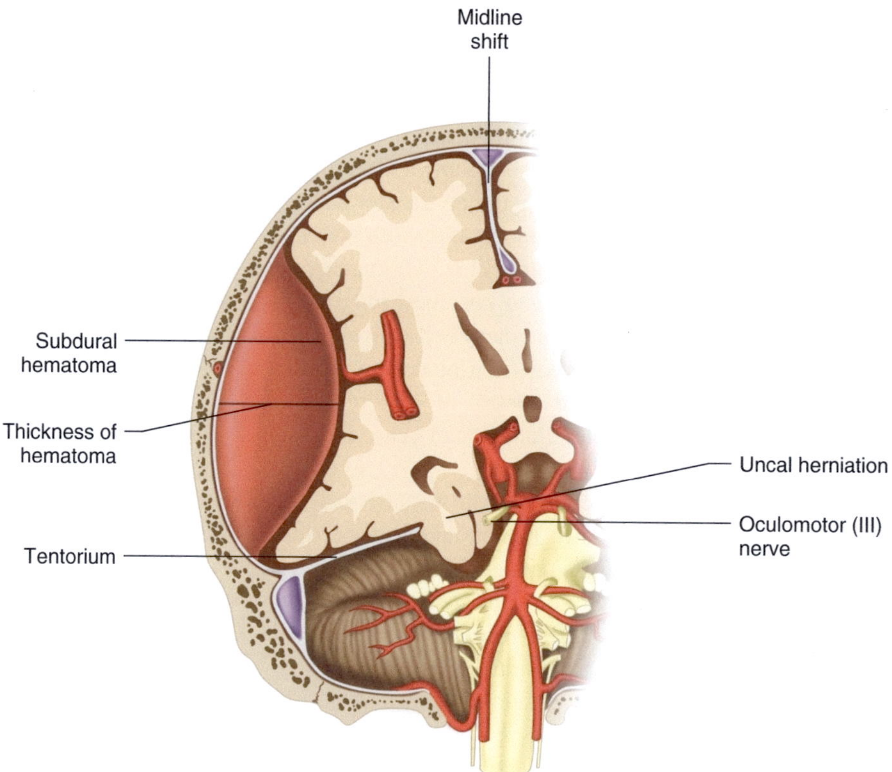

Fig. 22.2 Indications for surgery acute subdural hematoma

Timing of intervention for acute subdural hematomas:
Stronger correlation between time of onset of coma/deterioration to surgery than of time from injury to surgery
Surgery <2 h after onset of coma/deterioration improves outcomes
Surgery <3 h after clinical signs of herniation improves outcomes

Other Injuries

Indications for decompression of intracerebral hematomas, depressed skull fractures, penetrating injuries, etc.:
Midline shift >5 mm
Pupillary abnormalities
Deterioration of 2 or more points in GCS

Timing of intervention:

Stronger correlation between time of onset of coma/deterioration to surgery than of time from injury to surgery

Surgery <2 h after onset of coma/deterioration improves outcomes

Surgery <3 h after clinical signs of herniation improves outcomes

Preoperative Preparation

Preoperative evaluation and preparation is dependent upon the nature of the patient's injuries. Multisystem trauma patients should be managed by ATLS priorities to stabilize life-threatening injuries first. Even transient hypoxia or hypotension has a significant negative impact on neurologic outcomes for patients with TBI. Hypotension in multitrauma patients is most likely secondary to extracranial injury and rarely caused by TBI. Control of airway, respirations, and hemorrhage take priority over cranial decompression and should be dealt with first.

Patients requiring decompressive craniotomy should be treated with Mannitol (dose of 0.5–1.0 g/kg) preoperatively to help reduce intracranial pressure (ICP) and improve cerebral perfusion pressure. Other measures to reduce ICP include modest hyperventilation (only as a temporizing measure prior to surgery), hypertonic saline, and diuretics. The use of steroids is not indicated. Prophylactic antibiotics (usually Cefazolin) are used in our practice. As these patients are not typically mobile, they do have risk of venous thromboembolism (VTE). Mechanical VTE prophylaxis with sequential compression devices is certainly warranted. Pharmacologic VTE prophylaxis can be considered postoperatively on an individual case basis. The scalp is clipped with electric clippers immediately prior to surgery and skin preparation.

Patient positioning is important as well. Injury to a dural sinus (either from the trauma or intraoperative) can occur. In that event, raising the head as much as possible (reverse trendelenberg and/or sitting position) can significantly reduce the volume of bleeding. Angulation of the neck with resultant compression of the jugular veins can also increase venous backpressure. We prefer to have the ability to adjust the head position during the procedure (with cervical spine precautions) so we use a gel doughnut to hold the head. If the spine has been cleared radiologically, then position the patient's hips to allow a sitting position if needed. If the spine has not been cleared, then the patient must remain level from the hips up by flexing the bed at the hips. In the absence of clearance of the cervical spine (and associated abdominal or thoracic injuries requiring surgery) the patient may be placed in a lateral position to protect the cervical spine.

Operative Strategy

The principal goal of decompressive craniotomy is to reduce ICP and improve cerebral perfusion by adequate decompression of the brain and control of ongoing bleeding to prevent recurrence. This requires adequate exposure in order to accomplish these goals.

Secondary goals (but also of prime importance) are to prevent further progression of brain injury and secondary injury due to operative trauma.

Operative Technique

After induction of anesthesia, appropriate positioning, skin prep, and draping, a question mark incision is marked just anterior to the tragus. It is also a good idea to mark the midline to help avoid injury to the sagittal sinus. The incision should start at the level of the zygoma. The incision should be carried through the skin, galea, and down to the bone. It should be extended well posterior to the ear then curve a few centimeters lateral to the sagittal suture and continue forward to the hairline. The superficial temporal artery should be preserved if possible to improve blood supply to the flap. Bleeding from the skin incision (which can be significant) can be controlled by various means. Most common is the use of Raney clips (if available). If you have these, the incision can be made in segments and the clips applied to each segment before continuing the incision. More likely in a rural setting, you will not have access to these. We use the cautery (with coagulation set to 50) and have been able to achieve excellent hemostasis with this (Fig. 22.3a).

The temporal burr hole (also known as the key hole) (Fig. 22.3b) can then be made before raising the entire flap. In the event of rapid deterioration, this burr hole can quickly be enlarged to allow for at least partial decompression prior to proceeding with the craniotomy.

The next step is the muscle and soft tissue dissection. The musculocutaneous flap is developed and reflected anteriorly. This should be extended down to the root of the zygoma and as far below the keyhole as possible (Fig. 22.4).

After completion of the flap, several burr holes are made (3–5). The initial burr hole is the keyhole. In severe cases, the keyhole can be enlarged carefully with a rongeur and a cruciate dural incision can be made to provide partial drainage while completing the craniectomy (Fig. 22.5). The bone flap should be at least 10 × 15 cm in size in an adult patient to provide adequate exposure. The superior extent of the bone flap should be at least 1.5 cm below the midline to avoid injury to the sagittal sinus and granulations. Making the burr holes can be done with a powered self-arresting perforator (if available). If you do not have access

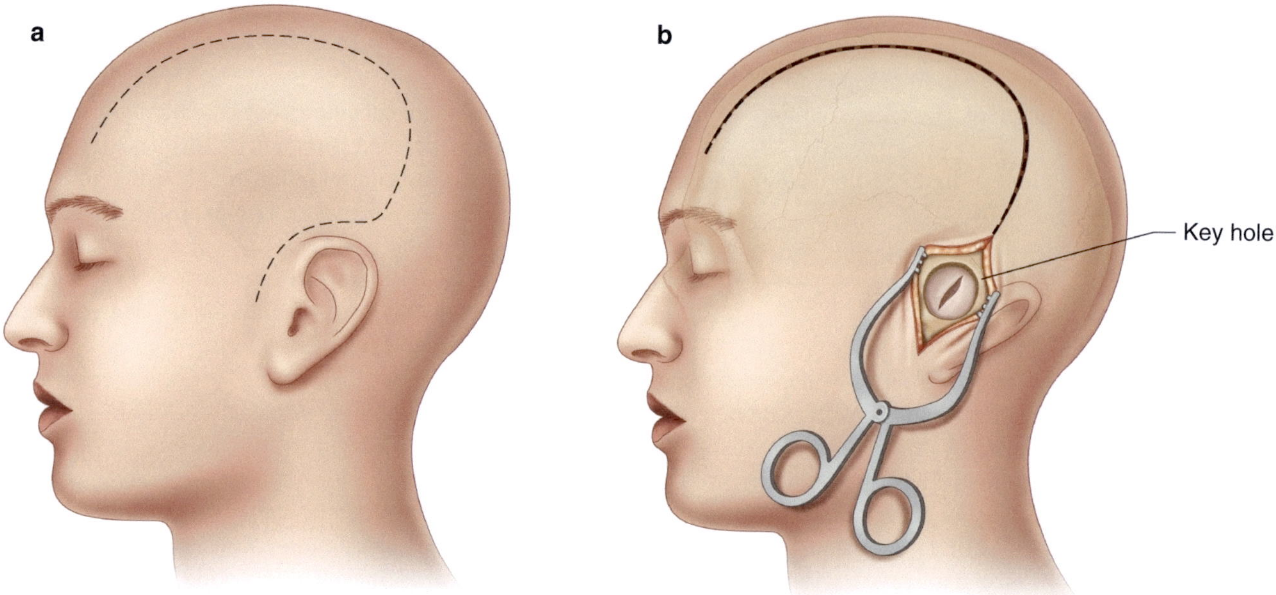

Fig. 22.3 (**a**) Skin incision for trauma craniotomy. (**b**) Keyhole incision

Fig. 22.4 Myocutaneous flap

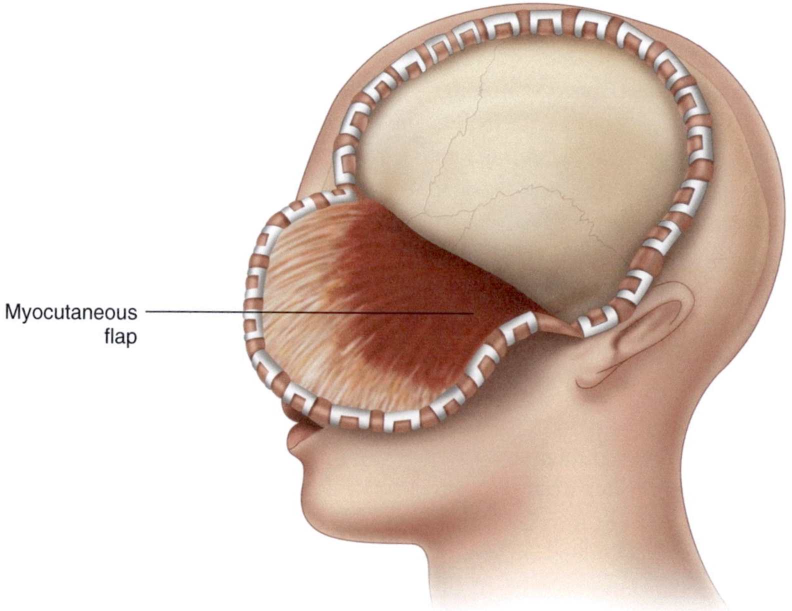

to a perforator, this can be done carefully with a hand drill. The dura is freed from the bone gently at each burr hole working in the direction of the next burr hole. This can be done with a Penfield No. 3 (a small malleable retractor can be used instead).

The burr holes are then connected either with a high-speed powered saw or a Gigli saw. The underlying dura and brain can be protected during this portion either with a Gigli guide or a narrow malleable retractor. Use of the Gigli makes a nice beveled cut in the bone and results in a more stable bone flap (if the bone is to be replaced). There are a few key tips in using the Gigli. The angle between the two sides of the saw blade should be as close to 180° as possible. A more acute angle results in bowstringing and can injure the underlying brain. Both hands should move gently back and forth simultaneously in the same direction (like using a two-handed scythe) rather than moving the hands rapidly in opposing directions (Fig. 22.6).

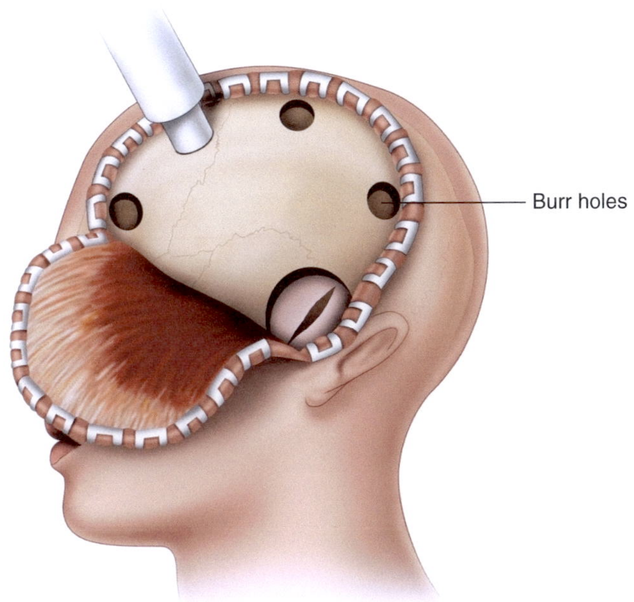

Fig. 22.5 Burr holes

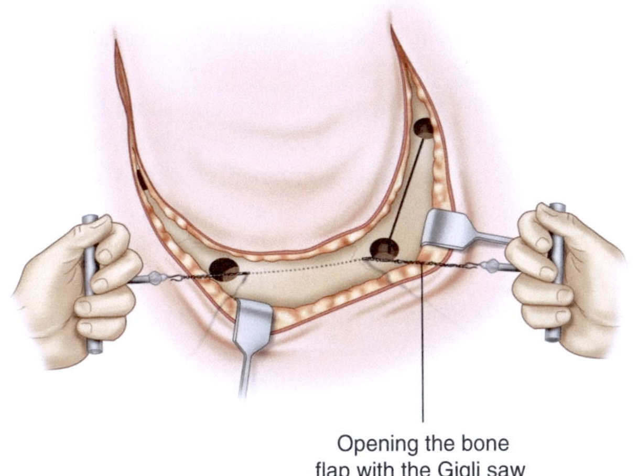

Fig. 22.6 Opening the bone flap with the Gigli saw

After removal of the bone flap, we then use a red rubber catheter and warm saline to irrigate any blood or clot off the dural surface. Any epidural bleeding is then controlled with suture ligation (we use a 5-0 proline on a vascular needle). Bleeding from the middle fossa may necessitate removal of addition temporal bone and exploration to control the bleeding. A rongeur can be used to remove additional temporal bone down to the floor of the middle fossa. One must take care with the rongeur to avoid twisting or torque as this may displace a basilar skull fracture and increase bleeding.

The dura is opened in a stellate manner (Y or X pattern) basing the superior dural flap in the superior sagittal sinus (Fig. 22.7). This should be done slowly and carefully. Rapid dural opening can result in cardiovascular collapse due to sudden reversal of elevated ICP and subsequent loss of the catecholamine support associated with the Cushing response. Adequate volume resuscitation can ameliorate or prevent this response. Care should also be taken to avoid (if possible) injury to the vein of Trolard or the vein of Labbé. If these must be sacrificed, then ligation should be accomplished away from the junction with the draining sinus to prevent bleeding from the sinus.

Again gentle irrigation with warm saline is used to remove blood and clot. Bleeding from the draining veins should be controlled with suture ligation. The bipolar cautery on a setting of 15–20 can be useful as well. Following control of bleeding and evacuation of hematoma, dural closure can be accomplished. If there is significant brain swelling, multiple small relaxing incisions can be made in the dura to allow closure. Duraplasty can be performed if necessary (as discussed in the next section). We place two closed suction drains through separate stab wounds remote from the skin incision in the subarachnoid and epidural spaces. With significant brain swelling, the skull flap can be left off to allow expansion (a craniectomy) and cranioplasty can be accomplished later. The skull flap may be preserved either by implantation in a subcutaneous pocket in the abdominal wall or cryopreservation (less widely available). Both methods have comparable (and acceptably low) subsequent infection rates.

If the skull flap is to be replaced, small holes can be drilled in the bone flap and the adjacent skull (protecting the underlying tissues with a small malleable) to permit suturing the bone flap in pace. The galea is then closed with multiple closely spaced absorbable sutures. The skin can be closed with staples or a running absorbable monofilament. While the latter closure takes a bit more time, it is more watertight and less prone to CSF leak through the wound.

Potential Pitfalls

Injury to a dural sinus can be a difficult problem encountered during this procedure. Elevation of the head as much as possible will decrease venous backpressure and reduce the rate of blood loss. Gentle direct pressure can be applied as well. The injury can either be sutured primarily or patched with temporalis fascia from the scalp flap to control bleeding. Attention to dural sinus anatomy when taking off the skull flap can reduce the likelihood on this problem (Fig. 22.8).

Bleeding from injury to the middle meningeal artery can occur within the base of the skull and give rise to an epidural hematoma. In this event, one must expose the foramen spinosum and plug the foramen to obtain control of the

Fig. 22.7 Dural incision

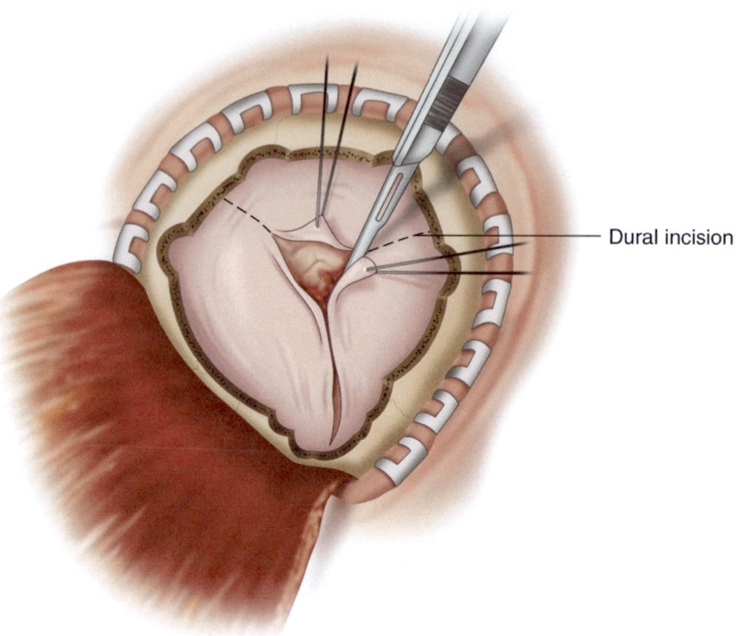

bleeding (Fig. 22.9). There is a plug (used by neurosurgeons) for this purpose. I suspect (as in our institution) that you will not have that plug available. We have had success with using fibrin glue, direct pressure over the ostia, and a small stainless steel screw from an orthopedic set to achieve control in this situation.

Incomplete re-expansion of the brain may allow an air gap between the brain and the skull, which will allow fluid to accumulate. This can result in recurrent compression of the brain. Volume expansion prior to closure can alleviate this problem. Dural replacements can be a biologic graft (not likely available in your facility if you do not have neurosurgery), calvarial periosteum, temporalis fascia, or fascia lata from the thigh. Another option is to leave the skull flap off and suture the temporalis fascia to the dural margins.

Oozing from the dura can also be an issue that can be difficult to control at times. Prominent bleeding should be controlled. Leaving the skull flap off and suturing the temporalis fascia to the dural margins can also control diffuse oozing. A closed suction drain in this space will get tissue adherence and reduce extradural fluid accumulation.

Contralateral skull fractures (opposite to the injury leading to surgery) can be associated with early postoperative epidural hematoma formation on the side opposite to the craniotomy and early postoperative herniation. Keep a high index of suspicion in this setting.

Postoperative Care

Postoperative care of the patient with TBI is complex and best accomplished in a trauma center with critical care and neurosurgery support.

These patients will need ICU care and should have ICP monitoring postoperatively. Most rural hospitals are not likely to have the necessary equipment or expertise to manage these patients effectively. Interim management while stabilizing the patient and awaiting transfer should be expected to be complex. We suggest involvement of your hospitalists or internists to facilitate management of the complex issues that frequently arise.

The Guidelines for Management of Severe Brain Trauma in suggested reading has an extensive discussion of management principles should transfer not be feasible in a short time frame.

Common Complications

The majority of morbidity and mortality associated with this procedure is due to the underlying injury. Morbidity of the procedure itself is mostly due to wound complication such as CSF leak or traumatic injury to the skin in the region of the incision.

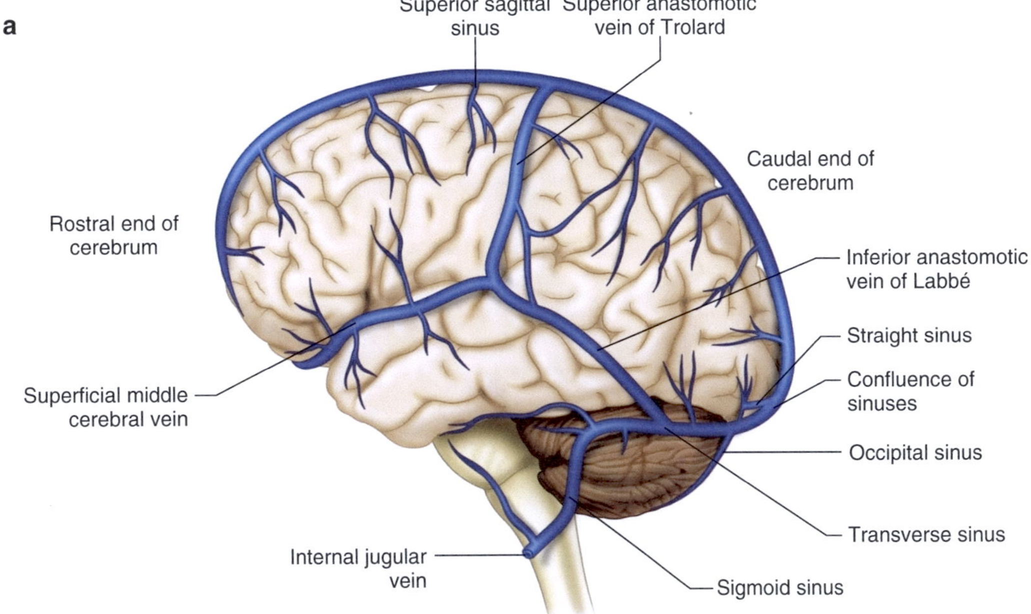

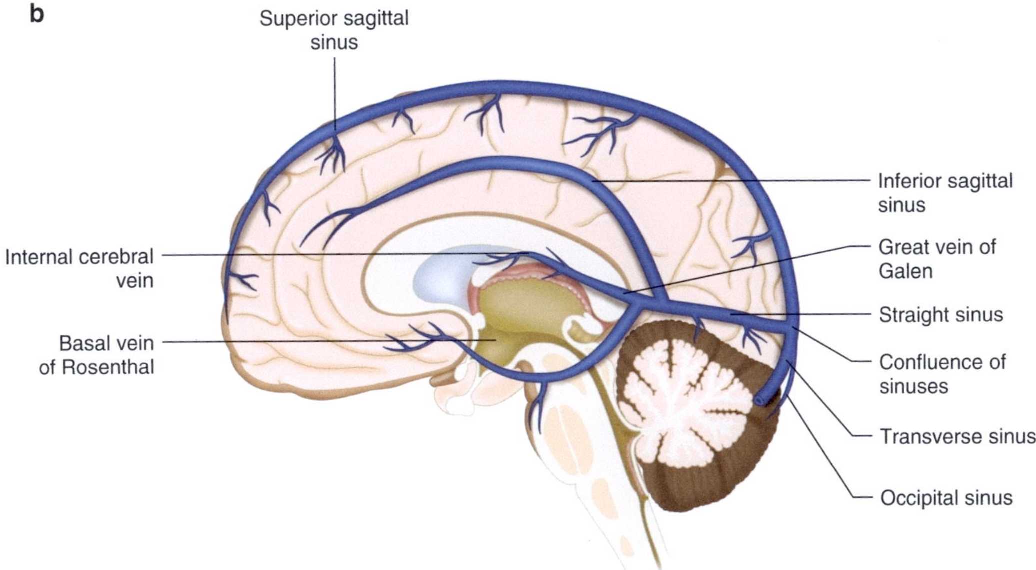

Fig. 22.8 Dural sinuses

Early complications:

Recurrent hemorrhage—best avoided, but if this occurs it may require re-exploration

Seizures—Phenytoin may be used in the first 2 weeks postop to reduce incidence of early posttraumatic seizures

SIADH—should be differentiated from central salt wasting syndrome

Neurogenic Pulmonary Edema—secondary to massive sympathetic discharge due to elevated ICP. Treatment is directed at reducing ICP; alpha blockers to control BP, and respiratory support

Elevated ICP—best managed with ICP monitoring

DIC—TBI is a risk factor for DIC

Neurologic defects—prolonged coma is not unusual

Infection

CSF leak

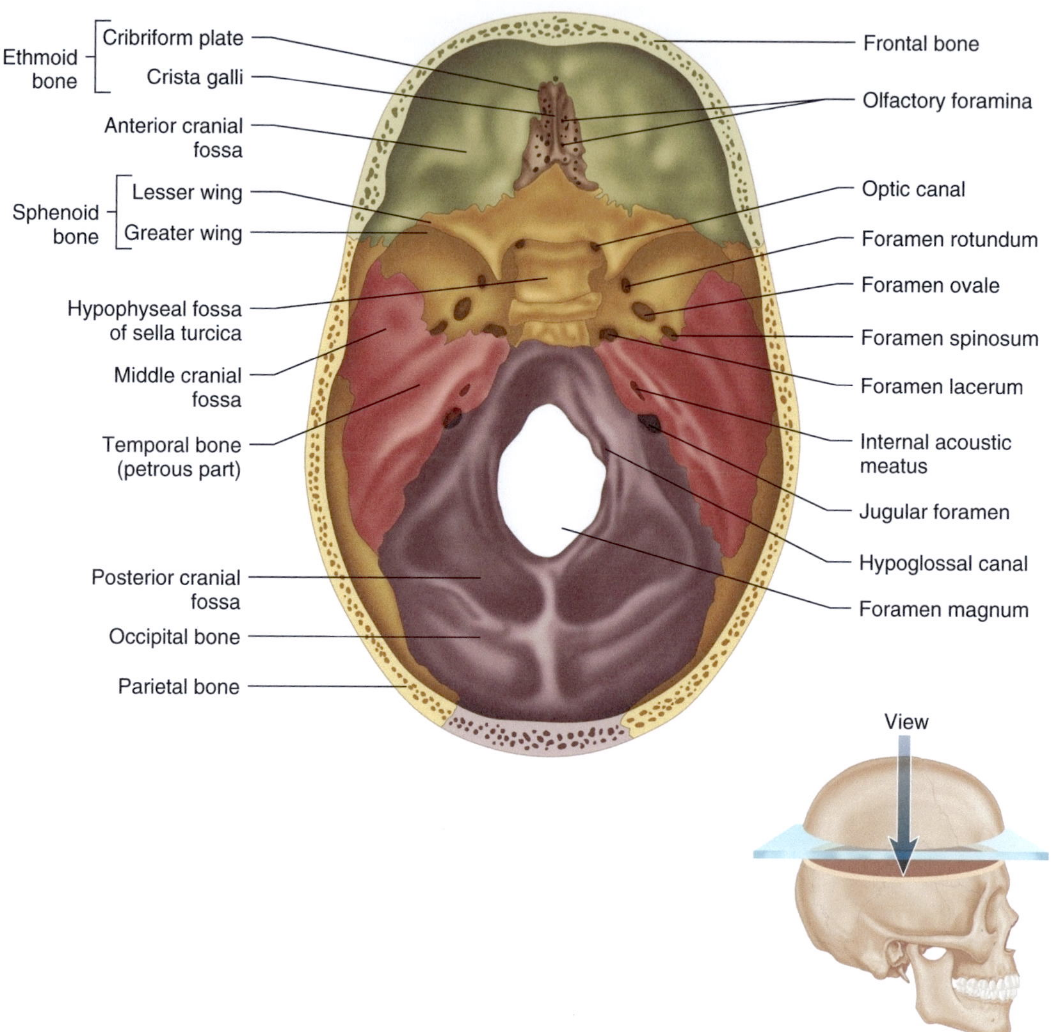

Fig. 22.9 Foramen spinosum

Late complications:

Late posttraumatic seizures—up to 50 % off penetrating injuries; ranging from 9 to 42 % in blunt trauma.

Neurologic deficits—prolonged or permanent deficits occur frequently

When to Transfer

Postoperative management of brain-injured patients is complex. Transfer should be initiated as soon after surgery as possible. These patients should be transferred to a trauma center with neurosurgical care. Ideally these arrangements can be made as part of the decision to perform the emergent craniotomy.

The majority of these patients will require ICP monitoring and appropriate therapy for elevated ICP to maximize brain perfusion.

It is our opinion that a rural surgeon contemplating this sort of intervention should spend some time developing a good collegial relationship with their consulting neurosurgical group where possible. Some time spent learning techniques for craniotomy (even if just observation of a few cases) should be considered a necessity. These operations are technically demanding and should not be undertaken lightly. The ability to consult the neurosurgeon (and electronically review films with your consultant) prior to intervention is extremely helpful. Ideally the consultants can assist with the decision whether to transfer the patient initially or to intervene prior to transfer.

Suggested Reading

The Brain Trauma Foundation. Guidelines for the management of severe traumatic brain injury [Internet]. 3rd ed. New York: The Brain Trauma Foundation; 2007. http://www.braintrauma.org/coma-guidelines/searchable-guidelines/.

The Brain Trauma Foundation. Guidelines for the surgical management of traumatic brain injury [Internet]. New York: The Brain Trauma Foundation; 2006. http://www.braintrauma.org/coma-guidelines/searchable-guidelines/.

Jandial R, McCormick P, Black P. Core techniques in operative neurosurgery. Philadelphia: Saunders; 2011.

Sakamoto GT, Shuer LM, Chang SD. Craniotomy in trauma. In: Jaffe RA, Samuels SI, Schmiesing CA, Golianu B, editors. Anesthesiologist's manual of surgical procedures. 3rd ed. Philadelphia: Lippincott Williams & Wilkins; 2009.

David C. Borgstrom

Indications

The primary indication for tracheostomy is prolonged pulmonary failure and the need for extended mechanical ventilation. Current literature is unclear as to the value of early tracheostomy mostly because of the difficulty with predicting the need for prolonged mechanical ventilation. A tracheostomy improves patient comfort and eases nursing care by facilitating the clearance of airway secretions. There is not a clear benefit from the standpoint of reduction of ventilator days or ventilator-associated pneumonia.

Cricothyroidotomy is indicated for the emergent management of an airway after failed attempts of nasotracheal or endotracheal intubation, most typically in a trauma setting, but it may be necessary at other times with loss of airway control.

Operative Strategy

It is important to start with adequate patient positioning. A small folded blanket behind the patient's shoulders provides gentle extension of the neck. It is important to avoid hyperextension of the neck (Fig. 23.1). In a patient with suspected cervical spine injury, the neck should remain immobilized to prevent spinal cord injury. Before starting a procedure it is important to have all necessary equipment available including electrocautery and adequate suction. Select the appropriate sized tube for the patient. A number 7 or 8 tracheostomy tube is suitable for the average adult. An endotracheal tube should be used for cricothyroidotomy. The flexibility of the tube facilitates ease of delivery into the trachea. The largest size that can fit through an adult cricothyroid membrane is a 6 endotracheal tube. Before starting, test the tube balloon

D.C. Borgstrom, M.D., F.A.C.S. (⊠)
Department of Surgery, Bassett Medical Center,
Cooperstown, NY 13326, USA
e-mail: david.borgstrom@bassett.org

and lubricate it with a sterile lubricant. Have a soft rubber suction catheter available on the sterile field for suctioning of the trachea after tube insertion. A properly placed incision and careful identification of anatomic landmarks are important for correct placement of tracheostomy or cricothyroidotomy (Fig. 23.2). Postoperative wound infections are rare and prophylactic antibiotics are generally not necessary.

Tracheostomy

Operative Technique

A transverse incision is made two finger breadths above the sternal notch. This transverse incision is taken down through the platysma and then all work subsequently is in the midline between the strap muscles (Fig. 23.3). The midline trachea is identified. The optimal placement is through the third tracheal ring, although this may be difficult in some patients based upon the length of their neck and their anatomy. Typically the isthmus of the thyroid is overlying the second and third tracheal ring. Division of the isthmus allows visualization of the third tracheal ring and mobilization of the thyroid gland off the trachea laterally. The isthmus is transected with cautery and then suture ligated with a braided suture on a robust needle (an MO-6 needle) (Fig. 23.4). This suture is then used for retraction of the soft tissues to gain better access to the trachea.

Stay sutures are placed around the third ring if possible, or the second if necessary. At this point in the procedure there is the risk of puncturing the endotracheal tube balloon. The risk of balloon perforation may be diminished by having anesthesia personnel untape the endotracheal tube and deliver the endotracheal tube deeper into the trachea so that the balloon will assuredly be below the level of the operative exposure. The stay suture should be placed with the same robust needle around the third tracheal ring as laterally as possible. The sutures that were used to retract the isthmus of the thyroid are then cut. An H-type incision is made through

A.L. Halverson and D.C. Borgstrom (eds.), *Advanced Surgical Techniques for Rural Surgeons*,
DOI 10.1007/978-1-4939-1495-1_23, © Springer Science+Business Media New York 2015

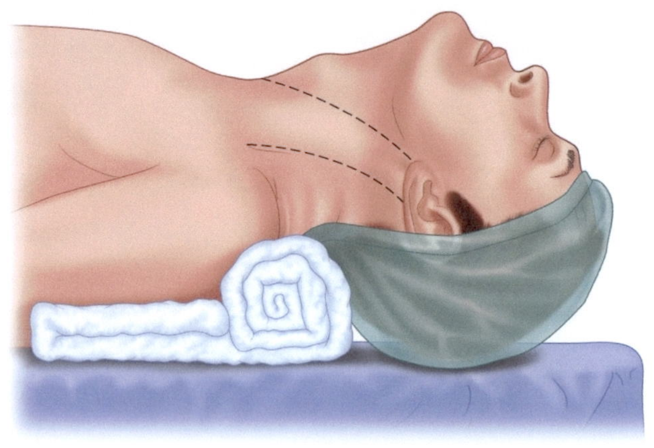

Fig. 23.1 Optimal patient positioning for tracheostomy

the third tracheal ring (Fig. 23.5). A tracheostomy spreader is then carefully used. The endotracheal tube is visualized and then slowly withdrawn. Once the endotracheal tube is pulled back to just proximal to the opening in the trachea, the tracheostomy tube is inserted. Some surgeons prefer to deliver the tube into the trachea when the angle is facing the patient's head and then rotate it 180° once it is in the trachea and deliver it down into the trachea (Fig. 23.6). The tracheostomy tube is then rotated into final position. When placing the tracheostomy tube, the only retraction necessary is the two stay sutures in the lateral trachea.

The ventilator is then hooked up to the tracheostomy tube and confirmed to be adequately placed with ease of ventilation and return of CO_2 by anesthesia. The stay sutures that were left in place of the third tracheal ring are then loosely

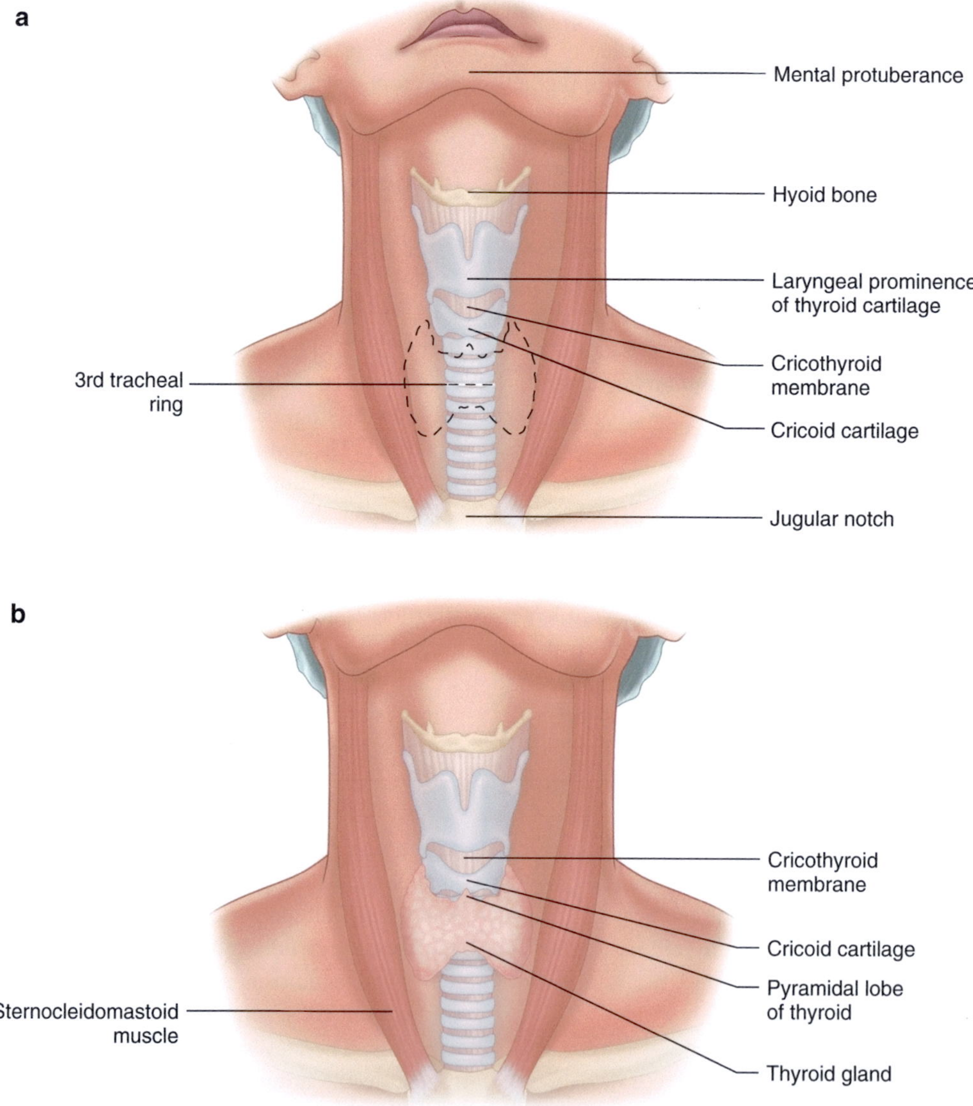

Fig. 23.2 Important neck anatomy for tracheostomy

Fig. 23.3 Transverse incision two fingers above clavicular notch

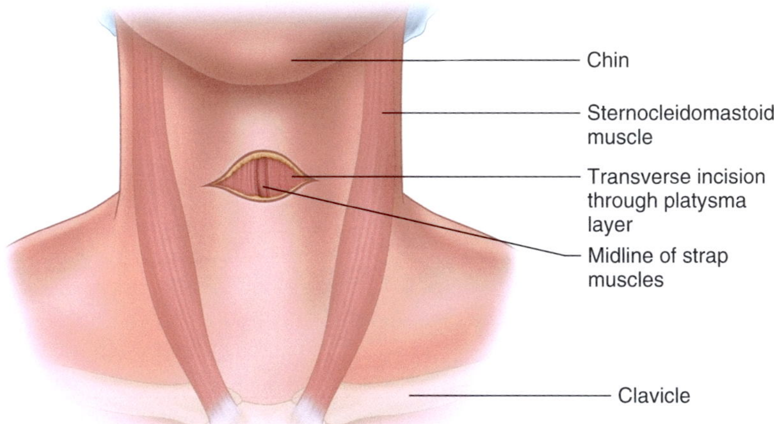

Fig. 23.4 Isthmus of the thyroid often must be divided

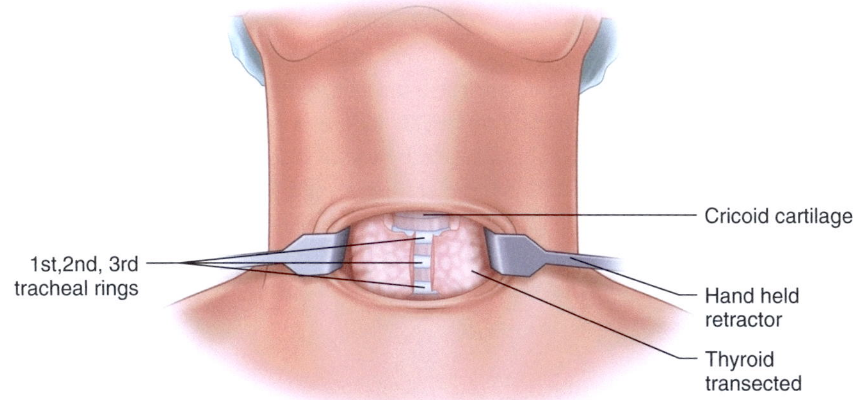

Fig. 23.5 H-type incision through third ring with stay sutures around lateral third ring

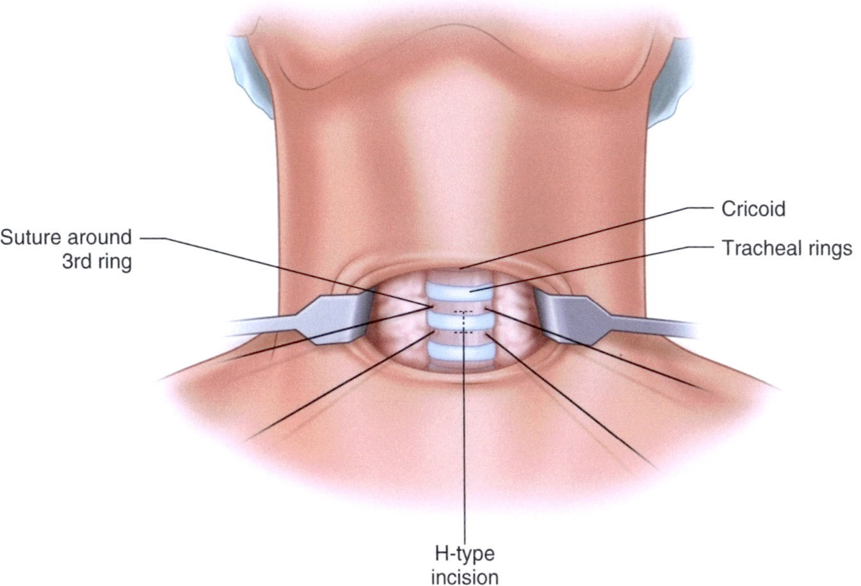

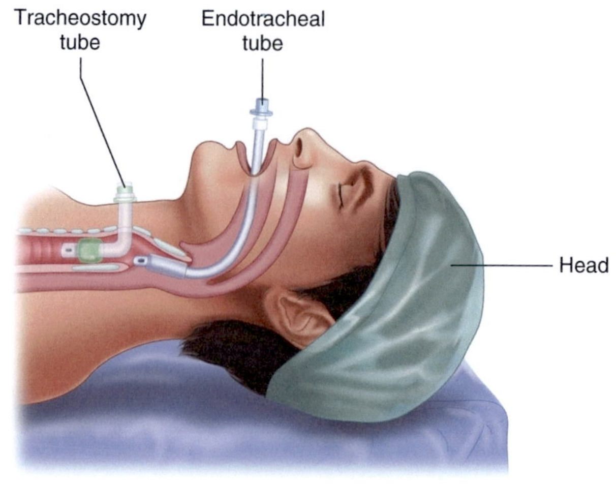

Fig. 23.6 Tracheostomy tube enters trachea best when oriented toward the head

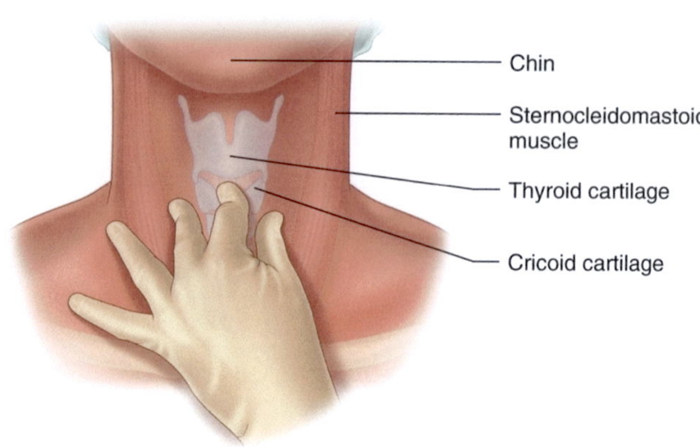

Fig. 23.7 Trachea is immobilized against the spine with the nondominant hand

taped with steri strips to the patient's anterior chest and tracheostomy tube is secured with sutures on the skin flange.

Complications of early tracheostomy cuff failure or inadvertent decannulation are readily managed by use of the stay sutures taped to the chest wall as these are usually the only retraction needed for tube placement. These are left in for about 7 days. Subsequent to that, tracheostomy tube change can easily be made without additional retraction or exposure.

Pitfalls of Tracheostomy

Pitfalls of tracheostomy are in getting away from the midline and not identifying the proper trachea anatomy. Stay sutures left in place for up to 1 week reduce the primary concern, which is tube dislodgement in the early postoperative period. Leaving these sutures in place makes the first tracheostomy exchange far easier.

Cricothyroidotomy

Operative Technique

It is important to understand that cricothyroidotomy should be done by feel. In the emergent setting it is often difficult to visualize all the layers and anatomy through the process. Since it is emergent, it needs to be done expeditiously.

Right-handed surgeons stand on the patient's left side, working with the right hand from the patient's head, facing down toward their body. Left-handed surgeons would stand on the patient's right. Prior to beginning it is important to have all the necessary tools.

Landmarks are identified with the nondominant thumb and middle finger, immobilizing the patient's trachea against their cervical spine. The nondominant index finger is used to identify the cricothyroid membrane. From this point forward the nondominant hand should remain in position to immobilize the patient's trachea and assure that continued dissection stays in the midline. The nondominant index finger is moved out of the way and a vertical incision is made in the patient's neck overlying the cricothyroid membrane using a 15 blade scalpel (Fig. 23.7). This incision must be big enough to easily facilitate airway access and may be extended if exposure is difficult. After an incision is made, the position is reconfirmed with the nondominant index finger, the dissection is continued in the midline until the superior and inferior edges of the cricothyroid membrane and the midportion of the membrane itself are clearly defined. The scalpel blade is used to create an opening in the cricothyroid membrane. The back end of the scalpel can then bluntly enlarge this opening (Fig. 23.8). The endotracheal tube is then delivered through the cricothyroid membrane into the trachea (Fig. 23.9). The nondominant hand is not released until appropriate placement is confirmed by anesthesia.

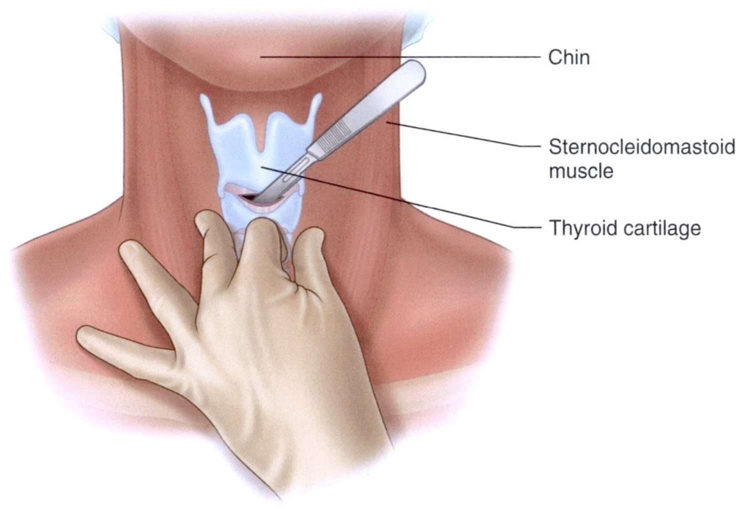

Fig. 23.8 Cricothyroid membrane incision is enlarged with the scalpel handle

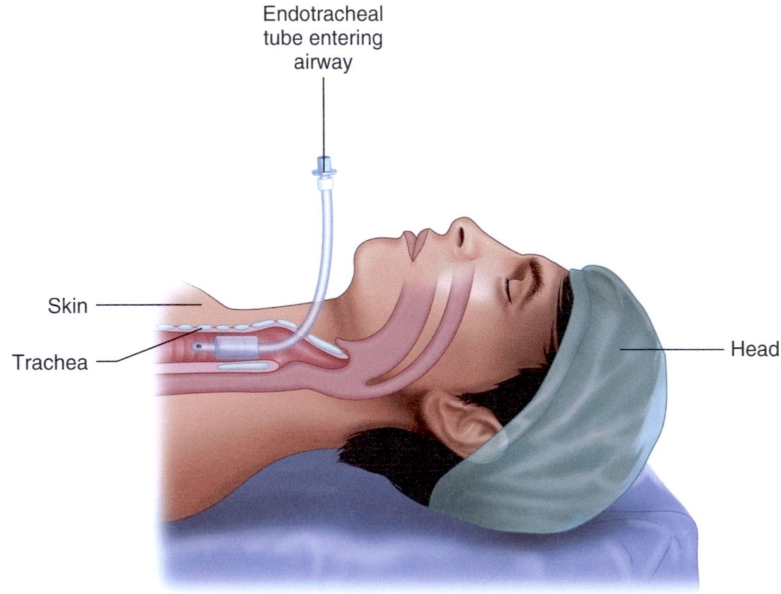

Fig. 23.9 Endotracheal tube is delivered into the trachea

Pitfalls of Cricothyroidotomy

The primary pitfall for cricothyroidotomy is getting away from the midline and expecting to visualize all the structures. It is easy to get away from the midline if you move your nondominant hand from its primary purpose of stabilization. In these circumstances blood of the patient and sweat of the surgeon often cloud easy visibility of the anatomy. It is therefore important to continue to make progress toward traversing the soft tissues overlying the cricothyroid membrane until it is confirmed by palpation.

Suggested Reading

Advanced trauma life support manual. 9th ed. Chicago: The American College of Surgeons; 2012.

De Leyn P, Lieven B, Marion D, et al. Tracheotomy: clinical review and guidelines. Eur J Cardiothorac Surg. 2007;32:412–21.

Hessert MJ, Bennett BL. Optimizing emergency surgical cricothyroidotomy in the austere environment. Wilderness Environ Med. 2013;24:53–66.

Carrico CJ, Thal ER, Weigelt JA, editors. Operative trauma management: an atlas. Stamford, CT: Appleton & Lange; 1998.

Eric K. Mooney

General Principles

Paramount among the general principles of managing soft tissue facial injuries is adherence to the principles of managing trauma. Attention is first turned toward airway assessment and management and ruling out c-spine injury (Fig. 24.1). Next, a detailed "secondary survey" of each region of the head and neck is performed, as missed injuries are a frequent source of complications in this region. Maintain a high level of suspicion as the face is an "anatomically dense" region (Fig. 24.2). Injuries of the forehead should trigger suspicions of frontal sinus injury. In injuries of the periorbita, rule out lacrimal system injuries, injuries to the globe or conjunctiva, and frontal branch nerve injuries (Fig. 24.3). In nasal injuries, septal hematoma should be sought out. Cheek injuries may entail parotid duct injury or facial nerve injury (Fig. 24.4). Tetanus prophylaxis is considered and appropriate imaging studies are obtained.

A prerequisite for managing facial injury is adequate anesthesia. For major injuries and those injuries in sensitive areas such as the periorbita, particularly in children, general anesthesia should be used liberally: there is no excuse for doing a less than rigorous repair. In adults, even large repairs can be performed with regional blocks in nearly every part of the face. Useful regional blocks include those of the supratrochlear/supraorbital, infraorbital, and mental nerves block (Figs. 24.5, 24.6, and 24.7). A regional block should be placed first, and only then supplemented with local infiltration. The eyes should be protected during injection and repair.

Adequate debridement with thorough wound inspection must be performed and this can only be done with good anesthesia. Foreign bodies are removed and "road rash" is scrubbed out (a surgical sponge will often do) to prevent

traumatic tattoo (Fig. 24.8). Actual debridement of nonviable tissue should be limited only to clearly nonviable tissue as the lavish blood supply of the face affords low infection rates and sometimes amazing recovery of tissues. The tissues are irrigated copiously but not vigorously (as with pulsed lavage) as this will obliterate tissue planes. An 18-gauge angiocatheter will suffice.

Lag time should not negate repair of facial tissues. The "golden rule" of 6 or even twelve hours does not apply to the face. Berk et al. found that healing rates of facial injuries were high even beyond 18 h. One should also be more liberal in closing contaminated wounds. The author routinely closes animal bites in a layered fashion.

Preoperative Preparation

Preoperative preparation is minimal in most cases and centers on educating the patient and providing proper anesthesia. The patient should be counseled that there will be scar but reassurance should be given that everything possible will be done to optimize it. There may be further revision surgery. When dealing with animal bites, the possibility of wound infection with subsequent conversion to open wound *with suture removal* is discussed. When these issues are dealt with in a straightforward, preemptive fashion, patients tend to accept them as opposed to dealing with them after the fact.

Repair with adequate lighting and magnification (loupes) with proper instrumentation should not be compromised.

Operative Strategy

Critical landmarks are realigned. These include natural curves such as the free margin of the ala and the lateral margins of the columella. The helical rim and antihelix are natural curves of the ear. Hairlines such as the brow, anterior forehead hairline, and sideburns are realigned (Fig. 24.9). Lacerations of the eyelid are repaired by realigning the gray

E.K. Mooney, M.D. (✉)
Surgery, Bassett Healthcare, Cooperstown, NY 13326, USA
e-mail: eric.mooney@bassett.org

A.L. Halverson and D.C. Borgstrom (eds.), *Advanced Surgical Techniques for Rural Surgeons*,
DOI 10.1007/978-1-4939-1495-1_24, © Springer Science+Business Media New York 2015

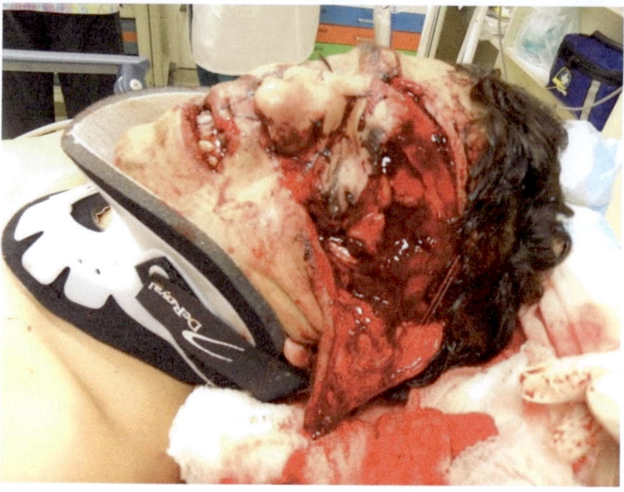

Fig. 24.1 The often disturbing appearance of facial injuries tends to be distracting. Attention must be paid first to proper trauma management including stabilization of the c-spine and airway management

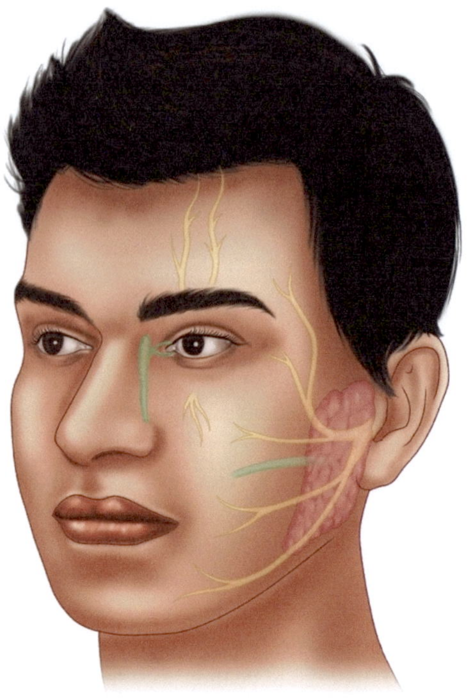

Fig. 24.2 The face is an "anatomically dense" region. A detailed secondary survey is aimed at identifying missed injuries and repairable structures such as nerves (*yellow*) and ducts (*green*)

line and lash line and, in doing so, preventing postoperative notching (Fig. 24.10). With lips, the vermillion border, wet/dry mucosal border, and free margin are all marked and aligned (Fig. 24.11). This can particularly help in lacerations of the oral commissure.

Operative Technique

In general, repair should proceed "from the known to the unknown," especially in extensive or geometrically complex wounds. First, the critical landmarks are marked before injection (as they may be obscured) and aligned. Angles within lacerations are inset. In this fashion, large avulsed wounds are gradually reduced to smaller open segments that are sequentially repaired. Repair is in a layered fashion, utilizing subcutaneous, muscle (ex. Orbicularis), and dermal stitches. Dermal stitches are placed in a buried fashion. This facilitates early removal of the superficial epithelial stitches without risking dehiscence (Fig. 24.12). Cyanoacrylate glue should not be used in areas of tension or in contaminated or abraded and thus exudative wounds.

Duct injuries, such as those of the lacrimal duct or parotid duct are repaired over a silastic stent, using magnification. The author uses an 8-0 nonabsorbable stitch such as nylon or prolene. Simple stenting alone without suture, however, may suffice. Nerve injuries, when repairable, are repaired with 8-0 or 9-0 nylon or polypropylene.

Potential Pitfalls

Perhaps the biggest pitfall is unrecognized deep structure injury, such as facial nerve damage or unrecognized fracture. As previously noted, the best way to avoid this is to maintain a high level of suspicion, do a thorough "secondary survey," and thoroughly explore the wound with adequate anesthesia (general, regional, etc.).

Postoperative Care

In general, most wounds are washed with mild soap and water daily and dressed with a moisturizing ointment. Patients are counseled to treat their wound "like chapped lips," that is, with a thin coating frequently enough so that it does not dry out. Antibiotic ointments may be used but are not necessary. They should not be used beyond a few days to prevent topical allergic reactions that may mimic cellulites. Once healed, sunscreen should be used as long as the scar is pink to prevent hyperpigmentation stimulated by the sun. Scar massage may be instituted after 2 weeks.

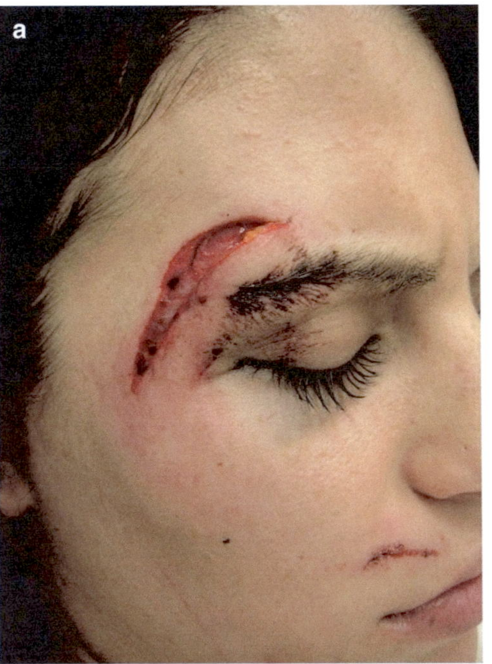

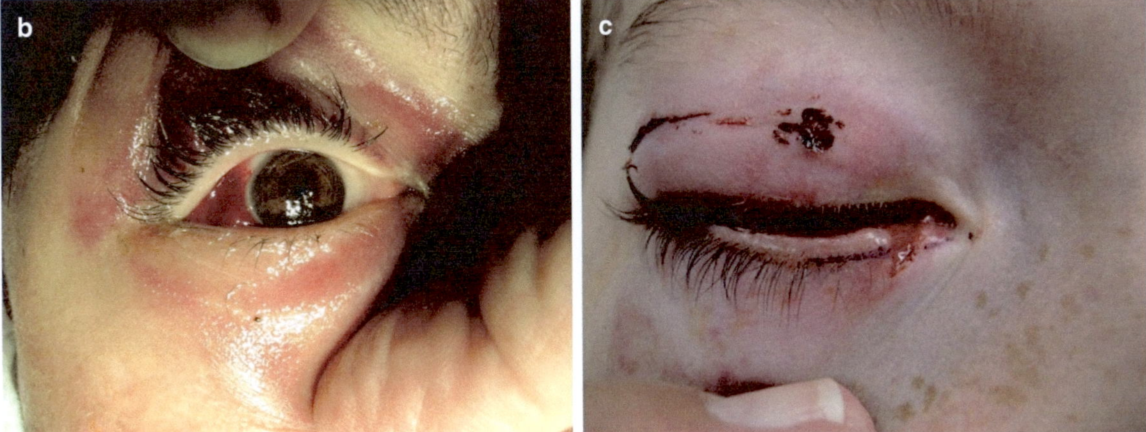

Fig. 24.3 Injuries of the periorbita may be those of the frontal branch of the facial nerve (**a**) and lacrimal duct (**c**). Suconjuctival hemorrhage may suggest zygoma fracture or orbital floor fracture (**b**)

Common Complications

Missed injury!

Cellulitis or abscess should be treated aggressively with early antibiotics. If there is no response, consider opening the wound, drainage, and irrigation. This is particularly true for periorbital cellulitis.

Remember, the repair of facial lacerations while the patient is on supplemental oxygen should be considered a fire hazard, particularly with nasal cannulas. When in the operating room, work with the anesthesia team to minimize this risk.

When to Transfer

Extensive injuries or those involving displaced facial bone fractures should be transferred. Of course, any transfer must first have a secured airway if there is any doubt whatsoever. Open facial fractures (such as open nasal fracture) do not necessarily require emergent ORIF. In this respect, they are not analogous to fractures of the extremities. Most often, the soft tissues are managed/closed and the facial fractures are dealt with at a later, timely date. Injuries requiring specialty skill such as injuries to the facial nerve or globe may also require transfer.

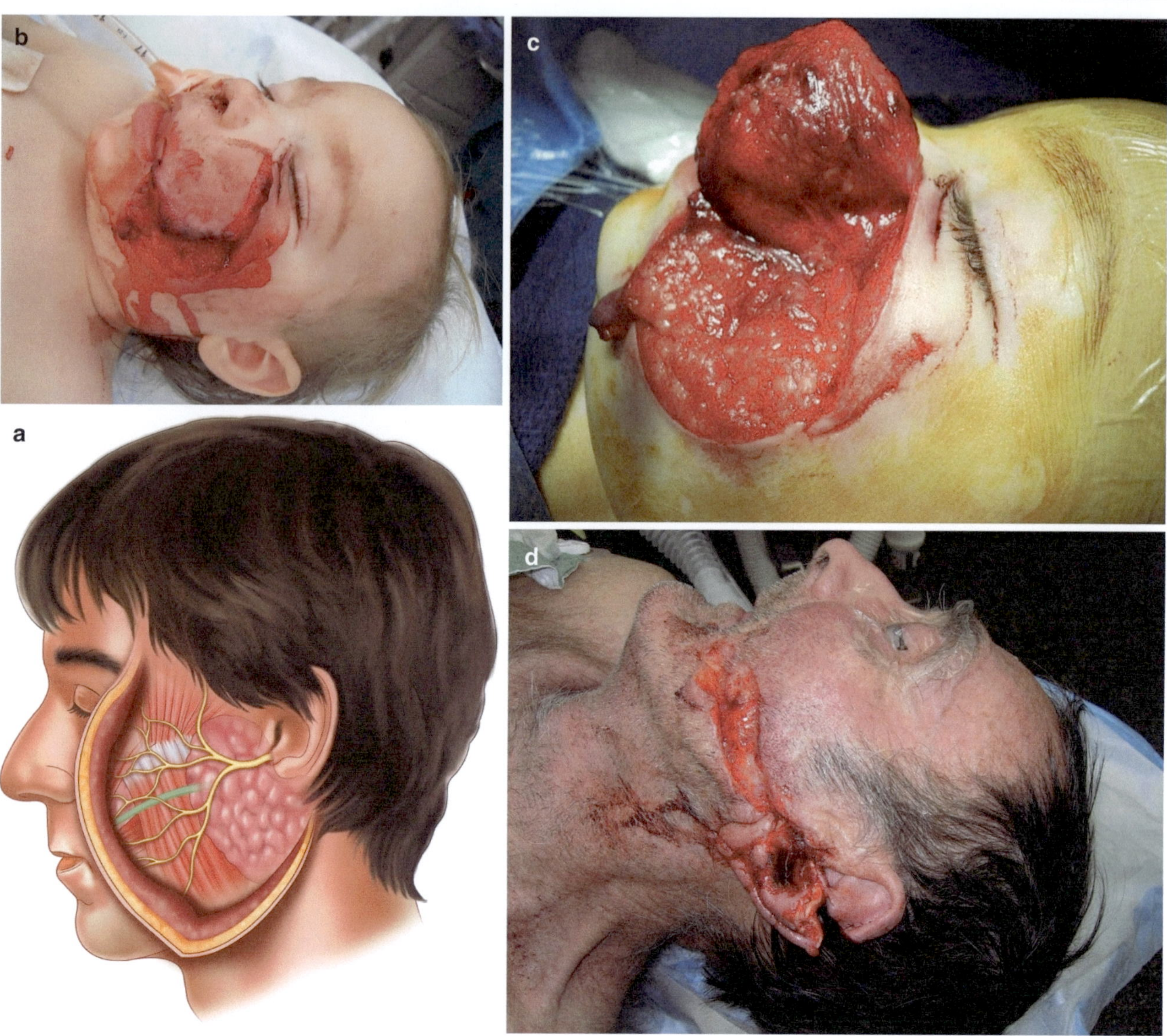

Fig. 24.4 (a) Cheek lacerations may involve the facial nerve or parotid duct (a). (b and c) A large dog bite to this baby's cheek involved the facial nerve buccal branches at the anterior margin of the masseter muscle. They were repaired. (d) A chainsaw laceration to the left cheek involved the facial nerve and parotid duct. The duct can be repaired over a stent

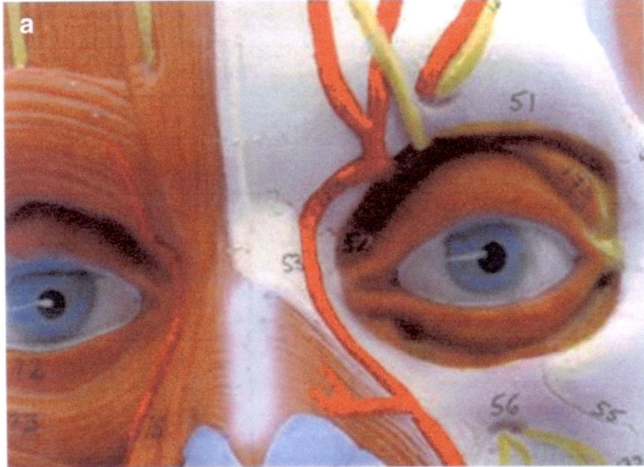

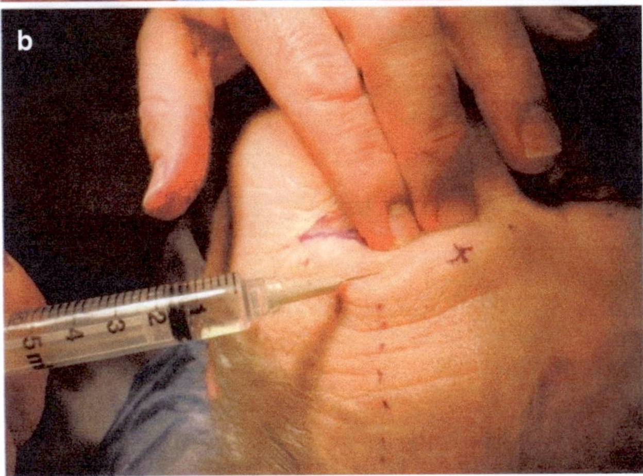

Fig. 24.5 (**a**) The supratrochlear and supraorbital nerves are blocked by injecting along the superior orbital rim. (**b**) While blocking the nerves, the supraorbital rim is palpated to protect the orbit. This block will block the forehead and anterior scalp

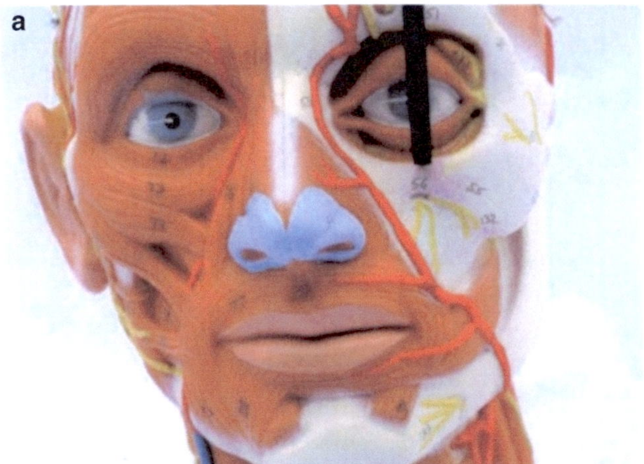

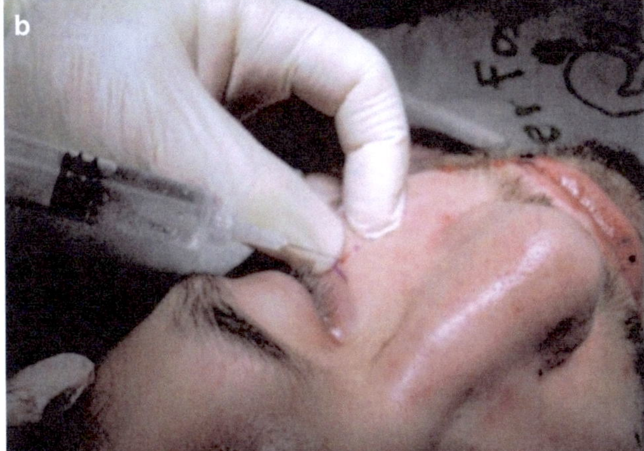

Fig. 24.6 (**B**) The infraorbital nerve is blocked by palpating and injecting the infraorbital foramen just below the inferior orbital rim. Alternately, the needle may be introduced at the alar base and directed up to the foramen. (**A**) The orbital rim is palpated while injecting at the foramen to protect the orbit. This block will anesthetize the upper lip and cheek 24 Repair of Soft Tissue Facial Injuries

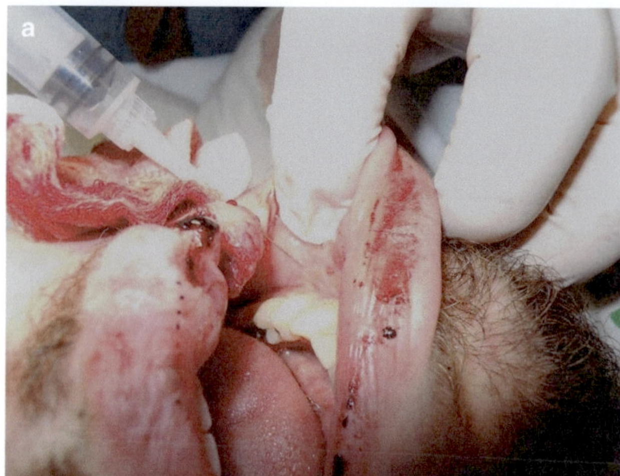

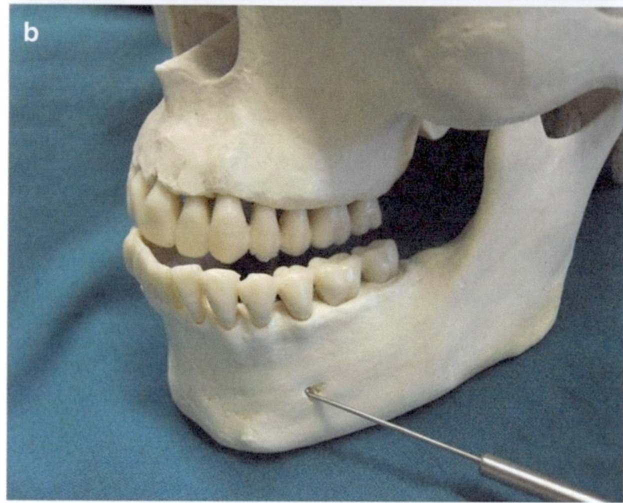

Fig. 24.7 (**a**) The mental foramen is located below the second biscuspid. (**b**) It may be blocked by injecting just beneath the mucosa of the labial sulcus at the second bicuspid. This will block the lower lip but not the chin

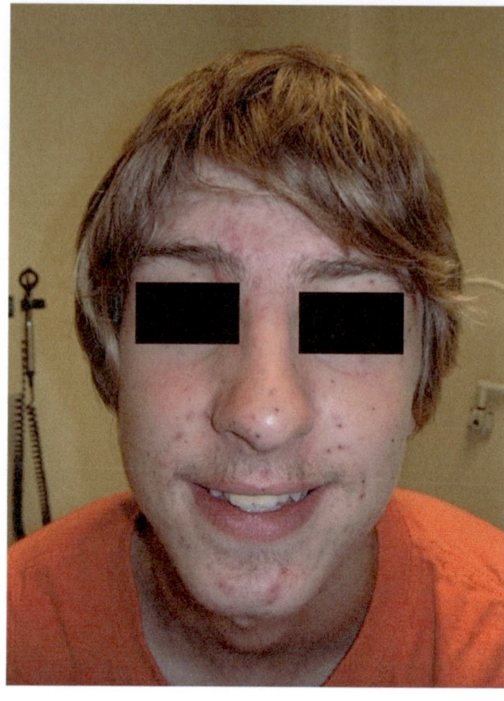

Fig. 24.8 Debridement of "road rash" can be done with a surgical scrub brush, a 19-gauge needle, a small curette, or even dermabrasion. This will prevent permanent traumatic tattooing

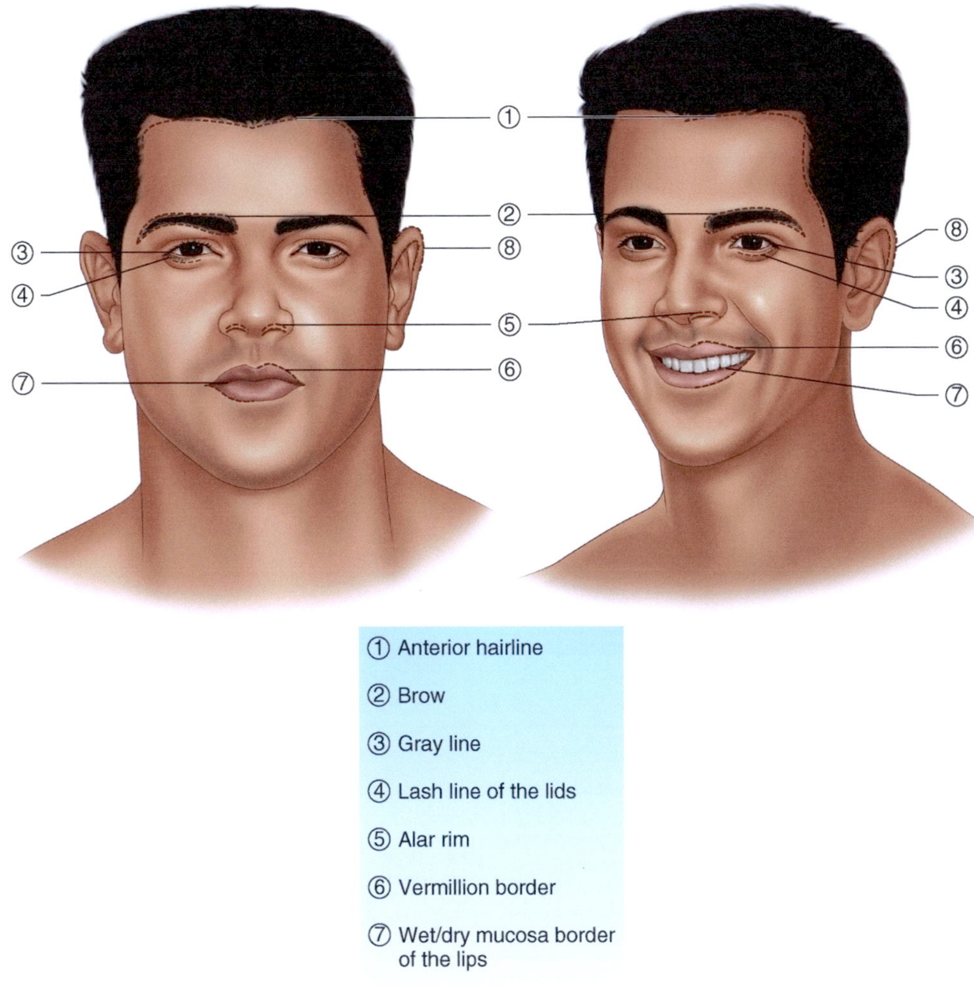

Fig. 24.9 Critical landmarks to be re-aligned are the anterior hairline (1), brow (2), gray line (3) and lash line (4) of the lids, alar rim (5), vermillion border (6) and wet/dry mucosa border (7) of the lips, and the helix of the ear (8)

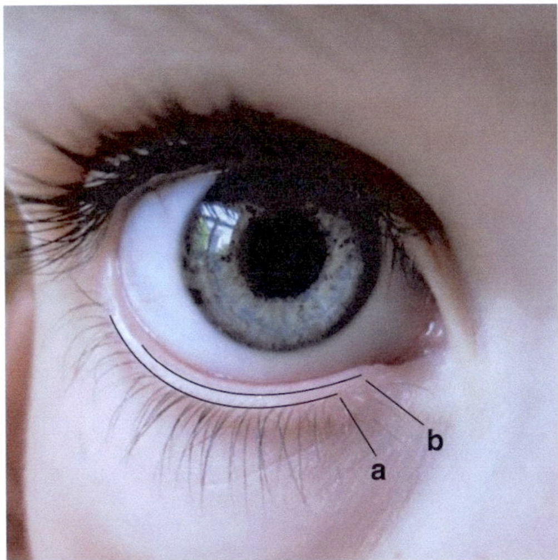

Fig. 24.10 Landmarks of the eyelids are the lashline (**a**), the gray line (**b**), and the free margin. Accurate alignment of these will prevent notching

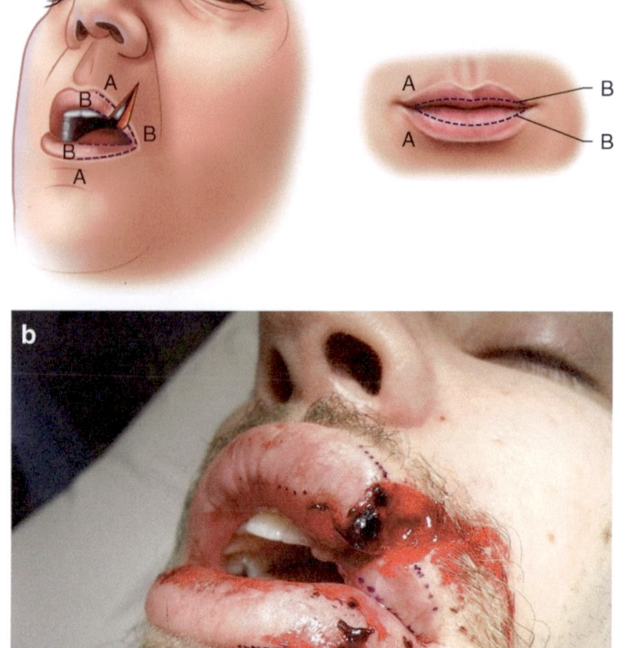

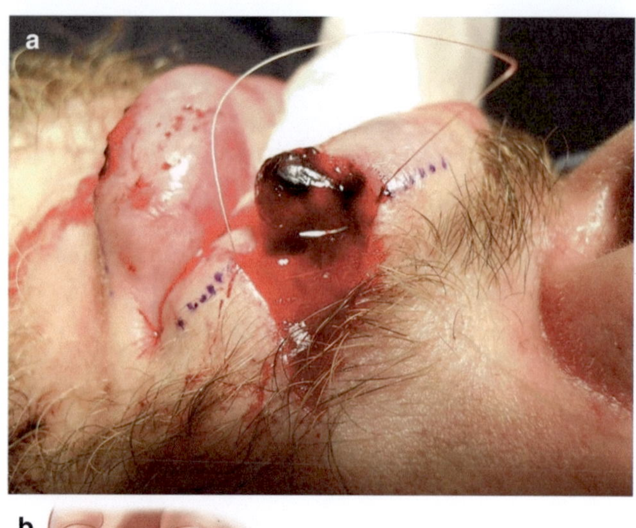

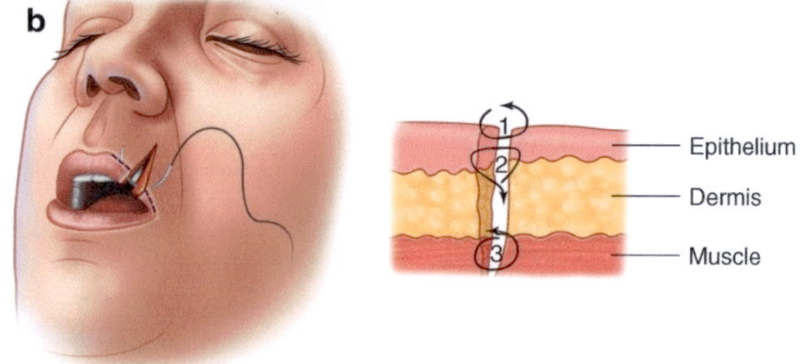

Fig. 24.11 Landmarks of the lips include the vermillion border (**a**), the wet/dry mucosa border (**b**), and the free margin. The muscle should be repaired as a separate layer to prevent grooving or a sulcus

Fig. 24.12 (**a**) A buried subcuticular stitch is placed to align the vermillion. (**b**) In general, the wound is closed in anatomic layers, including a buried dermal stitch for strength

Suggested Reading

Berk WA, Osbourne DD, Taylor DD. Evaluation of the golden period for wound repair: 204 cases form a third world emergency department. Ann Emerg Med. 1988;17(5):496–500.

Charles Carroll IV and Alan J. Micev

Indications

Upper extremity injuries are common in the emergency setting. Up to 20 % of all injuries presenting to an emergency room involve the hand. In our active urban, suburban, and rural worlds, finger injuries occur at home, work, during travel, and while engaged in sports. Fractures, dislocations, soft tissue injuries, and amputations can be found in various combinations. Each component of the injury may require primary care that ranges from observation to surgical reconstruction.

The primary goal of treatment is a painless fingertip with normal function and sensation. Secondary goals include maintenance of length, preservation of the nail, and cosmetic appearance. To meet these goals, careful consideration of padded soft tissue covering over bone is of paramount concern. Avoidance of neuromas with methodical dissection and a proper traction neurectomy can minimize bone and nerve pain. Preservation of the nail and supporting bone can minimize the risk of a hooked nail deformity and fingertip dysfunction with grasp and pinch. Appropriate hemostasis can minimize flap and skin graft slough and eventual loss. Methods of treatment include healing by secondary intention, debridement and closure, skin grafting, local flap coverage, or revision amputation. The attending surgeon should first consider the anatomy of the injured digit and work to restore functional anatomy and subsequent use. Careful planning and restoration of the anatomy available for reconstruction can lead to a reasonable and functional restoration of the injured fingertip. A careful amputation as part of one procedure may be better than multiple procedures with a

marginal and painful outcome may optimize an injured patient's return to a normal life.

In a rural setting, access to subspecialty care can be a challenge due to availability and distance. A finger injury may be amenable to immediate and local care without a need to consider triage and transfer to a tertiary facility. Careful consideration of soft tissue issues can allow for successful care and reconstruction in a primary care setting. To reconstruct an injured finger distal to the distal interphalangeal joint, a surgeon needs to consider the nature and the extent of soft tissue, vascular, neurologic, tendon, nail bed, bone, and distal interphalangeal articular injuries. Consider the injury and use a comparable finger on the patient as a visual guide for successful reconstruction. Anatomy directs and guides surgical decision making. Patient considerations and beneficence should be taken into account as consent is obtained for local emergent care or when considering a transfer to a tertiary facility.

Anatomy

The finger and hand are essential for grasping and experiential use in our world due to sensation and mobility. The opposition of the thumb allows the human to perform many of their daily tasks. On the brain motor homunculus, the thumb is well represented due to its importance in ape and human activities. Optimal treatment requires that the treating physician have a thorough understanding of fingertip anatomy.

The pulp of the fingertip has multiple fibrous septa and fat compartments that pad the volar distal phalanx and allows for compression with pinch. The nail and nail bed are contiguous with the dorsal distal phalanx (Fig. 25.1). The hyponychium forms the proximal border of the nail fold. The germinal matrix emanates from that anatomic area. The paronychium forms the radial and ulnar borders of the nail bed. The dorsal and volar creases over the distal interphalangeal joint allow for motion in flexion and extension. There is

C. Carroll IV, M.D. (✉)
Orthopedic Surgery, Northwestern University Feinberg School of Medicine, NOI NorthShore Orthopedics, Chicago, IL 60611, USA
e-mail: ccarrolliv@gmail.com

A.J. Micev, M.D.
Department of Orthopedic Surgery, Northwestern University Feinberg School of Medicine, Chicago, IL 60611, USA

A.L. Halverson and D.C. Borgstrom (eds.), *Advanced Surgical Techniques for Rural Surgeons*,
DOI 10.1007/978-1-4939-1495-1_25, © Springer Science+Business Media New York 2015

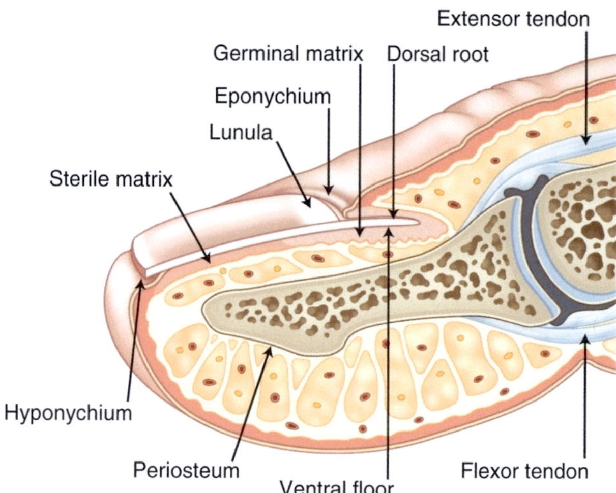

Fig. 25.1 Anatomy of fingertip in sagittal section. Lateral view of finger depiction dorsal aspect to volar aspect of nail, nail bed, distal phalanx, and volar tip from distal proximal phalanx to distal tip

more laxity of the skin over the dorsal aspect which allows for mobility as well.

The fingertip has a radial and ulnar digital nerve which has three distinct branches distal to the distal interphalangeal joint. The radial and ulnar digital arteries provide the dominant flow and are situated on the volar aspect of the finger and run with the digital nerves. The veins are predominantly dorsal and their location prevents venous congestion with pinch and grasp. The extensor tendon attaches to the proximal distal phalanx on the dorsal aspect. The flexor digitorum profundus tendon attaches to the proximal volar aspect of the distal phalanx. Injuries to any of these structures can warrant specialized care but most fingertip injuries do not require nerve or tendon care. An amputation proximal to the germinal matrix and nail fold requires neurectomies or tendon release as the flexor and extensor tendons should not be sewn together to prevent the quadregia effect and impair digital function.

Patient Evaluation

Evaluation of a patient with a fingertip injury begins with a thorough history which should include the mechanism of injury. A sharp and clean injury may be more amenable to an anatomic reconstruction than a dirty, crush, or avulsion injury. The presence or absence of the injured part determines whether replantation or use as a composite graft is possible. Patient factors to consider include hand dominance, age, occupation, recreational pursuits, history of previous injuries or hand problems. Medical comorbidities such as cardiac or vascular disease, diabetes, smoking, and alcohol consumption should also be assessed. A complete examina-

tion of the hand includes an assessment of the skin, vascularity, neurologic function and flexor and extensor tendon function. The injury is inspected with specific attention to the characteristics of the wound. Tetanus status should be assessed and cultures obtained in grossly contaminated injuries such as a barnyard injury. Intravenous antibiotics are indicated for patients with an associated fracture.

Inspection of the hand starts with color. Ischemia will cause a loss of the normal pink vascular appearance of the nail and volar tip. The nails should be smooth and the nail bed pink as well. Compression should cause a blanching that should clear in 1–3 s with a return to a pink color. Venous congestion can cause the tip and nail to turn blue and even darker in color. Infarcted or necrotic tissue is black. Hemorrhage in the nail bed can be a harbinger of fracture of the distal phalanx and a nail bed injury. The finger has a turgor to it that should be symmetric amongst all digits. The volar tip has a set of ridges that comprise our fingerprint. Each finger is unique with respect to the pattern of ridges (fingerprint) and care should be taken to minimize incisions and painful scars over the volar fingertip and pad.

After gross inspection of the soft tissue injury, radiographs of the hand and finger should be obtained to assess the change in the boney architecture. A clean amputation with bone involvement will have fewer possible issues to consider than a comminuted fracture involving the proximal distal phalangeal articular surface and possibly the middle phalanx distal articular surface.

Injury Patterns and Classification

Mechanisms of injury vary and range from clean sharp trauma to dirty blunt and crush injury. The mechanism of injury can be a guide to treatment. A sharp injury with an available soft tissue piece can be defatted and placed as a skin graft or sewn back on as a composite graft. If the soft tissue piece is gone and there is not any exposed bone, closure or hypothenar split thickness skin graft could be possible. An injury to bone and nail bed may require shortening and closure or a reconstructive local flap such as a V–Y flap or lateral Kutler flap. More complex techniques such as the vascular island flap, thenar flap, cross finger flap, or groin flap closure would likely require transfer to a hand surgical specialist.

Fingertip injuries can be divided into crushing injuries or clean amputations and can be classified based on the level of the amputation, the obliquity of the wound, and whether there is any exposed bone (Fig. 25.2). The Allen Classification is commonly utilized to describe fingertip injuries and can be used as a guide for treatment. Type I injuries are those in which only the pulp of the finger is involved without any exposed bone. Type II injuries are those in which there is both pulp and nail loss as well as exposed bone. Type III injuries are those in which there is partial loss of the distal phalanx as well as both pulp and nail loss. Type IV injuries are those in which the lunula of the nail is involved along with the pulp, nail bed, and distal phalanx. The obliquity of the amputation wound can be described as dorsal oblique, transverse, volar oblique, or lateral oblique (Fig. 25.3).

In Allen Type I injuries of the fingertip where there is loss of skin or pulp tissue without exposed bone, the wound may be allowed to heal via secondary intention or by performing a skin graft. Controversy exists as to which method is better, but most agree that wounds larger than 1 square centimeter are better treated with full-thickness skin grafting. In Type II and III injuries, with bone exposure, the wound may be closed primarily or a local flap may be utilized. Type IV injuries which are proximal to the lunula, can be treated by revision amputation, flap coverage, or microsurgical replantation. When bone is exposed, as in Type II–IV, the question becomes whether length should be preserved, necessitating coverage, or if sacrifice of length is appropriate.

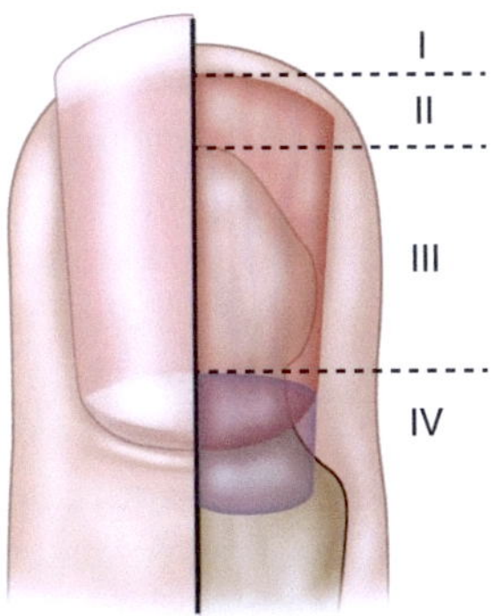

Fig. 25.2 Allen classification of fingertip Injuries

Preoperative Preparation

The patient should be carefully positioned with a hand table or appropriate substitute table to allow for placing the hand on a flat surface for exposure. The hand table can be a specialized table that allows for preparation and draping of a sterile field. A mayo stand or arm board may suffice if a hand surgery table is not available. Other injuries may require primary care as part of a primary and secondary survey. A digital or arm tourniquet should be available and used as necessary to minimize bleeding and optimize visualization. A good light source should be positioned. Adequate magnification may be helpful such as surgical loupes. The surgeon should consider a good irrigation and debridement of the wounds with a digital or wrist block anesthesia. Antibiotics should be administered and considered in the postsurgical period for 48–72 h. Open fractures and grossly contaminated wounds may require a longer period of up to 7–10 days. A sterile field should be set with adequate head, eye and mask coverage for the surgeon. Sterile hand washing, sterile gloves and perhaps a gown must be employed. Adequate instruments, suture, Adaptic, Xeroform, and dressings should be immediately available. Careful planning is essential if an assistant is not available to obtain materials as the reconstructive procedure moves forward.

After the evaluation of the patient and wound is completed, a treatment plan is formulated. If more than one option is available, the advantages and disadvantages of each should be discussed with patient, and the simplest method that accomplishes the desired result should be pursued. Most fingertip injuries can be managed in the emergency department, but complex regional flaps as well as more invasive procedures are more appropriately treated in the operating room.

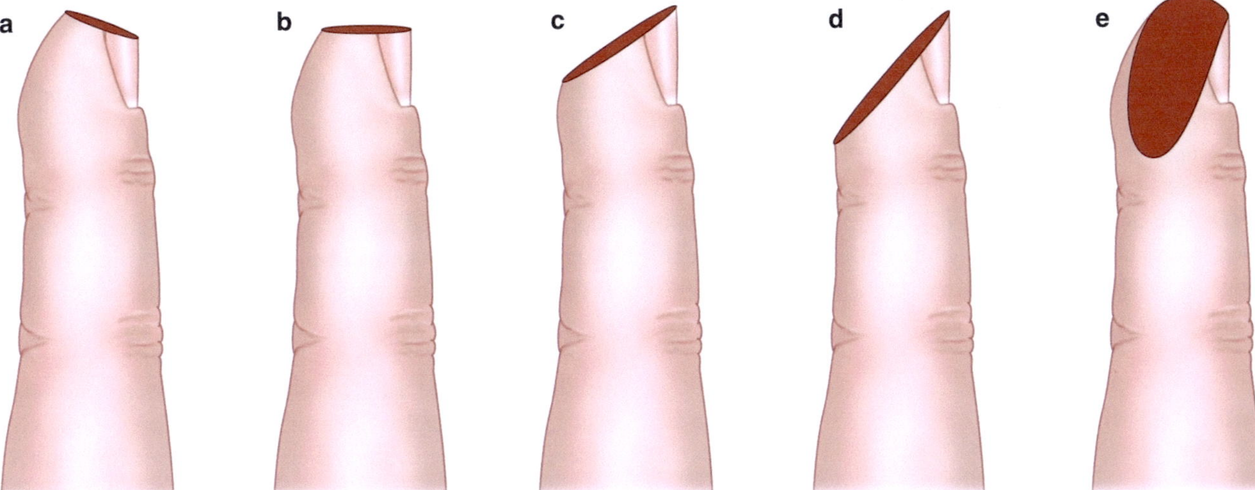

Fig. 25.3 Obliquity of the amputation

Facility and equipment availability requires consideration. Appropriate instruments including a freer elevator, rongeur, proper knife blades, and suture are necessary to technically perform the reconstructive procedure. A supply of dressings and splints are essential for postsurgical care. Access to follow-up care will optimize patient satisfaction and outcomes.

Debridement and Closure

Operative Strategy

Primary closure of a distal tip amputation of pulp may be an option where the location and amount of skin loss allow for closure without excessive tension. There must be adequate tissue for closure or shortening of the distal bone is necessary.

Operative Technique

The technique will differ depending on the nature of the injury and the complexity of the wound. In most cases, the digit may be anesthetized using a digital block. Four nerve branches, two dorsal and two volar, supply each digit. The dorsal nerves should be blocked only if the intervention will extend proximally from the distal interphalangeal joint. A 25-gauge with 10 cm^3 of 1 % lidocaine, or 0.5 % marcaine if longer duration is needed, can be inserted at the level of the distal palmar crease and 2.5 cm^3 of anesthetic can be injected on both sides of the metacarpal neck. A circumferential ring block at the base of the digit is not recommended because the subsequent pressure may result in ischemia to the digit.

The wounds should be effectively irrigated and debrided of devitalized tissue. A hematoma area 50 % of the size of the nail indicates a significant nail bed injury. Drainage with a sterile 18-gauge needle can alleviate pain. If a nail bed injury is present, the nail plate can be removed, and the sterile matrix should be re-approximated with 6-0 chromic gut or similar absorbable suture. After nail bed repair is completed, the nail plate should be placed into its native position to maintain the nail fold and protect the repair. The skin can be closed with a 4-0 or 5-0 nylon or similar sized non-absorbable monofilament suture. Absorbable sutures can be used in children or in places when removal may be a challenge. A sterile non-adherent dressing is applied. The finger should be immobilized.

Potential Pitfalls

The nail plate should not be disposed. Failure to identify a nail bed injury could result in a painful ridged or split nail.

Postoperative Care

The dressing is removed after 5 days. The nail bed repair is protected and the finger is immobilized for the first 3–4 weeks. After this time, the sutures are removed. Distal phalanx fractures are followed by radiographic evaluation after 2–4 weeks as well as clinical resolution of pain. The fracture will usually heal over 3 months and the nail regenerates over 4–6 months.

Common Complications

Common complications include infection, cold intolerance, dysesthesias and sensitivity over the fingertip, and deformities of the nail.

Skin Grafting

Operative Strategy

Skin grafts can be applied to larger wounds greater than 1 cm^2 without exposed bone or tendon. The graft should be full thickness because they are more durable, less tender, contract less, and achieve better sensation than split thickness skin grafts. A full-thickness skin graft as large as 2 cm in width and 6 cm in length is taken from the hairless hypothenar area of the hand with minimal scarring and morbidity. This is the preferred donor site as it is convenient and provides durable skin with similar color and quality to the skin of the pulp. The donor site is closed primarily and the graft is sutured over the defect.

Operative Technique

After wrist block or axillary anesthesia, an appropriately sized graft should be selected based on the nature and size of the wound. The area is outlined over the hypothenar in an ellipsis which can be closed primarily using interrupted 4-0 or 5-0 nylon sutures (Fig. 25.4). Lidocaine without epinephrine is injected under the skin to be taken. The skin is taken as a full-thickness skin graft leaving behind as much as fat and subcutaneous tissue as possible. The graft is completely defatted because that will otherwise act as a barrier to prevent vascularization. The graft is then tailored to match the area of skin loss and sutured into the defect exactly with 5-0 nylon or absorbable sutures. A sterile non-adherent dressing is applied and the finger is immobilized with a padded aluminum splint or short arm splint with the finger protected.

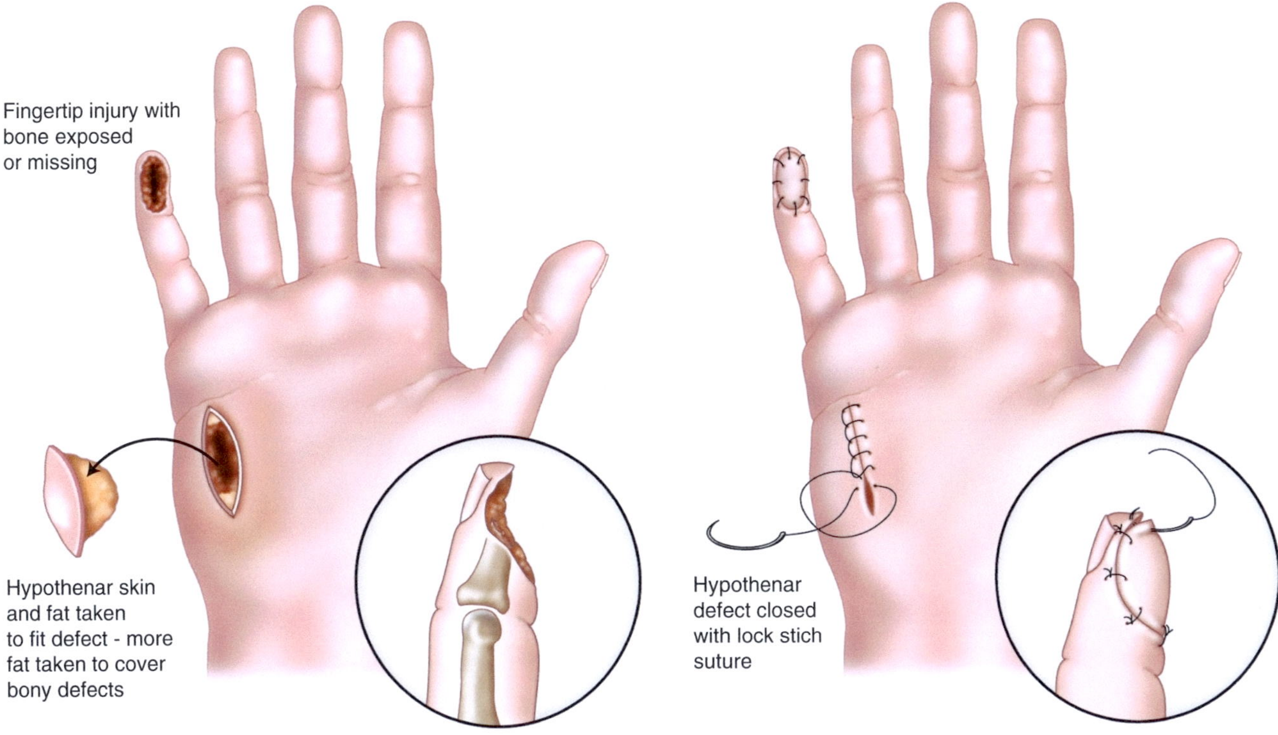

Fig. 25.4 Hypothenar skin graft

Potential Pitfalls

During the defatting process, it is critical to avoid removing the dermal layer of skin which in effect would convert the graft to split thickness.

Postoperative Care

The dressing and splint are removed after 4–6 days at which point range of motion exercises is begun. Sutures are removed at 2–3 weeks.

Common Complications

Potential complications include donor or recipient site infection, graft failure, fingertip hypersensitivity, or donor site scar hypersensitivity.

V to Y Advancement

Operative Strategy

When bone is exposed, satisfactory soft tissue coverage must be obtained. In cases where there is insufficient local tissue available for primary closure and preservation of length is desired, coverage by a local flap is indicated. The triangular volar V–Y advancement flap is indicated for transverse or dorsal oblique amputations. It is contraindicated in cases of volar oblique amputations where there is more palmar skin loss than dorsally. The distal edge of the flap can be advanced only about 1 cm. The flap is designed with the distal edge of the wound as the base of a triangular flap. The apex is a point in the midline of the distal interphalangeal crease.

Operative Technique

After induction of digital anesthesia, a Penrose drain is used to exsanguinate the digit and is clamped with a hemostat to serve as a tourniquet. The wound is thoroughly irrigated and debrided of devitalized tissue. Any protruding bone from the distal phalanx may be trimmed using a rongeur to allow for advancement of the flap. Outline a triangular V-shaped flap to cover the defect. The base of the triangle is the distal cut edge with the apex being at the distal interphalangeal joint crease (Fig. 25.5). The skin and subcutaneous tissue are then incised, with great care being taken not to damage the neurovascular bundles. Do not undermine the flap because it will devitalize the flap. Advance the flap over the defect and suture it to the remaining nail or nail bed with either 5-0 or 6-0 chromic gut absorbable sutures. To adequately mobilize the flap, all the fibrous septa that anchor the pulp tissue to the periosteum of the distal phalanx must be divided. The tourniquet can be

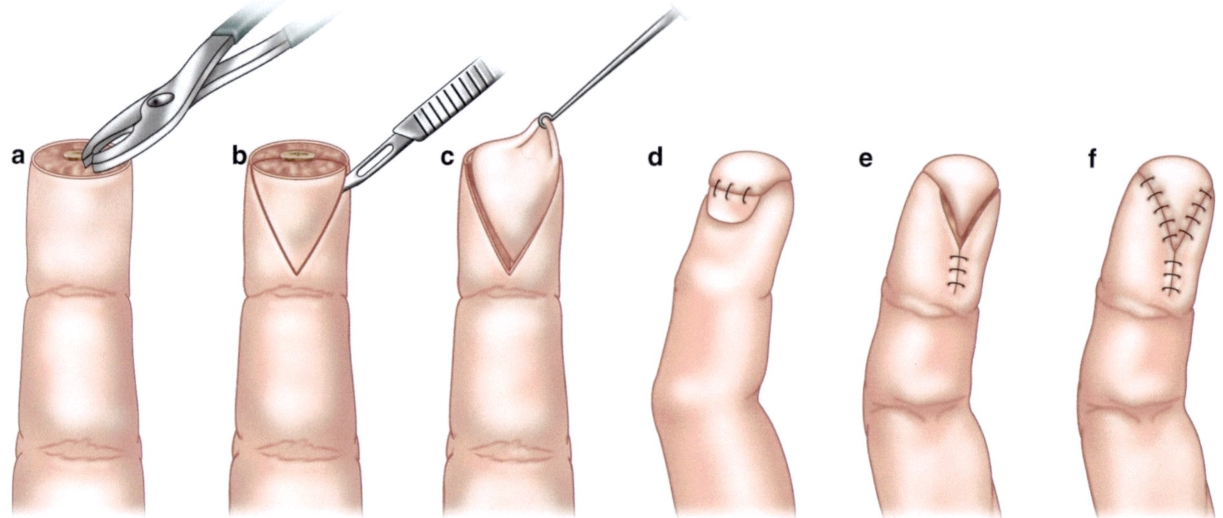

Fig. 25.5 V to Y advancement flap

removed at this point to inspect the vascularity of the flap. If capillary refill is delayed, it is usually because there has been inadequate mobilization and the vessels are under tension. The apex of the flap is closed primarily converting the triangular "V" incision to a "Y" shape. The skin should be closed without tension. A loose closure will minimize flap ischemia. A sterile non-adherent dressing is applied and the finger is immobilized to protect the flap.

Potential Pitfalls

During dissection it is critical to avoid iatrogenic injury to adjacent digital nerves and blood vessels. Care should be taken to spread gently during flap preparation to prevent ischemia and flap loss.

Postoperative Care

The dressing is removed after 7 days. The finger is immobilized for 2 weeks. Sutures are removed after 10–14 days at which point the patient is allow to progressively return to active motion. A small tip protector splint can be fashioned by an occupational hand therapist. Desensitization of the tip may be necessary.

Common Complications

Complications include infection, flap necrosis, cold intolerance, and hypoesthesia or dysesthesia over the fingertip.

If the flap shows no vascularity at the conclusion of the procedure, it should be left in place to serve as a biologic dressing.

Lateral Kutler Flap

Operative Strategy

Kutler described the use of dual triangular flaps for distal transverse, volar oblique or lateral oblique amputations with exposed distal phalanx. Triangular flaps are designed on each side of the tip, with the bases being the distal edges of the wound and the apices more proximal. The disadvantage of this technique is that the flaps are small, may be difficult to advance for an adequate tension free closure, and leave a sagittal scar on the tip of the finger.

Operative Technique

After induction of digital anesthesia, the tip of the digit is debrided of devitalized tissue and copiously irrigated. It is reasonable to trim any protruding bone from the distal phalanx using a rongeur to allow for advancement of the flaps. Two triangular flaps are developed from the midlateral aspect of each side of the digit. As in the V–Y advancement flat, the bases of the triangles are the cut edges of the wound. The dorsal edges of the two flaps begin 1–2 mm volar to the edge of the fingernail. The apex of the flap sits just distal to the distal interphalangeal joint crease. An incision is made down through the dermis, and the subcutaneous tissue is mobilized

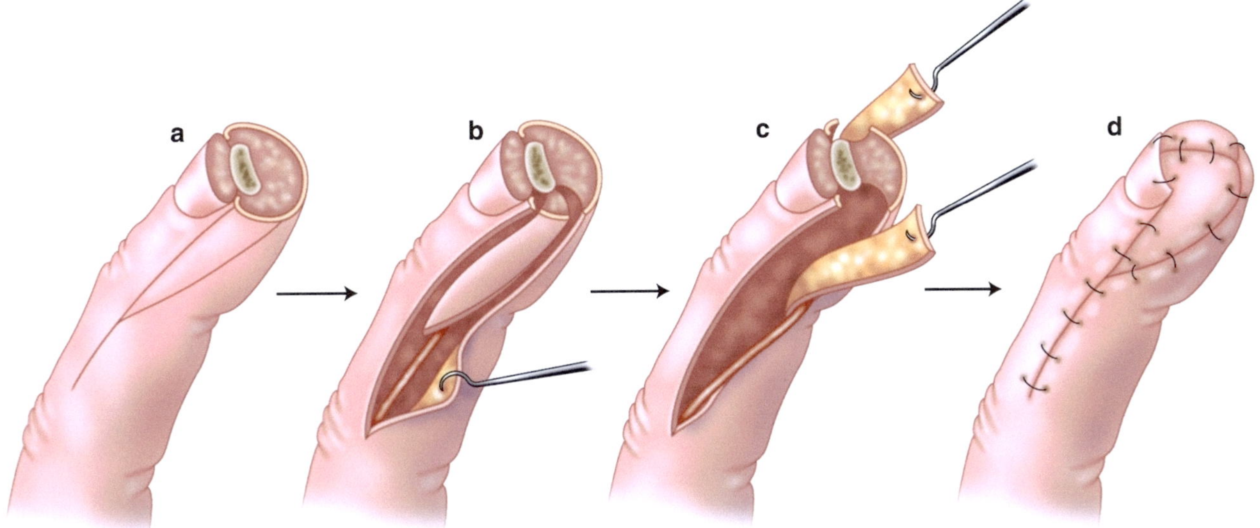

Fig. 25.6 Kutler lateral advancement flap

from the phalanx in a deep plane. The apex of the triangle is closed in a "Y" fashion, and the surrounding edges and nail bed, or nail, are carefully sutured to the distal edges of the advanced flaps with either 5-0 or 6-0 nylon or absorbable suture (Fig. 25.6). It is not necessary to close the skin centrally over the fingertip as long as there is good soft tissue coverage over the exposed distal phalanx. A sterile nonadherent dressing is applied and the finger is immobilized with a padded aluminum splint or short arm splint to the finger and perhaps adjacent digits.

Potential Pitfalls

The flap should not be undermined because this will devitalize the flap. Gentle and careful mobilization will minimize the risk of flap ischemia.

Postoperative Care

The dressing and splint are removed after 7–10 days at which point range of motion exercises are begun. Sutures are removed at 10–14 days. A tip protector can be applied as well by the occupational therapy team. Desensitization should follow 3–4 weeks post surgery.

Common Complications

Potential complications can include infection, cold intolerance, tenderness on percussion, as well as slight hypoesthesia or dysesthesia over the fingertip. Tissue sloughing may occur if the skin is closed under tension.

Revision Amputation

Operative Strategy

Shortening and primary close of fingertip injuries is indicated in adults when less than 5 mm of sterile matrix remains to produce an adherent stable nail, in patients with significant soft tissue trauma not amendable to flap or local coverage, or in cases where preservation of length is not required to preserve function.

Operative Technique

After induction of digital anesthesia, the digit is exsanguinated and a tourniquet is applied. Available skin flaps for primary closure are outlined. Distal traction is applied to the flexor and extensor tendons, which are then transected and allowed to retract. The tendons should not be sutured as this could compromise function to the remaining digits. The prominent volar condyles of the head of the middle phalanx are removed with a rongeur to avoid any bony prominence. It is essential that the digital nerves are identified, mobilized a short distance, and transected under tension about 1 cm from the wound edge to prevent the occurrence of a painful neuroma (Fig. 25.7). The germinal and sterile matrices must be adequately removed to prevent the formation of a hook nail or retained nail horn. At this point the tourniquet may be release, and the digital vessels can be ligated to avoid excess bleeding. The palmar skin is then brought over the end of the bone and sutured to the dorsal skin using 4-0 or 5-0 nylon sutures. The closure should be tension free. Excess skin may need to be trimmed to obtain satisfactory contour. A soft bulky non-adherent dressing is applied.

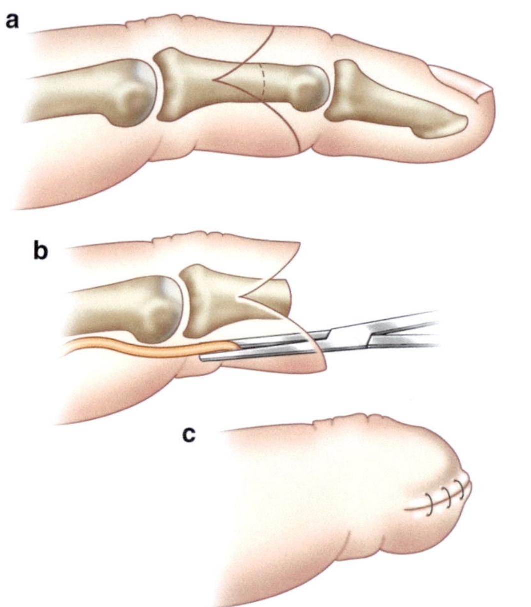

Fig. 25.7 Revision amputation. The image demonstrates identification of the digital nerve and appropriate resection technique

Potential Pitfalls

To obtain a painless and functional stump certain principles must be observed. The volar skin flap should be long enough to cover the volar surface, the tip, and osseous structures to join the dorsal flap without tension. The ends of the digital nerves should be dissected carefully from the volar flap and resected at least 6 mm proximal to the flap to avoid painful neuroma formation at the distal stump. A sharp traction neurectomy should be performed with a #15 blade. The nerves should be allowed to retract proximally. The end of the bone must be padded well. The flexor and extensor tendons should be drawn distally, divided and allowed to retract proximally. If the amputation is proximal to the lunula, the sterile and germinal matrices should be carefully resected by thoroughly scraping the dorsal cortex of the distal phalanx with a curette to prevent the formation of nail horn, which can be a frustrating complication and require further surgery.

Postoperative Care

The dressing is removed in 5–7 days at which point digital motion therapy is initiated. Stitches are removed at 2–3 weeks. A tip protector and occupational therapy can facilitate recovery.

Common Complications

Common complications include painful neuroma formation, a hook nail deformity, as well as poor cosmetic appearance. Recurrence of nail horns can also be a problem requiring additional surgery.

When to Transfer

Microsurgical replantation is indicated in cases of thumb amputations, multiple digit amputations, and any amputation in children. The amputated part should be expeditiously prepared under the guidance of the treating hand surgeon. In most cases, the amputated part can be wrapped in saline soaked gauze in a plastic bag which can be placed on ice. The amputated part should never be frozen or placed directly on ice. Maximum ischemic time varies with the level of amputation.

Suggested Reading

Allen MJ. Conservative management of finger tip injuries in adults. Hand. 1980;3:257–65.

Atasoy E, Ioakimidis E, Kasdan ML, Kutz JE, Kleinert HE. Reconstruction of the amputated finger tip with a triangular volar flap: a new surgical procedure. J Bone Joint Surg Am. 1970;52(5):921–6.

Blair JW, Moskal MJ. Revision amputation achieving maximum function and minimizing problems. Hand. 2001;17:457–71.

Chow SP, Ho E. Open treatment of fingertip injuries in adults. J Hand Surg Am. 1982;7:470–6.

Das SK, Brown HG. Management of lost finger tips in children. Hand. 1978;10:16–27.

Fassler PR. Fingertip injuries: evaluation and treatment. J Am Acad Orthop Surg. 1996;4:84–92.

Green DP, Hotchkiss R, Pederson WC. Green's operative hand surgery, vol. 2. London: Churchill-Livingstone; 1998.

Hwang E, Park BH, Song SY, Jung HS, Kim CH. Fingertip reconstruction with simultaneous flaps and nail bed grafts following amputation. J Hand Surg. 2013;38A:1307–14.

Kumar VP, Satku K. Treatment and prevention of "hook nail" deformity with anatomic correlation. J Hand Surg Am. 1993;18(4):617–20.

Kutler W. A new method for finger tip amputation. JAMA. 1947;133:29–30.

Schenck RR, Cheema TA. Hypothenar skin grafts for fingertip reconstruction. J Hand Surg Am. 1984;9:750–3.

Damage Control Laparotomy

David H. Livingston and Tim Schwartz

Introduction

The term "damage control" laparotomy for trauma was popularized by Rotondo et al. [1] to describe techniques that address abbreviated treatment of major intraabdominal hemorrhage, contamination from hollow viscera followed by some sort of temporary closure. More definitive treatment would occur following a period of resuscitation and warming in the intensive care unit. The term damage control was borrowed from the navy describing the scenario where a ship is severely crippled and the crew provides what urgent and often temporary repair is needed to get it to port for subsequent definitive and permanent repairs. Thus, damage control should be thought of more as a concept than technique and its reintroduction into modern trauma care has been credited for increased survival in severely injured patients. Damage control techniques have also advanced beyond laparotomy alone and have been advocated and described for thoracic, orthopedic, and vascular trauma as well as non-trauma indications such as intraabdominal sepsis. The concept and mind-set necessary to embark on damage surgery is ideal for the rural surgeon where resources and collegial support may be limited or readily exhausted. In fact, in institutions with limited resources, damage control may be the only realistic option in many cases. This chapter will outline and describe the three likely situations (hemorrhage control for trauma, intraabdominal sepsis, and intraoperative consultations) where it may be necessary for the rural surgeon to employ damage control principles and techniques to achieve successful patient outcomes.

Preparation

Similar to elective surgery, the success of damage control begins with preoperative preparation and planning. In this case, it is not the steps of the operation you are going to perform but rather what "tools are available in your toolbox" at that moment in time. How much blood does my blood bank have and more importantly how much can they supply to the operating room at 2 a.m.? What about fresh frozen plasma and platelets? Which surgical colleagues (vascular, thoracic, etc.) are in town and who will be available to help? Knowing these data is of paramount importance to successful outcomes.

Patients who require damage control procedures following trauma or for the treatment intraabdominal sepsis are generally in extremis where there is little time for extensive preoperative work-up and evaluation. After a rapid primary survey the patient usually needs to be urgently transported to the operating room. Control of airway is usually required and only limited attempts at the correction of vital signs should be undertaken as it is impossible to fully correct physiology without taking care of the primary problem in the operating room. In the setting of trauma, blood should begin as soon as possible and the blood bank should be alerted. In fact, the only blood sample that is absolutely necessary in this circumstance is for type and cross-match. Fluid resuscitation as well as vasopressor agents if necessary should be rapidly instituted for patients in septic shock. In both cases, direct communication with anesthesia is necessary to ensure that the patient is optimally resuscitated, coagulopathy is addressed, and hypothermia is avoided.

Damage Control for Trauma

Indications

There are several points in the care of injured patients where a surgeon may decide to proceed with a damage control approach. Sometimes it is obvious from the outset.

D.H. Livingston, M.D., F.A.C.S. (✉) • T. Schwartz, D.O.
Department of Surgery, Rutgers-New Jersey Medical School,
University Hospital M234, Newark, NJ 07103, USA
e-mail: livingst@rutgers.edu

A.L. Halverson and D.C. Borgstrom (eds.), *Advanced Surgical Techniques for Rural Surgeons*,
DOI 10.1007/978-1-4939-1495-1_26, © Springer Science+Business Media New York 2015

The presence of hypotension, hypothermia, and acidosis on presentation are all obvious markers for abbreviated laparotomy. Following injury, any hypotension in the presence of multiple body system injuries should be a tip off that damage control approach may be warranted. Acidosis and high lactate levels on arterial blood gas analysis and the need for emergent transfusion are also indicators of deranged physiology where a damage control approach may be necessary. More insidious is the patient that "doesn't look too bad" upon presentation but rapidly deteriorates in the operating room. It is here where ongoing discussion with anesthesia regarding the patient's temperature, acid–base status, and need for intermittent vasopressor support should indicate that the patient's physiology is deteriorating and a shift in mind-set to damage control is needed. Other intraoperative signs are increasing bowel edema, cold tissues, and diffuse oozing, especially in areas that were formerly hemostatic. Lastly, certain injuries by themselves or in combination with others are better served by abbreviated laparotomy. High grade liver injuries, combination of major abdominal vascular and intestinal injuries, intraabdominal injuries in the setting of a massive pelvic fracture are among those frequently discussed in the literature as indications for damage control procedures.

Pitfalls and Danger Points

There are times when the source of hemorrhage is not straightforward. In patients with penetrating thoracoabdominal wounds, the source of hemorrhage may be in the chest, the abdomen, or both cavities. In addition, massive bleeding from the chest could actually be coming from an intraabdominal source when the diaphragm is lacerated. Making that assessment early with chest radiography and cardiac ultrasound will help in operative planning. Patients with blunt trauma and hemoperitoneum who have an associated pelvic fracture may have substantial retroperitoneal hemorrhage in addition to intraabdominal bleeding. This particular group of patients will be discussed in the following sections.

Operative Strategy

Damage control laparotomy begins with rapid access and wide exposure followed by control of bleeding and contamination in that order. Rapid control of hemorrhage followed by resuscitation with blood, plasma, and platelets in a 1:1:1 ratio is designed to prevent the lethal triad of hypothermia, acidosis, and coagulopathy. Again, constant communication with your anesthesia colleagues is of paramount importance. One needs to be aware of not only patient's vital signs that you can see on the monitor but also of other physiological parameters such as temperature, base deficit, blood transfusion requirements, and need for vasopressor and ionotropic support.

The patient needs to be prepped and draped from neck to the knees. Enter peritoneal cavity through midline incision from xyphoid to pubis using a scalpel or curved mayo scissors. Large volumes of blood coming from the peritoneal cavity render the electrocautery useless in this circumstance. We preferentially go around the umbilicus on the left as it avoids having to take down the falciform ligament. We also advocate opening the skin, subcutaneous tissue, and fascia widely prior to entering the peritoneal cavity as the rapid egress of blood through a small hole in the peritoneum can obscure vision and opening the remaining incision difficult. The peritoneal cavity can be ideally accessed just superior to umbilicus where peritoneum is the thinnest. Once inside, incise the remaining peritoneum taking down the preperitoneal fat along the left side with scissors taking care to avoid injuring underlying intestines, left lobe of the liver, and transverse colon superiorly and bladder inferiorly.

Four quadrant packing is the first step in damage control laparotomy. This requires that the scrub team should have 20–30 large laparotomy pads opened and ready to go. They should be handed to surgeon completely open as time is truly of the essence. Prior to packing blood and clot must be scooped from the peritoneal cavity. Suction is NOT useful in this circumstance. Clots and liquid blood should be removed manually and with the aid of lap pads. There is also no time to worry about neatness or the mess you are making on the field or the floor. The scrub team should provide the surgeon with a large basin to aid with removal of blood and clots but this is not an absolute either. Once the clots are removed you are ready to pack. At this point one may get an idea of which quadrants are bleeding. The left upper quadrant is packed from the right side with the assistant pulling up in the abdominal wall. The spleen should be palpated and 3–5 laparotomy pads will fit into the space. Conversely, the liver and right upper quadrant is best packed from the left by placing several pads above the liver. Liver is then pressed against the packs and diaphragm and the subhepatic space packed cephalad. Again the liver should be palpated and the identification of any liver injuries made at that time. One has to be careful not to compress the inferior vena cava (IVC) when packing the liver and right upper quadrant. Again, communication with anesthesia is the key here. The lower quadrants are packed by grasping the omentum and transverse colon cephalad and eviscerating the small intestine up and to the patient's right. Identification of a zone III hematoma in the face of a pelvic fracture can be made at this time. Lap pads are placed into the pouch of Douglas and along each gutter. With small intestine out of the way, packing is much more effective as it is almost impossible to pack the lower quadrants with the small bowel in place. Eviscerating the small bowel also allows the identification and clamping of any mesenteric vascular injuries. Careful and systematic packing works to arrest, at least temporarily, venous and most lower volume arterial bleeding, but it is unlikely to arrest substantial arterial hemorrhage from named vessels. Nonetheless it cleans the field and temporizes the situation. It also allows anesthesia to resuscitate the patient and the surgeon to call for any needed equipment and catch their breath so that the abdomen can be fully explored in a more organized way. Setting up a self-retaining retractor system can be extremely helpful when extra assistance is not available. While it may take several minutes to set up, it will likely result in less hemorrhage down the line, provide far better exposure, and is well worth the setup time.

Once the abdomen has been packed, even if the extent of all injuries has not been determined the surgeon will have gained significant amount of information. Most importantly, did the packing and initial evaluation arrest the hemorrhage? If not and the packs are "bleeding through," there is likely uncontrolled arterial hemorrhage that needs to be immediately addressed. Even though it has not controlled all hemorrhage, what packing has done in this instance is guide the surgeon to a specific quadrant or area. If the packing has been successful it is now time to unpack. There is great temptation to immediately attack areas or quadrants that contained the obvious injuries. Resist this urge at all cost and unpack those quadrants where no obvious injuries were identified. A tightly packed abdomen results in limited exposure. Unpacking uninjured quadrants allow significantly improved exposure and ability to move the viscera around. It is also during this step where a more formal exploration of the bowel can be performed.

The small bowel should be run from the ligament of treitz to the ileocecal valve, inspecting mesenteric and antimesenteric surfaces. Any hematomas should be considered suspicious and explored. This is especially true in the face of penetrating trauma. Mesenteric hemorrhage can be controlled with clamps or sutures. Bowel perforations can be controlled with either a Babcock or intestinal clamp or tied with umbilical tapes until the extent of repairs and resections can be determined. Retroperitoneal colonic surfaces, posterior aspect of transverse colon, as well as hepatic and splenic flexures need to be carefully examined. The increased amount of fat on the colonic wall can hide significant perforations and any hematoma must be carefully unroofed and explored. The anterior stomach is easily explored but any injury encountered mandates the surgeon to carefully explore the posterior surface by entering the lesser sac and mobilizing the stomach from the pancreas by lysing the avascular gastropancreatic attachments. It is easy to miss injuries high up along the greater or lesser curves of the stomach near the gastroesophageal junction.

Identification of liver injuries is straightforward. You can not only see it but also feel it by running your hand over surface of the liver. The best advice for many liver injuries is to leave lacerations that are not bleeding alone. Other minor injuries that were controlled by packing can often be controlled with electrocautery, argon beam coagulation, or topical hemostatic agents. Hepatorrhaphy, preferably with omental packing, is a technique to handle more extensive injuries. The initial packing of the liver in a sandwich of 8–10 laparotomy pads from above and below may be the only hemostatic maneuver required. In the instance where a damage control procedure is going to be performed and hemostasis has been accomplished with packing, the surgeon must resist the strong temptation to "peak" one more time at the injury. This maneuver will only result in increased hemorrhage and coagulopathy and repacking the second time may not be as effective. If packing the liver as described has not been effective the next step is to control the inflow by performing controlling the portal triad (Pringle maneuver). A Pringle maneuver can be accomplished with a vascular clamp through the foramen of Winslow or by encircling the portal triad and using a Rummel tourniquet. If using a vascular clamp, we prefer a long handed angled Satinsky clamp with the handle positioned down toward the left lower quadrant. This will keep the clamp away from the surgical field in the right upper quadrant. Control of hemorrhage with a Pringle clamp indicates arterial hemorrhage or an injury to a major portal vein branch. In this instance the liver must be explored in order to control the bleeding. Another adjunct that may prove useful is using balloon tamponade for bleeding deep in a tract in the liver. These can be controlled using a Blakemore tube by inflating esophageal balloon inside the tract and gastric balloon outside. Alternatively and only if the capabilities exist, taking the patient for angiographic embolization with a Pringle clamp in place until the angiographer has the catheter in place is a possibility.

If despite packing and effective Pringle there is still bleeding, it is important to distinguish bright red arterial bleeding from dark venous bleeding. In the former you may be dealing with anomalous hepatic artery and supraceliac aortic clamping is a reasonable option. If on the other hand there is dark blood coming from either behind or from within deep liver wound, you must prepare for retrohepatic IVC or hepatic vein injury. Occasionally these injuries can be controlled with careful packing and compression; however, if they have already bled through your packing and Pringle maneuver it is likely that you will need to attempt surgical control. It is in these circumstances that additional surgical assistance if available is invaluable. Anesthesia must also be ready for the potential of rapid blood loss. Rapid mobilization of the liver and direct "attack" is the only way to salvage these very difficult injuries.

The only damage control option for splenic injury is splenectomy. In patient in extremis there is no time or indication to attempt splenic salvage. The spleen should be rapidly mobilized and delivered to the midline. Once the spleen is in your hand, apply large clamps sequentially across the hilum and short gastric vessels and ligate sequentially as close to the spleen as possible to avoid injury to the tail of the pancreas and stomach, respectively. Following removal, either at the first or subsequent operations, the greater curve of the stomach should be carefully examined to see if a piece of stomach was caught in one of the short gastric camps placed during the emergency splenectomy. Any area of the stomach that is questionable should be imbricated with Lembert sutures.

Options for dealing with perinephric hematomas in the face of damage control laparotomy boil down to: (1) leave them alone or (2) nephrectomy. The choice is usually easy to make and a rapidly expanding hematoma especially with bright arterial bleeding from the renal hilum is an indication for nephrectomy. While many have advocated vascular control prior to opening Gerota's fascia, this recommendation is doomed to fail and will result in exaggerated blood loss. A long incision should be performed into the retroperitoneal hematoma through Gerota's fascia and the kidney grasped in the surgeon's hand and brought medially. The hilum should be pinched between the thumb and fingers. The surgeon should now have a relatively nonbleeding kidney in their hand. Hilar vessels can then be ligated either individually or en masse with heavy ties. The ureter is stripped down toward the bladder and divided wherever it is convenient. While palpation of the contralateral kidney prior to nephrectomy is advocated, this recommendation is meaningless in damage control situations with a shattered kidney.

Hemorrhage from the retroperitoneum especially that which bleeds through the initial packing usually indicates major arterial or venous hemorrhage which will require control to allow the patient to be stabilized for transport to another institution or later reoperation. For the successful evaluation of the retroperitoneum, the surgeon must be familiar with two key maneuvers to provide exposure. Right medial visceral rotation or the Cattel-Braasch maneuver includes mobilization of hepatic flexure and ascending colon and complete Kocherization of the duodenum follows. To complete full right-sided medial visceral rotation, incise small bowel mesenteric attachments from the posterior peritoneum. You can now have access to IVC, infrarenal aorta, bilateral iliac vessels, renal arteries and veins, superior mesenteric vessels, and third and fourth portion of the duodenum. Left-sided medial visceral rotation, also known as the Mattox maneuver, involves mobilizing descending colon along the white line of Toldt. Continue superiorly in the same plane and rotate spleen, distal pancreas toward the midline. The left kidney may be mobilized or left in place depending upon the injury pattern. A completed left medial visceral rotation provides exposure to the abdominal aorta, celiac axis, superior mesenteric artery, left renal artery, and left iliac artery and vein.

Detailed control of each possible vascular injury is beyond the scope of this chapter and a thorough knowledge of anatomy and exposure are keys to successful outcomes. However in a damage control laparotomy, control of hemorrhage can roughly be divided into knowing which vessels need to be repaired and which ones can be safely ligated. Almost all veins with the exception of the suprarenal IVC and the superior mesenteric vein can be ligated if necessary. On the arterial side, the internal iliac arteries can be ligated, even bilaterally if necessary with little morbidity. If simple suture repair of major arterial and venous injures cannot be performed during damage control, then temporary intravascular shunting should be employed. Almost all types of temporary conduits have been employed depending upon the size of the vessel including the various types of carotid shunts, chest tubes, and even nasogastric tubes. Systemic heparinization, especially in the acute phase is not needed in patients who are shunted.

Patients with significant and displaced pelvic fractures who have an indication for laparotomy either after positive FAST or DPL are a challenge. The surgeon must exercise caution when entering peritoneal cavity as to not release pelvic hematoma. Therefore, supraumbilical upper midline incision should be used for the intraabdominal portion of the case. Since packing the pelvis from inside the abdomen is ineffective, a preperitoneal approach is utilized. This can be done via lower midline or Pfannenstiel incision. After opening the fascia, pack the pelvis on each side of the bladder taking care not to disturb peritoneum. It may require three or more packs on each side. In order for preperitoneal packing to be effective, some sort of pelvic stabilization must be in place. It may be either an external fixator applied by the orthopedic team or a C-clamp.

Patients with thoracoabdominal penetrating injuries also pose a special challenge since there are several cavities and therefore several potential sources of hemorrhage. Thoracoabdominal region extends from the nipple line in males and inframammary fold in females to costal margin. Both pleural spaces, mediastinum, upper abdomen, and retroperitoneum are potential sources of bleeding in patients with penetrating injuries to that anatomic region. Bullet trajectory can be informative when faced with the decision of which cavity to explore first. Preoperative radiographs of chest and abdomen can be very helpful in that regard. During exploratory laparotomy, certain clues such as unexplained hypotension, elevated peak airway pressures, and elevated central venous pressure may lead you to suspect bleeding in the chest. To rule out cardiac tamponade, pericardial window through the abdomen will be diagnostic. Keep in mind that chest tubes can be clogged or kinked and the surgeon and the anesthesia team need to be observant and maintain high index of suspicion regarding the function of chest tubes. Damage control packing of the chest and even mediastinum with temporary closure has been employed with and without concomitant damage control laparotomy.

Control of enteric spillage during damage control procedures is usually done in two stages. Early in the exploration and packing phase, gross spillage is accomplished by clamping, whip stitching, or tying the segments off with umbilical tape. The goal is to merely control gross enteric spillage until hemorrhage control can be dealt with. If clamps are utilized, babcocks or other noncrushing intestinal or vascular clamps are preferred. However, any clamp can be utilized in an emergency. Following control of life-threatening hemorrhage, dealing with enteric injures is next stage in a damage control laparotomy. The extent of all gastrointestinal injuries needs to be identified. Hematomas, especially those on a fatty colonic surface need to be explored to ensure that they are not hiding a full thickness injury. Conceptually, the care of intestinal injuries in damage control surgery follows the dictum simple is better. Injuries that can be easily closed should be repaired primarily. Multiple sequential injuries of the small bowel, even if they could be repaired, are usually better treated as a single resection. Even small bowel injuries that appear separated by sufficient intervening normal intestine should be treated by a single resection if the intervening bowel length is less than 15–20 cm. Colonic injures that are not amenable to simple repair should be resected. During the initial damage control operation, no anastomosis should be performed and no ostomy brought out the abdominal wall. These procedures are part of the later reconstructive phases of damage control and should not be considered during the first operation.

Temporary Abdominal Closure

There are a number of ways to obtain temporary abdominal closure after damage control laparotomy ranging from simple skin closure with a running suture or towel clips to commercially available negative pressure systems to a combination of techniques. The basic principles are to isolate intraabdominal viscera, prevent abdominal compartment syndrome, and provide adequate drainage of the effluent. One simple way is to place sterile X-ray cassette cover or an open 3 L IV bag inside the abdomen, tuck it into right and left paracolic gutters and the pelvis, cover with rolls of gauze, place two nasogastric tubes, and cover with adherent plastic drape. Nasogastric tubes are then connected to suction. There are commercially available devices that serve the same purpose. Sutures should NOT be placed on the fascia at this time, nor should any drains or ostomy exit the abdominal wall.

Damage Control for Intraabdominal Sepsis

Although as outlined earlier, damage control laparotomy has been traditionally described for use following severe injury, the concept and technique of an abbreviated laparotomy are applicable in emergency general surgery. The most common indications for damage control in these circumstances are intestinal ischemia, peritonitis, and massive upper or lower gastrointestinal bleeding. Similar to the treatment of intestinal injuries, ischemic or perforated sections of bowel should be quickly resected. No attempts at anastomosis should be undertaken at this time. The abdomen should be irrigated free of gross spillage and a temporary closure with a cassette cover or a commercially available device should be performed. These cases are not amenable to suture closure. Patients with massive lower gastrointestinal bleeding are best handled by subtotal colectomy. Those with upper gastrointestinal tract bleeding require control of hemorrhage and closure of gastrotomy or duodenotomy as simply as possible.

Damage Control for an Intraoperative Consultation

Occasionally the rural general surgeon will be asked to come into the operating room for consultation during a colleague's case. While the majority of these are elective and deal with unexpected pathology or findings, at times it may be due to a misadventure or complication usually resulting in hemorrhage. Examples from our own practice are major vascular injuries during spine surgery or secondary to trocar insertion during laparoscopy. It is in these circumstances that damage control concepts need to remembered and employed. Exposure is a key principle. In the instance where the operation was being performed in an open fashion, extension of the incision is almost always required and the blood is usually at the far edge of the field. In laparoscopic cases, a generous incision similar to an acute trauma case needs to be utilized. Unlike the trauma situation, the quadrant of injury is usually obvious. But again, packing to gain control remains the first step. In many of these cases, anesthesia will have to obtain additional large bore IV access and the blood bank will have to be notified to have more blood available than was anticipated for the original case. The conduct of the case should then proceed as outlined for trauma. These cases do not only test the ability but may also the professionalism of the surgeon. The original surgeon may not think they need an incision "that big" or if they just did "x" it will be all better, especially once the bleeding is controlled. An even demeanor and gentle moving the case along without yelling or rancor is the key to successful outcome both for the patient and the professional relationship between colleagues.

Conclusion

Damage control concepts and techniques need to be part of every surgeons "tool box" and may be more applicable to rural surgeons than those working in resource "rich" environments. Successful damage control laparotomy begins with appropriate patient selection, whether preoperatively or during the operation itself. We cannot stress enough the importance of good communication between the surgeon, anesthesiologist, nurses, blood bank, and the potential accepting facility. Things to keep in mind in preparation for damage control are awareness of your experience as a surgeon and capabilities of your institution. The conduct of the operation itself adheres to basic damage control principles.

Rapid access and exposure, control of hemorrhage and contamination, and temporary closure are three basic steps of damage control laparotomy. The same steps can be applied to emergency general surgery and during intraoperative bleeding complications. While technique is undoubtedly important, embracing damage control as a mind-set and approach will lead to successful patient outcomes.

Reference

1. Rotondo MF, Schwab CW, McGonigal MD, Phillips 3rd GR, Fruchterman TM, Kauder DR, Latenser BA, Angood PA. 'Damage control': an approach for improved survival in exsanguinating penetrating abdominal injury. J Trauma. 1993;35:375–82.

Siobhan Hayden and Anouk R. Lambers

Indications

Cesarean delivery is indicated when labor is contraindicated, refused by the patient or for the safety of the mother and/or fetus. The most common indications for a Cesarean section in industrialized countries are repeat Cesarean deliveries and those performed for labor dystocia (failure to dilate or failure of fetal descent). Although the indications are numerous, 85 % of cesarean deliveries are performed because of non-vertex presentation, prior Cesarean delivery, labor dystocia, or non-reassuring fetal status [4]. There is a national standard to be able to proceed with Cesarean section within 30 min of decision [8].

Preoperative Preparation

Type and screen.
CBC.
Check with your state regarding mandatory requirements for admitted obstetric patients, such as RPR (syphilis testing).
Surgical site antibiotic skin prophylaxis given prior to incision.
Lower extremity pneumatic compression devices should be placed unless contraindicated.
Supine positioning with leftward lateral tilt (approximately 15°).
Foley catheter.
5 % chlorhexadine or iodine skin prep.
Allis clamp test prior to incision in patients under regional anesthesia.

S. Hayden, M.D. • A.R. Lambers, M.D. (✉)
Obstetrics and Gynecology, Bassett Medical Center,
Cooperstown, NY 13326, USA
e-mail: anouk.lambers@bassett.org

Operative Strategy

Once the decision has been made to proceed with Cesarean section, rapid transition to an operating room should occur. A transverse skin incision should be used in the majority of cases. Strict hemostasis upon entry into the uterus is not critical, as delivery of the baby in a timely fashion is the primary goal. It is helpful to have some idea of placental location and fetal position and presentation prior to incision to be better able to anticipate potential complications during the surgery.

Operative Technique

Anesthesia

There are two categories of anesthesia for cesarean section: general and regional anesthesia. Regional anesthesia includes both spinal and epidural anesthesia. Regional anesthesia is the preferred mode of anesthesia for a cesarean section as general anesthesia may cause severe uterine atony as well as neonatal depression. However, in the case of a true emergency regional anesthesia may take too long to accomplish and in that case, general anesthesia is preferable. It is very important to have the patient prepped and draped prior to proceeding with general anesthesia and proceed with the cesarean section expeditiously once the induction of anesthesia is complete.

As with most surgical procedures, there is no standard technique for Cesarean section. Many variants of previously described techniques are currently being utilized. They include transverse and vertical incisions. The transverse incision (Pfannenstiel, Joel-Cohen) is preferred secondary to less postoperative pain, greater wound strength, and improved cosmetic results [6]. There are occasional instances that require a vertical skin incision. These include a potential need to access the upper abdomen in some morbidly obese patients.

A.L. Halverson and D.C. Borgstrom (eds.), *Advanced Surgical Techniques for Rural Surgeons*,
DOI 10.1007/978-1-4939-1495-1_27, © Springer Science+Business Media New York 2015

Skin Incision

The Pfannenstiel Incision (Fig. 27.1)

A 10–12 cm curvilinear convex incision 2 cm above the symphysis pubis is made with a scalpel. The subcutaneous tissue is then incised and brought down to the fascia. The fascia is exposed and incised transversely. The incision is extended laterally with heavy curved Mayo scissors. The superior edge of the fascia is grasped with Kocher clamps and elevated. The underlying muscles are separated from the fascia by sharp and blunt dissection. Once the fascia is dissected, the rectus muscles are separated with finger dissection. Any perforating vessel is electrocoagulated or suture ligated. The peritoneum is incised sharply and the incision is extended vertically. The rectus muscles are then pulled manually in a transverse direction to increase exposure [7].

The Joel-Cohen Incision (Fig. 27.1)

A 10–12 cm straight incision is made through the skin 3 cm below the level of the anterior superior iliac spines with the scalpel. The subcutaneous tissues and the fascia are opened only in the midline. Both subcutaneous tissues and the fascial incision are extended transversely by blunt finger traction and the peritoneum is opened. Finger traction is carried out to separate the rectus muscles in the midline and all layers of the abdominal wall are stretched manually to the extent of the skin incision.

A bladder blade is inserted into the abdomen and the vesicouterine peritoneum is identified, and entered sharply with the Metzenbaum scissors. This incision is extended laterally, and a bladder flap is created digitally by blunt dissection (Fig. 27.2). The bladder blade is reinserted [7].

Uterine Incisions

Transverse Incision

The incision of choice, and therefore the most common incision, is a transverse incision made in the lower uterine segment. The advantages of this incision include greater ease

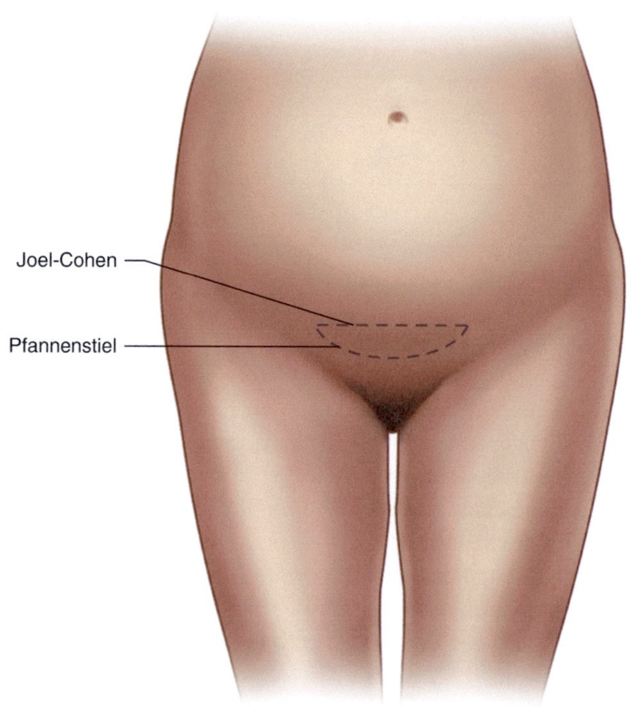

Fig. 27.1 Joel-Cohen and Pfannenstiel incisions

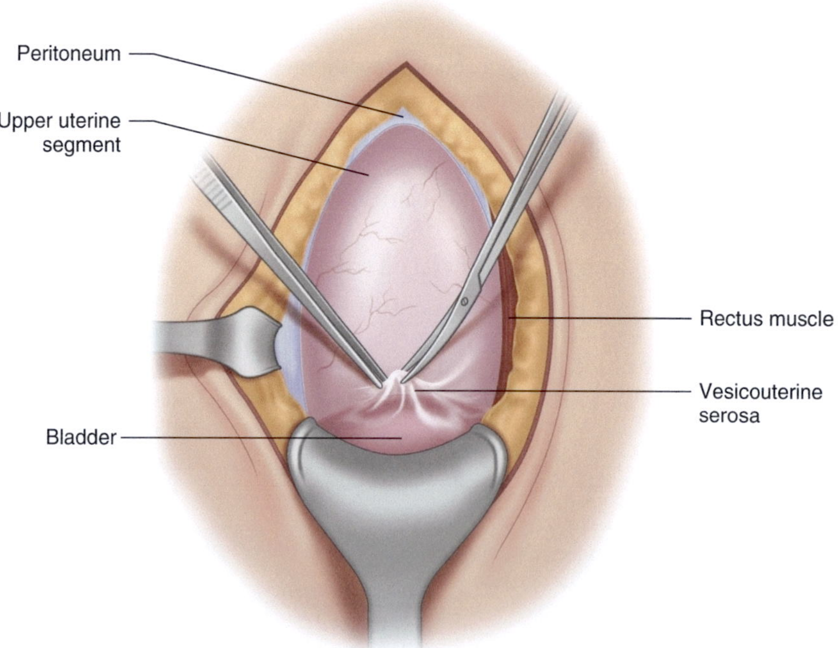

Fig. 27.2 The vesicouterine peritoneum is identified and entered sharply with the Metzenbaum scissors

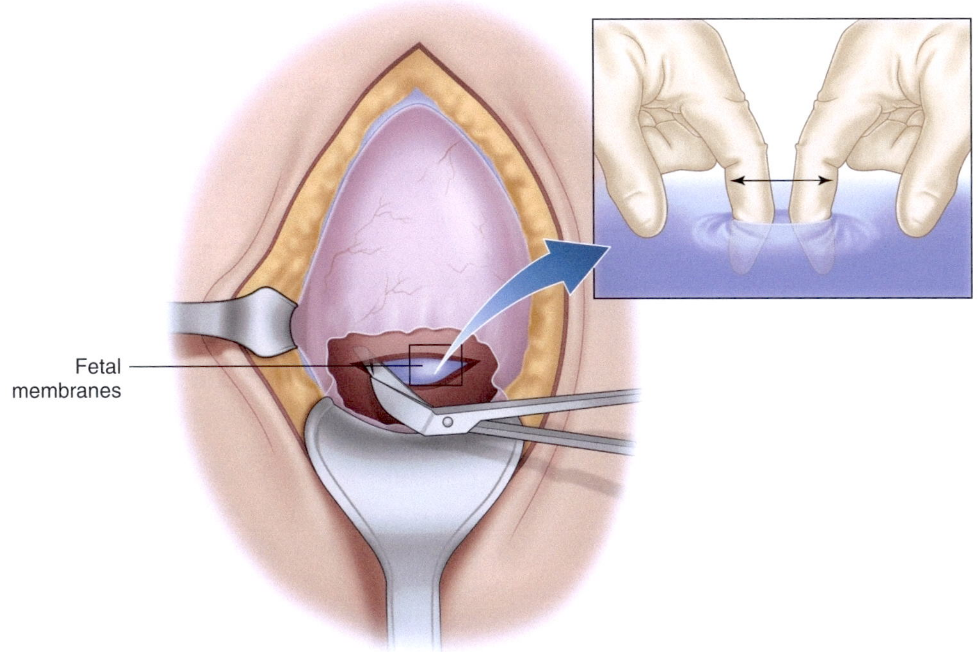

Fig. 27.3 Uterine incision extended with the bandage scissors or manually

of repair, a location that leads to less chance of rupture with subsequent pregnancies and less chance of bowel or omentum adherence [6]. A 1–2 cm transverse incision is made with a scalpel with a #10 blade approximately 1 cm below the upper margin of the peritoneal reflection in the midline. This should be placed higher in women who have achieved advanced or complete dilatation so as not to inadvertently enter the vagina and to avoid extension to the lateral vessels [4]. Great care should be taken to avoid injury to the fetus with laceration, which is the most common fetal injury seen [5]. The incision is extended with the Bandage scissors (Fig. 27.3a) or manually (Fig. 27.3b) in a lateral and upward fashion.

Care is taken not to extend the cut into the lateral uterine vessels. It is very important to make the uterine incision large enough to deliver the fetus intact without trauma. If the placenta is encountered, it must be retracted or incised, necessitating rapid delivery of the fetus. If the incision needs to be extended this can be accomplished by extending the lateral edges of the uterine incision upward or by a midline, vertical, inverted "T" incision. The amniotic sac is then ruptured using an Allis clamp.

Vertical Incision

A vertical, or classical, incision is used in certain situations to gain improved access to the uterine cavity, such as in the case of inadequate exposure of the lower segment due to adhesions, myoma or obesity, multiple gestations, or a fetus in a non-vertex presentation, especially if it is large and in a transverse, back-down position. This type of incision may also be necessary for the delivery of a preterm fetus, when the lower segment is not developed enough, thus not wide enough, to accomplish delivery atraumatically through a transverse incision. A vertical uterine incision is carried out by incising the uterus with a scalpel beginning in the lower uterine segment and extending upward using bandage scissors until it is of sufficient length to allow for atraumatic delivery of the fetus.

Fetal Extraction

Cephalic

Delivery of the fetus is accomplished by passing a hand in the uterine cavity between the symphysis pubis and fetal head. The fetal head is then carefully elevated through the incision while the assistant provides mild fundal uterine pressure (Fig. 27.4). If there is difficulty with delivery of the fetal head, consideration of an inadequate incision size at either the skin, fascia, rectus muscles, or uterus should be evaluated and corrected, if necessary. If the incision is assessed to be an adequate size and the head cannot be delivered, application of a vacuum device should be considered. After delivery of the head, the mouth and nares are cleared of amniotic fluid and mucus with a bulb syringe. The remainder of the fetus including shoulders and body are delivered by gentle traction and fundal pressure. The umbilical cord is doubly clamped and cut. The infant is handed off to the awaiting designated attendant who can perform resuscitative efforts if necessary, preferably a pediatrician or someone certified in neonatal resuscitation. Umbilical artery blood gas and blood samples are obtained from the umbilical cord.

Breech

It is very important to make the uterine incision larger prior to attempting to deliver the fetus to minimize unnecessary traction on the after-coming head. The breech fetus may be delivered in frank breech presentation (buttocks presenting with hips flexed and legs extended above the head) (Fig. 27.5a), complete breech presentation (one or both knees are flexed) or footling breech presentation (one or both feet are the lowest presenting part).

Frank Breech Extraction

At the point of hip flexion, the fetus is grasped with a finger bilaterally and gentle downward traction is placed on the hips (Fig. 27.5b) until the legs are completely delivered and the fetus has been delivered to the level of the scapulas. Both hands are then placed over the bony pelvis and a moist cloth is placed under the body of the fetus to provide support. Each humerus is palpated until the elbow is reached. The humerus is supported and the arm is swept downward without force or traction taking care not to rotate the fetal spine. The head is then delivered gently without pressure from above, taking care to make sure the head remains flexed, preventing neck hyperextension.

Complete or Footling Breech Extraction

Prior to puncture of the amniotic sac, the fetal feet are identified and grasped in one hand. The amniotic sac is ruptured

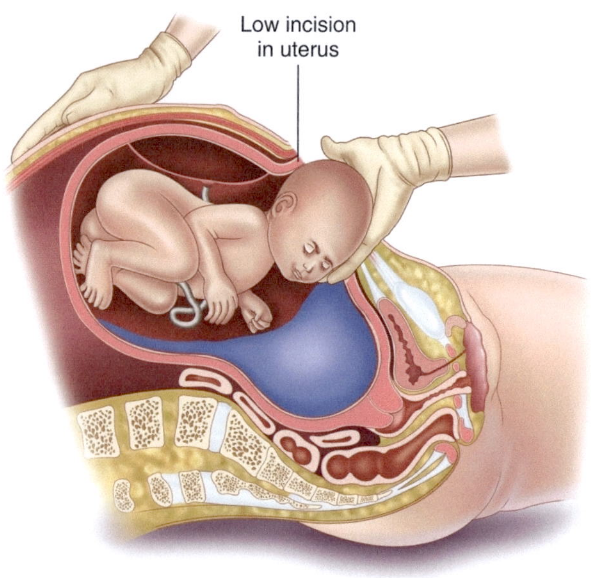

Fig. 27.4 Fetal head is carefully elevated through the incision

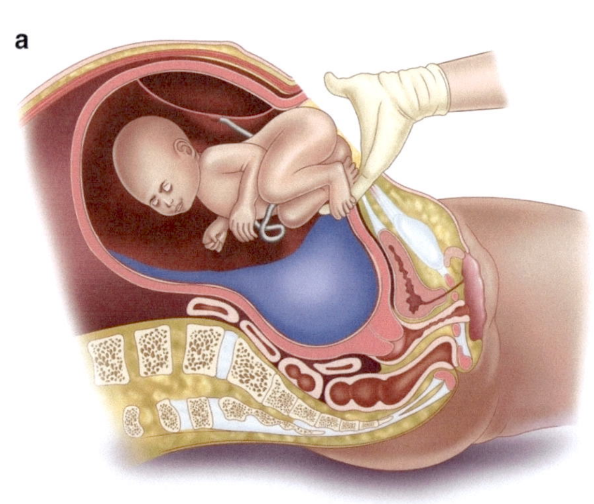

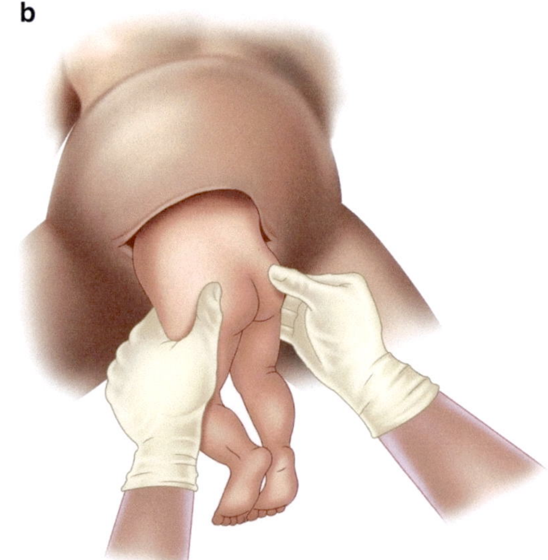

Fig. 27.5 (**a**) Frank breech presentation. (**b**) Gentle downward traction on fetal hips

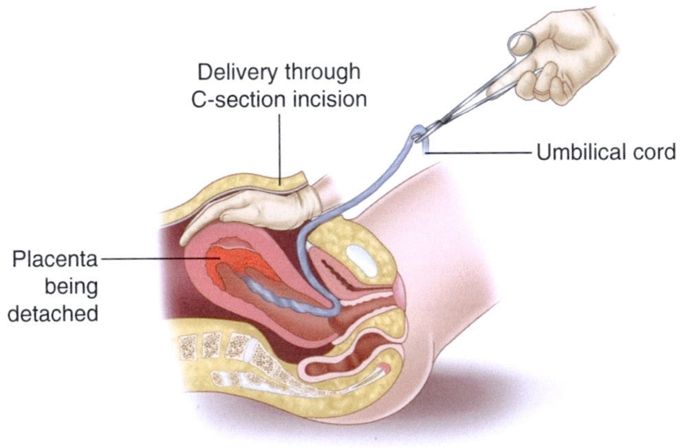

Fig. 27.6 Technique for placenta delivery

and using gentle downward traction on the fetal legs, the fetus is delivered to the level of the scapulas. The remainder of the delivery is as described above.

Placental Delivery

Immediately after delivery of the fetus, an intravenous infusion of oxytocin 20 U in 1,000 mL of crystalloid solution bolus should be started until adequate uterine tone is achieved, at which time the rate can be decreased. The placenta is removed by gentle massage of the uterine fundus and gentle traction of the umbilical cord. All placental contents including amniotic membranes should be removed which can be accomplished with the use of a Kelly clamp to slowly dissect the amnion from the uterine wall (Fig. 27.6).

Uterine Repair

The placenta is handed off and the uterus is grasped at the fundus and delivered out of the incision and placed on the maternal abdomen. Although some surgeons prefer to repair the uterus in situ, the advantages of exteriorizing the uterus include immediate assessment of uterine tone, increased ease in identifying and repairing bleeding sites and ability to visualize the adnexa for any abnormalities or for performing tubal ligation. The sole disadvantage is potential increase in discomfort to the patient [4]. The uterine fundus is then covered with a moist laparotomy pad. A sweep of the uterine cavity is performed with a dry laparotomy pad in order to ensure complete removal of all clots and possible placental debris. Any brisk bleeding from the uterine incision is clamped with T-clamps (broad based Allis clamps) until the incision is repaired. The uterine incision is closed with a continuous 0 delayed-absorbable suture in a running, locked fashion beginning at one angle of the incision through the full thickness of the myometrium. It is important to identify the uterine vessels and place them between thumb and index finger prior to placement of the needle into the myometrium.

A Kelly clamp is placed on the suture end on each angle of the incision as a means to manipulate the uterus. A second imbricating layer of suture of the same material is carried out. Once the needle has been placed it should not be withdrawn to minimize bleeding. There is no evidence to suggest that there is any benefit to closure of the bladder flap. If uterine vessels appear to be lacerated, an O'Leary stitch should be placed promptly to minimize blood loss (described under "Complications").

For repair of a vertical incision, a deep suture of continuous, interlocking 0 delayed-absorbable suture should be placed, incorporating half of the depth of the incision. A second layer with the same suture is placed incorporating the remaining superficial portion of the incision. Inward manual traction of the incisional edges by an assistant may be necessary to facilitate adequate closure and minimize tension on the suture line during closure. The uterine serosa, if not already incorporated, may be reapproximated with a 2–0 delayed-absorbable suture [4].

Abdominal Closure

Once hemostasis and adequate uterine tone is established, the uterus is carefully returned to the abdomen. The gutters are cleared of all blood clots and hemostasis is again assured by inspecting the uterine scar after elevating it to the abdominal incision. The sutures are then cut and the uterus is left in place.

Needle, lap, and instrument count should be correct prior to proceeding with closure of abdominal wall. Closure of the peritoneum with a running suture of 2–0 delayed-absorbable suture can be performed if there is distended bowel impeding safe closure, although otherwise it is not necessary. As each layer is closed, bleeding sites are cauterized or suture ligated. The rectus muscles are then left to fall into place and the subfascial space is thoroughly inspected for hemostasis.

The rectus muscles can be approximated in the midline with a single mattress suture of 2–0 delayed-absorbable suture material. The overlying fascia is reapproximated with running suture of 0 delayed-absorbable suture material. The subcutaneous tissue should be repaired for a depth of >2 cm using interrupted sutures of 2–0 delayed-absorbable suture material [3]. The skin is closed by subcuticular closure with 4–0 delayed-absorbable suture material and subsequent application of skin adhesive or adhesive strips. When the risk is increased for the development of post surgical infections, such is the case of morbidly obese patients or those with a diagnosis of chorioamnionitis, placement of skin staples is advised.

All drapes are then removed from the patient's abdomen and uterine massage is carried out to clear the uterine cavity of all blood clots and to ascertain that uterine tone is still adequate before leaving the operating suite. A second and last count should be carried out prior to taking the patient to the recovery room. In the case of an emergent cesarean section, an instrument count can be deferred with the performance of an abdominal-pelvic X-ray at the completion of the case.

Pitfalls and Danger Points

Delay in decision to proceed with Cesarean section leading to potential fetal injury

Fully dilated patient with a prolonged second stage (pushing)

Nonvertex presentation

Multiple gestation

Anteriorly located placenta

Need for general anesthesia which can lead to uterine atony and fetal depression

Careful entry into uterus to prevent fetal laceration

Avoid extension of uterine incision inferiorly and laterally which can lead to hemorrhage

Uterine atony

Intrapartum Complications

Complications that may arise at the time of Cesarean section include hemorrhage, bladder (1.4 per 1,000), ureteral (0.3 per 1,000) or bowel injury, fetal injury, and complications from anesthesia [4]. Obesity increases all of these risks. The most commonly identified injury at cesarean delivery is fetal laceration, and its incidence has been reported to be as high as 3 % [12]. Cesarean section can lead to increased postpartum morbidity including puerperal infection (wound, urinary tract, and uterine), thromboembolism, and future obstetric and surgical complications related to abnormal placentation, which increases the risk for peripartum hysterectomy [2].

Postpartum Hemorrhage

Postpartum hemorrhage is defined as a total blood loss of more than 500 mL, as estimated after the delivery of the placenta. The average blood loss following an uncomplicated Cesarean delivery is estimated at 800–1,000 mL. "Near term, it is estimated that 600 mL/min of blood flows through the intervillous space. With separation of the placenta, there is separation of the many uterine arteries and veins that carry blood to and from the placenta" [4]. Causes of postpartum hemorrhage following a Cesarean delivery include uterine atony, retained placental tissue, placenta accreta, uterine artery laceration, inadvertent uterine incision extension, and coagulation defects. Bleeding may be massive, or a steady continuous flow that persists and may not be recognized until severe hypovolemia ensues. In pregnancy, most often large amounts of blood loss have occurred before the pulse and blood pressure show any change [4].

Uterine Atony

Risks factors for atony include prior history of postpartum hemorrhage, use of oxytocin in labor, prolonged labor, grand multiparity (more than four previous deliveries) or an overdistended uterus such as with large fetuses, excessive amniotic fluid (polyhydramnios) or multiple gestation [4]. There are both medical and surgical options available for the treatment of uterine atony.

Medical Management of Uterine Atony

There are several effective medications to increase uterine tone and should be the first line of treatment in uterine atony (see options below) when uterine massage/bimanual compression fails (Table 27.1) [10].

Surgical Management of Uterine Atony

If medical management fails, there are several surgical options, including uterine compression sutures, arterial ligation, uterine packing, and radiologic interventions. Peripartum hysterectomy is reserved for those cases refractory to other interventions or when the chance of mortality is high due to massive blood loss.

B-lynch technique: Close the lower uterine segment in the usual manner (Fig. 27.7). Using a #1 delayed-absorbable suture, place the initial bites on the right side of the uterine

Table 27.1 Medication options for management of postpartum hemorrhage

Medication	Dose/route/frequency	Contraindications	Side effects
Oxytocin	10–40 units IV bolus in 1 L NS or LR	Maximum dose	Undiluted rapid IV infusion may cause severe
	10 units IM into myometrium	Of 60 units	Hypotension or cardiac arrest
Methylergonovine	0.2 mg IM every 2–4 h	Hypertension	Hypertension
Misoprostol	800–1,000 µg PR once		
15-Methyl PGF2α	0.25 mg IM every 15–90 min × 8 doses	Asthma	Diarrhea, hypertension, fever, flushing tachycardia
Dinoprostone	20 mg PV or PR every 2 h	Hypotension	Hypotension

Modified from ACOG Practice Bulletin #76, postpartum hemorrhage, October 2006, reaffirmed 2013

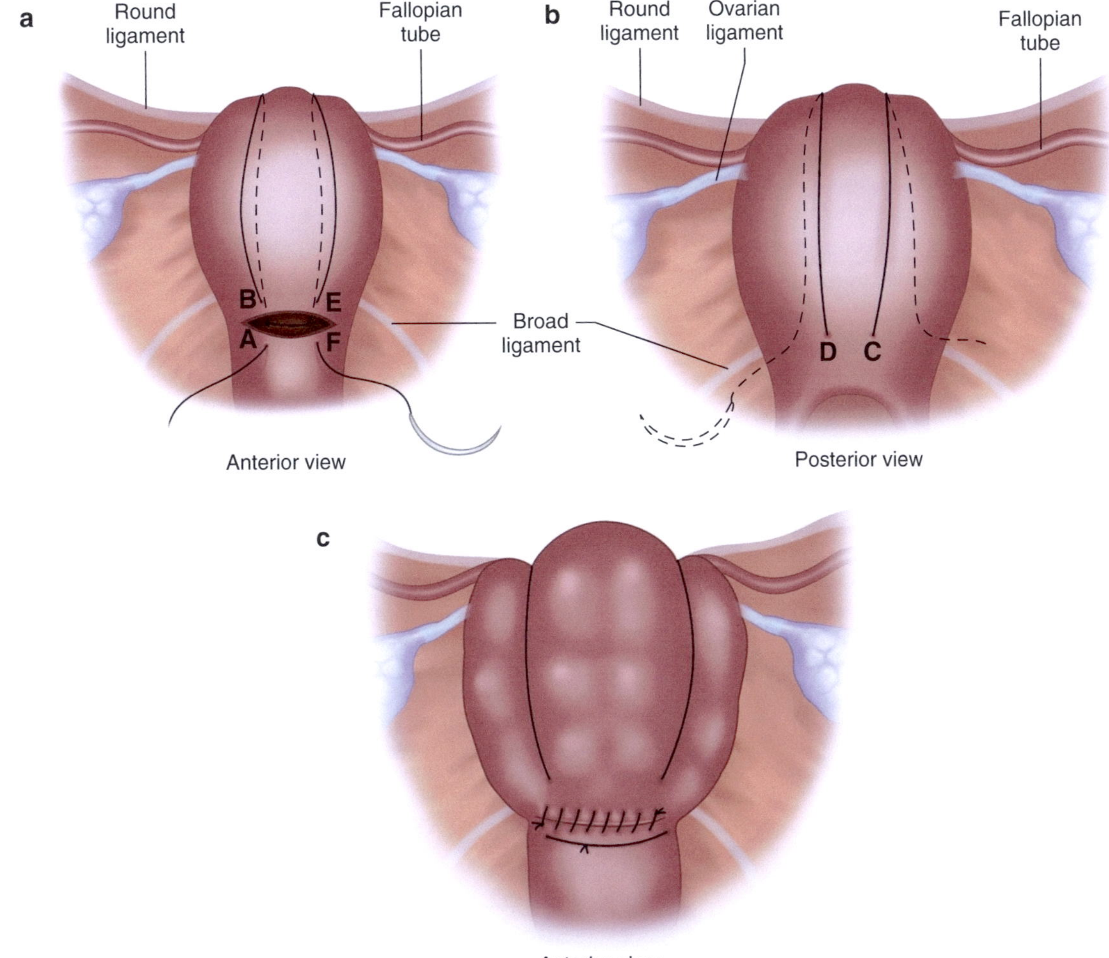

Fig. 27.7 B-Lynch suture

incision approximately 3 cm below and then above the hysterotomy incision (A and B). Loop the suture around the fundus and reenter the uterus through the posterior uterine wall at point C, which is directly behind point B. Pull the suture tightly, but do not tear into the myometrium. Exit the posterior wall of the uterus through point D. Loop the suture over the uterine fundus. Anchor the suture in the lower uterine segment by taking bites on either side of the left edge of the uterine hysterotomy incision (E and F) at the same height as the contralateral sutures were placed. Pull the two ends of the suture tight while an assistant simultaneously squeezes the uterus to aid compression. Place a surgical knot while the assistant continues to compress the uterus [1].

Uterine artery ligation (O'Leary stitch): A #1 needle 0 delayed-absorbable suture material is passed through and into the myometrium from anterior to posterior 2–3 cm medial to the uterine vessels and 2–3 cm below the closed uterine incision but above the reflected bladder flap to avoid ligating the ureters. The needle is then brought forward through an avas-cular area in the broad ligament lateral to the uterine artery and vein. The suture is tied anteriorly. When done bilaterally, this results in a 90 % reduction of the uterine blood supply. Collateral circulation and revascularization will reestablish within 6–8 weeks. This has a success rate of 95 % [9].

Uterine packing: Several techniques are described such as the use of 24 F Foley catheter with a 30 cm^3 balloon placed into the uterine cavity, use of an SOS Bakri Tamponade Balloon Catheter, and direct packing of the uterine cavity with laparotomy pads [4].

Placenta Accreta

Placentation abnormalities occur in 0.2 % of pregnancies [13]. Placenta accreta is defined as any placental implantation in which there is abnormally firm adherence to the uterine wall, related to an absence or incomplete development of Nitabuch layer. The placenta may attach to the myometrium (accreta), invade the myometrium (increta) or extend through the myometrium into surrounding structures (percreta). The risk is higher with a history of prior Cesarean delivery, with an incidence of 1 in 2,500 deliveries. This is a tenfold increase over the past 50 years, most likely due to the rise in the rate of Cesarean section. A placental accreta should be highly suspected in such patients who are also found to have a placenta previa, defined as a placenta that is located over or very near the internal cervical os, as this increases the risk of an accreta 54-fold [4]. If an accreta is suspected, Cesarean delivery should be performed in a tertiary care center due to the high risk of hemorrhage and potential for massive hemorrhage and need for peripartum hysterectomy.

Surgical Management of Placenta Accreta

- Placement of sutures in the myometrium in the area of placental adherence
- Uterine artery ligation (O'Leary stitch, as described above)
- Hypogastric artery ligation (only for those who are experienced and is successful in less than half of the patients in whom it is attempted)
- Uterine packing
- Uterine artery embolization by interventional radiologist
- Peripartum hysterectomy

Postoperative Care

Foley catheter to drainage until ambulatory and hemodynamic stability confirmed
DVT prophylaxis based on published guidelines
Frequent uterine fundal checks in the first 4 h to assess for uterine atony
Monitoring for excessive vaginal bleeding

Postoperative Complications

Infection
Ileus
Thromboembolism

References

1. Barbieri F. A stitch in time: the B-Lynch, Hayman and Pereira uterine compression sutures. OBG Manag. 2012;24:12.
2. Cesarean delivery on maternal request, ACOG Committee Opinion 559; 2013.
3. Chelmow D, Rodriguez EJ, Sabatini M. Suture closure of subcutaneous fat and wound disruption after cesarean section. Obstet Gynecol. 2004;103:974.
4. Cunningham FG, et al. Williams obstetrics. 22nd ed. New York: McGraw-Hill; 2005, 591–9, 824–33
5. Gerber AH. Accidental incision of the fetus during cesarean section delivery. Int J Gynaecol Obstet. 1974;12:46–8.
6. Haeri AD. Comparisons of transverse and vertical incisions for cesarean section. S Afr Med J. 1976;50:33–4.
7. Hofmeyr JG, Novikova N, Mathai M, Shah A. Techniques for cesarean section. Am J Obstet Gynecol. 2009;201:431–4.
8. Mooney SE, Ogrinc G, Steadman W. Improving emergency caesarean delivery response times at a rural community hospital. Qual Saf Health Care. 2007;16(1):60–6.
9. O'Leary JA. Stop ob hemorrhage with uterine artery ligation. Contemp Obstet Gynecol. 1986;28:13–6.
10. Postpartum Hemorrhage. October 2006, reaffirmed 2013. ACOG Practice Bulletin #76.
11. Rajasekar D, Hall M. Urinary tract injuries during obstetric intervention. Br J Obstet Gynaecol. 1997;104:731.
12. Wiener JJ, Westwood J. Fetal lacerations at cesarean section. J Obstet Gynaecol. 2002;22:23–4.
13. Wu S, Kocherginersky M, Hibbard JU. Abnormal placentation: twenty-year analysis. Am J Obstet Gynecol. 2005;193:1458–61.

Suggested Reading

ACOG website, www.acog.org
Cunningham FG, et al. Williams obstetrics. 22nd ed. New York: McGraw-Hill; 2005.
Dahlke JD, Mendez-Figueroa H, Rouse DJ, et al. Evidence based surgery for cesarean delivery: an updated systematic review. Am J Obstet Gynecol. 2013;209:294–307.
Hofmeyr JG, Novikova N, Mathai M, Shah A. Techniques for cesarean section. Am J Obstet Gynecol. 2009;201:431–44.
Mathai M, Hofmeyer GJ. Abdominal surgical incisions for cesarean section. Cochrane Database Syst Rev 2007;(1):CD004453.

Gary H. Lipscomb

General Indications for Surgery

Hemodynamically unstable patients with suspected ectopic pregnancy

Ruptured ectopic pregnancy

Stable ectopic pregnancy not desiring future fertility or medical management

Preoperative Preparation

The rural surgeon may be required to provide the initial diagnostic workup for ectopic pregnancy or verify the diagnosis made by non-surgeons. An accurate diagnostic workup prevents inappropriate treatment of a viable intrauterine pregnancy. Early diagnosis of unruptured ectopic pregnancies also allows for the use of more conservative tubal-preserving treatment options. In fact, in selected patients, surgery may be avoided entirely and replaced with medical management.

Since the protocols for diagnosing ectopic pregnancies can be cumbersome and complex, the orderly and logical use of diagnostic tests can be difficult, particularly for individuals who do use these protocols on a regular basis. As such, diagnostic algorithms have been developed to simplify the management of suspected ectopic pregnancies. An example of such an algorithm is presented in Fig. 28.1. Although the algorithm is straightforward, pitfalls do exist where the algorithms are inaccurate or may not apply such as with potential twin pregnancies, pregnancies conceived with assisted reproductive techniques, patients with renal failure and when phantom hCG may exist. Practitioners are encouraged to

exercise caution when these situations exist. A detailed discussion on all the nuances in the diagnosis of ectopic pregnancy is beyond the scope of this chapter but more detailed sources are provided in the references.

In patients with hemodynamic instability or hematoperitoneum without a strong indication of an ectopic pregnancy, the possibility of other causes such as a ruptured ovarian cyst should be considered. In these cases, the use of an intrauterine manipulator during laparoscopy should be avoided to avoid interruption of an early intrauterine pregnancy. If needed a single-tooth tenaculum placed on the cervix can usually provide adequate uterine manipulation without risk.

Operative Strategy

The primary goal of all surgeries for ectopic pregnancy is to control bleeding, if present, and to remove the ectopic pregnancy. Secondary goals include preservation of fertility in those patients desiring for more children. Traditionally these surgeries were performed via laparotomy, but are now generally performed with laparoscopic techniques. Laparotomy remains the operative route of choice in situations where laparoscopy is unfeasible, or unavailable.

After operative exposure is obtained via laparotomy or laparoscopy, one must determine whether to attempt conservation of the affected tube in those patients desiring fertility. In patients with extensive tubal damage or uncontrolled bleeding, tubal removal is advisable. Likewise, unstable patients may be better served with tubal removal if tubal conservation will require prolonged surgery or continued blood loss.

In patients that are otherwise candidates for tubal conservation, the condition of the contralateral tube and the location and size of the ectopic pregnancy are determining factors. Expert opinions are divided on appropriate candidates. Salpingostomy may increase subsequent overall pregnancy rate at the expense of an increased ectopic rate. On the other hand, even normal appearing tubes may suffer from the same

G.H. Lipscomb, M.D., F.A.C.S. (✉)
Department of Family Medicine, University of Tennessee Health Science Center, Memphis, TN 38119, USA

Department of Obstetrics and Gynecology, University of Tennessee Health Science Center, Memphis, TN 38119, USA
e-mail: garyhlipscomb@gmail.com

A.L. Halverson and D.C. Borgstrom (eds.), *Advanced Surgical Techniques for Rural Surgeons*, DOI 10.1007/978-1-4939-1495-1_28, © Springer Science+Business Media New York 2015

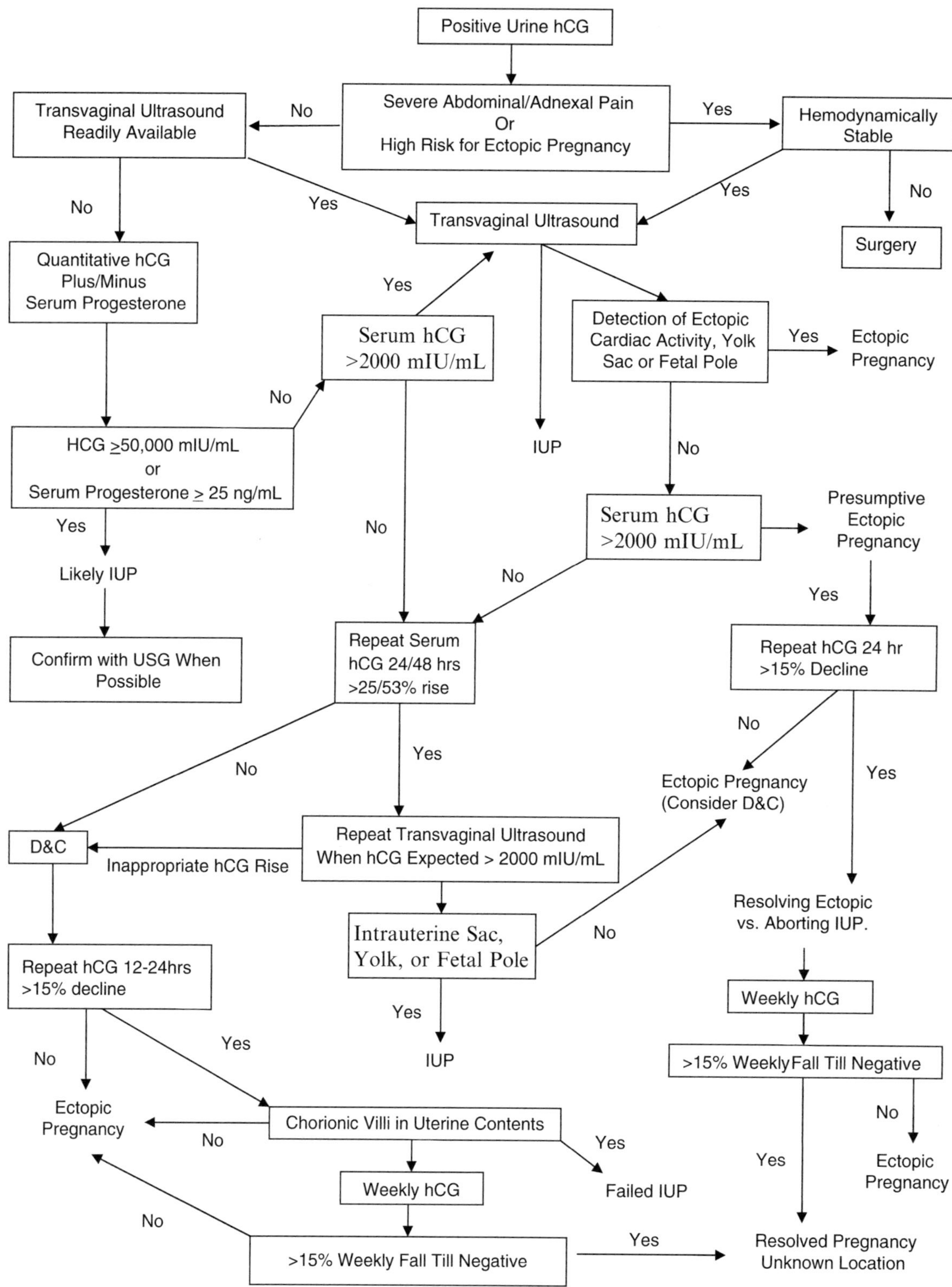

Fig. 28.1 Algorithm for diagnosing ectopic pregnancy

disease process as affected tubes as evidenced by the 15–20 % recurrent ectopic rate in patients with prior salpingectomy. As a rule, if the contralateral tube appears normal, salpingectomy may be a more appropriate option. The decision is based on the condition of the contralateral tube, the location of the ectopic pregnancy in the tube, and the ease of salpingostomy.

When feasible, laparoscopy is considered the preferred method for all but those with absolute contraindications or hemodynamically unstable. Even patients with massive hematoperitoneum that have been stabilized are frequently amenable to laparoscopic management. Particularly in patients with uncertain diagnosis, laparoscopy should be considered for diagnostic confirmation even if laparotomy will be required for treatment.

Potential Pitfalls

Ectopic pregnancy is frequently associated with dense pelvic adhesions that predate the ectopic pregnancy or result from intense inflammatory reactions seen with more chronic ectopic pregnancies. Laparotomy may be required to safely manage some cases. Injuries to surrounding structures may not be avoidable even with the best of surgical techniques but careful dissection and attention to anatomy should minimize these complications.

The most common general pitfalls are accidental ligation of the arterial supply to the ovary or removal of the ovary with the ectopic pregnancy. Preservation of the ovary is not always possible as the ovary may be the site of the ectopic pregnancy or become so encased in adhesions that safe removal of the ectopic pregnancy requires removal of the ovary as well. Although uncommon, ureteral injury can occur when the ectopic pregnancy is adherent to the pelvic sidewall. If necessary, the ureter can generally be identified above the disease process and dissection performed to free the ureter from the ectopic mass. Vascular injuries to the external and internal iliac can occur under similar conditions.

Postoperative Care

Postoperative care is generally straightforward and similar to that of any laparotomy or laparoscopic case. Unique aspects that may occur are discussed under those particular procedures.

Common Complications

Although not technically a complication, required removal of the affected tube when continued fertility is desired is not uncommon. This possibility should be discussed with the patient prior to surgery unless emergent surgery prevents full discussion. Persistent trophoblastic disease may require additional surveillance measures as well as further medical or surgical treatment and also should be discussed with the patient as part of the consent process or prior to discharge depending on circumstances. Additional details may be found in the subsequent sections.

When to Transfer

The presentation of an ectopic pregnancy is quite variable. With current diagnostic tools, ectopic pregnancy may be diagnosed in completely asymptomatic patient. Likewise, the patient may present with severe hypovolemic shock. In the latter, transfer is not an option and emergent surgery is required to preserve life. However, even when hypovolemic shock is present, many patients with ectopic pregnancy will stabilize rapidly to fluid and blood replacement. Transfer may still be possible in selected cases. The decision to transfer will depend on the facilities available, the training of the surgeon, the stability of the patient, and the distance to the accepting medical facilities. The emergent treatment of the typical ectopic pregnancy is within the skill set of any surgeon who performs routine abdominal surgery and should be possible at any facility that performs these surgeries/a surgery.

Salpingectomy (Figs. 28.2, 28.3, and 28.4)

Indications

Patient does not desire future fertility
Patient desires complete tubal removal
Extensive tubal damage discovered at the time of surgery

Operative Strategy

Salpingectomy is the simplest and most rapid of the surgical procedures for the treatment for ectopic pregnancy. Thus it remains the procedure of choice in unstable patients and those with excessive ongoing bleeding. This procedure is easily performed by both laparotomy and laparoscopy. The ovary and its blood supply, the infundipulopelvic ligament are identified to avoid accidently removing the ovary or

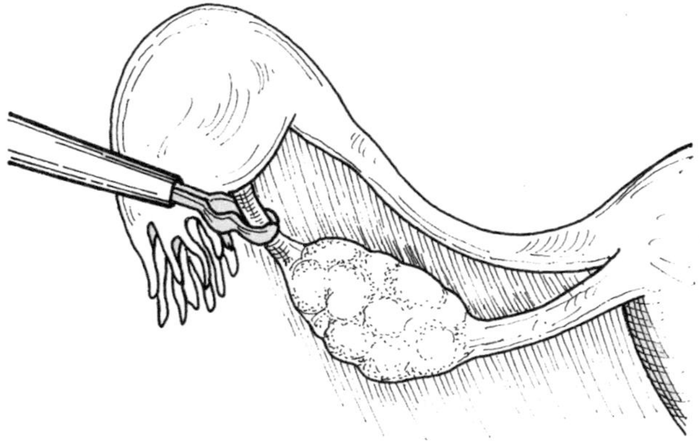

Fig. 28.2 Laparoscopic division of mesosalpinx of fallopian tube

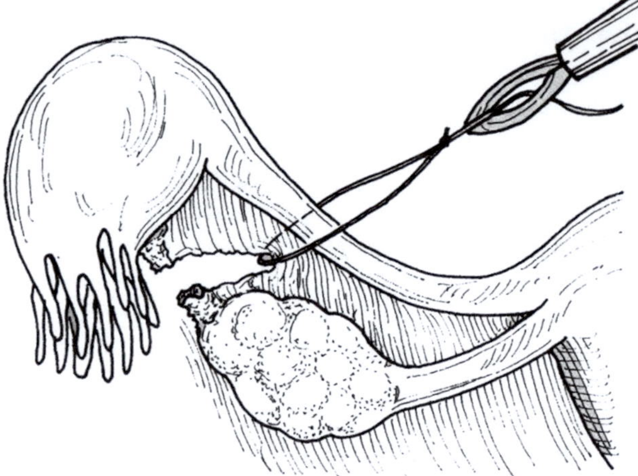

Fig. 28.3 Laparoscopic ligation of fallopian tube

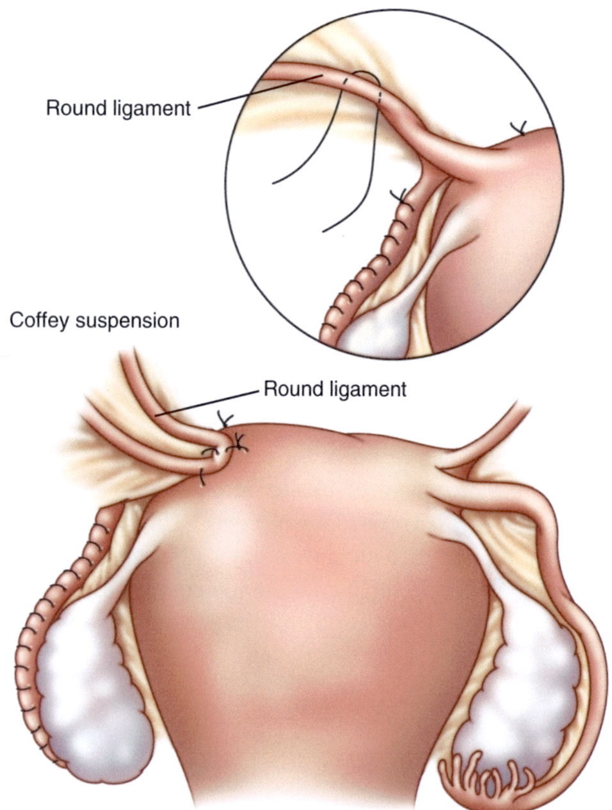

Fig. 28.4 Coffee suspension to cover cornual resection of uterus

interrupting its blood supply. The mesosalpinx is divided by any of the several methods followed by transection of the proximal fallopian tube.

Operative Technique

The pelvis explored and the ectopic pregnancy identified. Rarely bilateral hematosalpinx are present and the exact location of the ectopic pregnancy is not obvious. In these cases, the tube may be opened as discussed in the section on salpingostomy to confirm the tube containing the ectopic pregnancy. The fallopian tube is retracted medially and the location of the ovary and the infundipulopelvic ligament is identified. If the surgery is performed via laparotomy, the mesosalpinx is sequentially clamped and divided with each pedicle suture ligated. The final clamp is placed across the proximal fallopian tube. If the surgery is performed via laparoscopy, segmental coagulation and division of mesosalpinx and fallopian tube is performed starting at the distal end of the fallopian tube. This may be performed with minimal instrumentation using a bipolar coagulation instrument and division with laparoscopic scissors or placement of suture endoloops around the fallopian tube followed by excision with laparoscopic scissors. Alternatively, any of the combination coagulation and division instruments may also be used. Laparoscopic stapling devices can be used; however, even with vascular loads, the thin mesosalpinx is prone to bleeding. The fallopian tube and products of conception are then removed within an endoscopic pouch.

The above sequence of coagulation and division may be more easily performed in reverse order starting at the proximate end of the fallopian tube if the distal end is densely adherent to the ovary or adjacent tissue.

In the past, removal of a portion of the interstitial segment of the tube (cornual resection) was also recommended. Some surgeons further advised suturing the round ligament to the posterior surface of the uterus (modified Coffey suspension) to cover the peritoneal defect produced by cornual resection. This has not been shown to reduce future ectopics and may predispose to uterine rupture in future pregnancy.

Partial Salpingectomy

Indications

Patient desires future fertility *AND* more conservative methods are not possible.

Uncontrolled bleeding after salpingostomy and patient strongly desires fertility AND contralateral tube is absent or severely damaged.

Isthmic location of ectopic pregnancy AND contralateral tube absent or severely damaged.

Operative Strategy

This procedure is generally performed when future fertility is desired and more conservative procedures are not possible due to extensive damage or continued bleeding after salpingostomy. A partial salpingectomy should not be performed unless reanastomosis is planned either immediately or as a second procedure at a later date, since repeat ectopic pregnancy in the blind distal tubal segment is possible unless the patient uses some form of contraception.

Because of the low tubal patency rate following linear salpingostomy for isthmic ectopic pregnancies, partial salpingectomy has been advocated as the most appropriate conservative procedure for this type of ectopic pregnancy. However, other authors believe that the tubal patency rate following isthmic linear salpingostomy is acceptable. Given the need for a second surgery for reanastomosis as well as the inability of many patients to afford a surgery that is generally not covered by health insurance in the United States, many surgeons are reluctant to perform a partial salpingectomy unless immediate reanastomosis is planned.

Operative Technique

After exploration and identification of the ectopic pregnancy, the fallopian tube is elevated and location of the ovary and the infundipulopelvic ligament is identified. If the surgery is performed via laparotomy, surgical clamps are placed across the fallopian tube and across the mesosalpinx to isolate the tubal segment containing the ectopic pregnancy. The segment is excised free and the pedicles suture ligated. If the surgery is performed via laparoscopy, the segment of affected tube is removed in a similar manner as for a salpingectomy. This may be performed with any of the instruments previously discussed in the salpingectomy section including bipolar coagulation devices and laparoscopic scissors, suture endoloops, combination coagulation, and division devices and laparoscopic staplers.

The fallopian tube and products of conception are then either directly or laparoscopically using an endoscopic pouch.

Pitfalls

As previously mentioned partial salpingectomy should not be performed unless reanastomosis is planned either immediately or as a second procedure at a later date, since repeat ectopic pregnancy in the blind distal tubal segment is possible unless the patient uses some form of contraception.

Reanastomosis is generally not covered by health insurance in the United States, and should only be performed when all these issues have been addressed preoperatively.

Salpingostomy

Indications

Patient desires future fertility

Preoperative Preparation

Same as general preoperative preparation except if performed laparoscopically, then availability of a 1.5 in. or longer 18 gauge needle and a long 25 gauge spinal needle is needed.

Operative Strategy

Opening the fallopian tube and removing the products of conception is the most common conservative surgical therapy for management of an ectopic pregnancy. The tubal incision may be closed with fine-caliber suture (salpingotomy), or allowed to heal by secondary intention (salpingostomy). Intrauterine pregnancies have been shown to occur earlier after salpingostomy than with salpingotomy. In addition, the presence of sutures may also favor adhesion formation. Therefore, it is generally recommended that the tubal incision be left open.

The basics of linear salpingostomy involve the use of a scalpel, needle-point electrode, or laser to incise the antimesenteric border of the fallopian tube over the ectopic pregnancy. The products of conception are then gently removed with laparoscopic graspers or thumb forceps. Vigorous removal is not recommended as this may lead to increased bleeding and damage to the tubal epithelium. The use of pressurized irrigation fluid has been suggested by some surgeons as a method of flushing additional trophoblastic tissue from the tube without increasing the risk of bleeding.

The injection of vasopressin (10 units in 20–50 mL of saline) prior to the linear salpingostomy can be used to markedly decrease bleeding. Injections are made in the antimesenteric portion of tube over the ectopic pregnancy, in the mesosalpinx beneath the ectopic and/or the region of the fimbica-ovarica, where branches of the ovarian blood vessels enter the mesosalpinx to supply the tube. These injections can be performed laparoscopically with special laparoscopic instruments or by using standard spinal needles passed

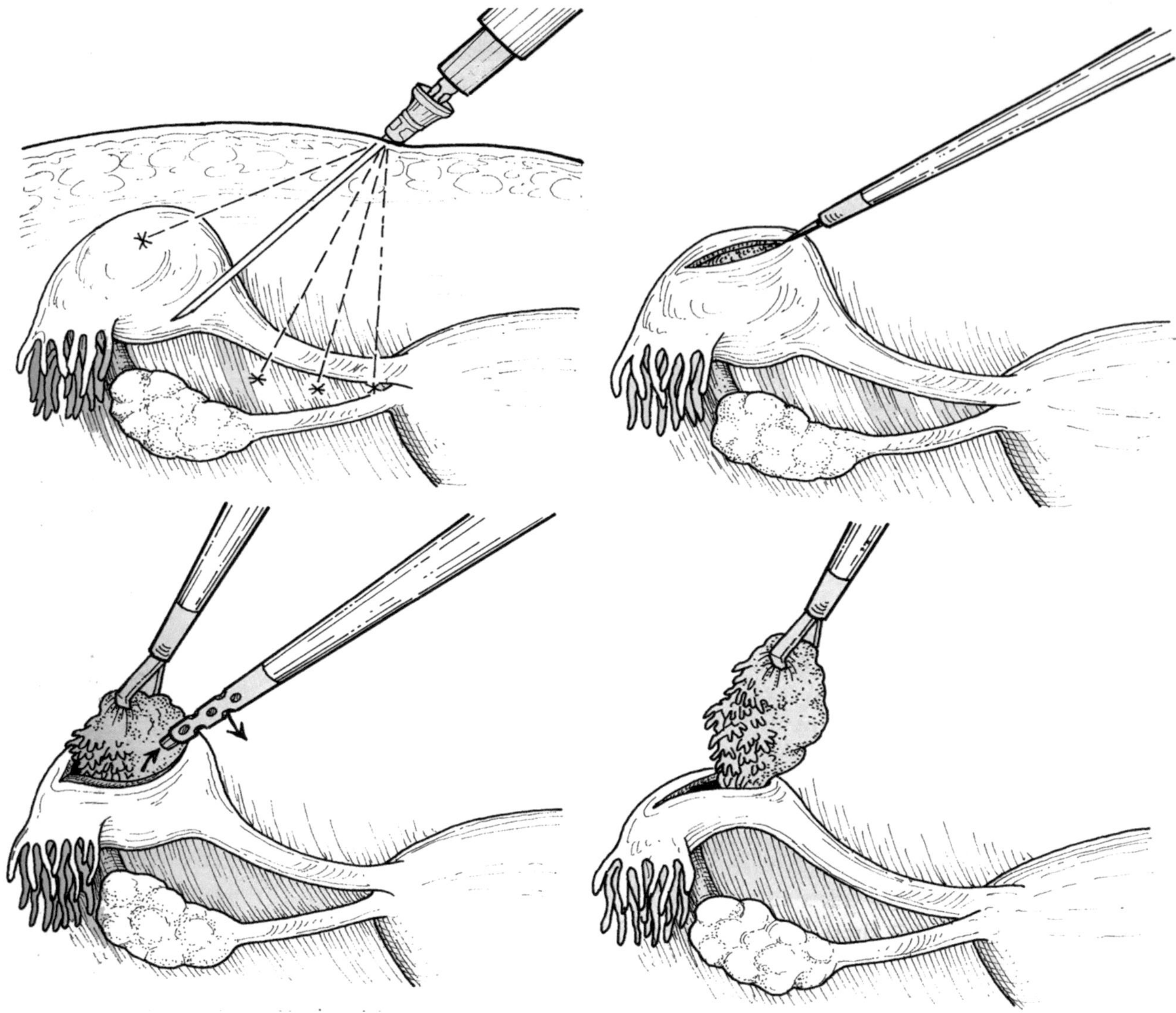

Fig. 28.5 Techniques for laparoscopic salpingostomy for ectopic pregnancy

transcutaneously. A 25-gauge spinal needle inserted using a shorter 18- or 20-gauge needle as an introducer will maintain optimal maneuverability, yet easily penetrate the tubal wall without the use of the excessive counter tension on the tube that is frequently needed with the use of larger needles.

Operative Technique

The involved fallopian tube is elevated and location of the ovary and the infundipulopelvic ligament is identified. If performing the surgery laparoscopically, insert the 18 gauge needle through abdominal wall over the ectopic pregnancy. Insert the 25 gauge spinal needle through the 18 gauge needle.

Direct the smaller needle by manipulating the hub of the larger gauge needle. Inject vasopressin 20 units diluted in 40 cm³ sterile water into the antimesenteric portion of tube over the ectopic pregnancy and if possible into the tubal mesentery under ectopic pregnancy (Fig. 28.5a). Incise the antimesenteric portion of tube with nonmodulated (cut) current using an electrosurgical laparoscopic needle point, spatula, or opened tip of laparoscopic scissors starting at the point of maximal dilatation on the proximal fallopian tube (Fig. 28.5b). Remove the products of conception from tube with graspers and/or with alternating suction irrigation using a standard laparoscopic suction irrigator (Fig. 28.5c, d). Remove all products of conception from abdomen directly or using an endoscopic pouch.

Potential Pitfalls

Persistent trophoblastic disease is the continued growth of trophoblastic tissue in the fallopian tube of the abdominal cavity following surgical treatment for ectopic pregnancy or after reimplantation elsewhere in the abdomen of tissue fragments dislodged during the removal attempt. Untreated, persistent trophoblastic tissue may lead to tubal rupture and life-threatening intra-abdominal hemorrhage.

The incidence of persistent trophoblastic disease after salpingostomy ranges from 3 to 20 % and is increased with gestations greater than 7 weeks, ectopic size larger than 2 cm, hCG > 3,000 mIU, with rapidly rising hCG levels.

Postoperative Care

If salpingostomy is performed, monitoring with weekly hCG concentrations until normalization is required. If hCH concentrations fall less than 15 % between levels or begin to increase then treatment with systemic methotrexate or salpingectomy is required.

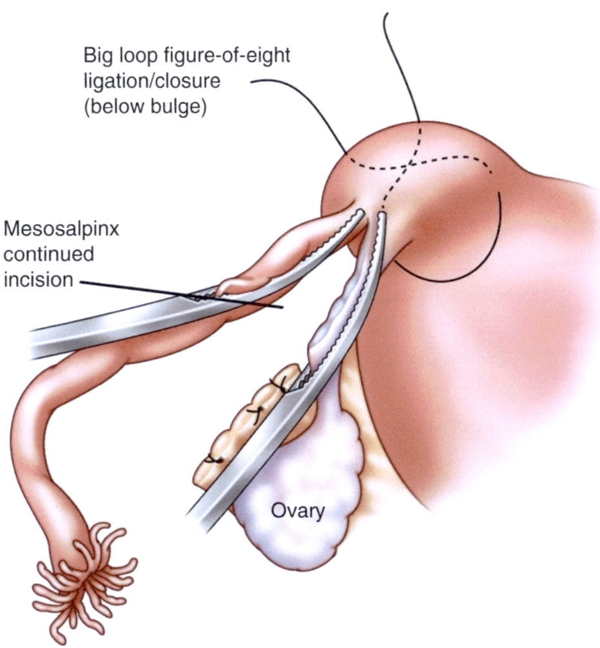

Fig. 28.6 Techniques for excision of cornual ectopic pregnancy

---

Cornual Resection for Cornual Ectopic (Fig. 28.6)

Preoperative Preparation

Cornual ectopic pregnancies have the greatest potential for intraoperative blood loss and preparation for this should be made. Surgery can be performed by skilled laparoscopic surgeons but conversion to laparotomy should be made promptly if the procedure exceeds the skills of the surgeon or uncontrolled hemorrhage ensues. Hysterectomy to control hemorrhage may be needed and a surgeon comfortable performing hysterectomy should be readily available.

Operative Strategy

The potential for massive hemorrhage dictates much of the operative strategy. Several prophylactic measures have been suggested to prevent massive bleeding. Placement of a figure of eight stitch under the pregnancy to ligate some of the blood supply may be helpful. Likewise, placement of several deep interrupted untied sutures under the planned area of resection that can be quickly tied after ectopic removal may also be useful. Additional prophylactic methods include ligation of the ascending uterine artery on the side of the ectopic pregnancy. Placement of an endoloop at the base of a cornual pregnancy that is primarily outside the myometrial has also been described as a hemostatic method. Personally I have found liberal injection of dilute vasopressin solution circumferentially beneath the cornual pregnancy frequently results in almost bloodless surgery and allows laparoscopic resection to be performed with minimal blood loss.

Operative Technique

The fallopian tube is elevated and the ovary and the infundipulopelvic ligament are identified. The selected prophylactic measures for hemostasis are now performed. If vasopressin is used, it is diluted as previously described and injected circumferentially under the ectopic pregnancy to produce a vasospastic tourniquet. The previously described techniques using an 18 gauge introducer to place a 25 gauge needle may be used. However it is often easier to use an 18 gauge needle alone to penetrate the thicker tissue of the uterus. Segmental coagulation and division of mesosalpinx of tube performed with any of the previously described methods. The ectopic pregnancy is resected en block using standard electrosurgical instruments.

If the procedure is performed via laparotomy and the cornual pregnancy is primarily outside most of the myometrial tissue, heavy hysterectomy clamps may be able to be placed completely under the ectopic pregnancy. If this is possible the ectopic mass is excised and the tissue pedicles are then suture ligated in a standard fashion. If the mass has been resected with electrosurgery, the resulting defect is sutured closed in one or more layers. The use of barbed suture or laparoscopic suturing devices greatly simplifies suturing if the procedure is performed laparoscopically.

Potential Pitfalls

Failure to adequately perform prophylactic hemostatic measures may result in uncontrollable uterine bleeding and may occasionally necessitate hysterectomy. Care must be taken to remove all products of conception. Cornual ectopic pregnancies may extend deep into the uterus and require full thickness uterine resection to remove.

Postoperative Care

Monitoring with weekly hCG concentrations until normalization is required if there is any uncertainty that all products of conception were removed. If hCH concentrations fall less than 15 % weekly or begin to rise then treatment with systemic methotrexate or repeat surgery is required. If more than superficial myometrial resection is performed, most authorities would recommend treating the patient similarly to a previous classical cesarean section if subsequent pregnancy occurs. Vaginal delivery would be contraindicated Cesarean section should be performed at 36–37 weeks gestation to prevent the possibility of catastrophic uterine rupture.

Common Complications

With cornual ectopic pregnancies the possibility of operative hemorrhage is greatly increased. Appropriate blood products should be available. Although increasingly uncommon, hysterectomy may be required to control hemorrhage.

When to Transfer

Because of their location, cornual ectopics frequently are of greater gestational age with greater vascularity than tubal ectopic pregnancies. They have the greatest potential for profuse hemorrhage that can be difficult to control and may require hysterectomy. Fortunately they frequently are diagnosed prior to rupture. If diagnosed early and hemodynamically stable, these pregnancies should be managed by surgeons comfortable with uterine surgery and hysterectomy. Ideally these pregnancies can be managed laparoscopically by skilled laparoscopic surgeons.

Suggested Reading

1. DeCherney AH, Romero R, Naftolin F. Surgical management of unruptured ectopic pregnancy. Fertil Steril. 1981;35:21.
2. DeCherney AH, Boyers S. Isthmic ectopic pregnancy: segmental resection as the treatment of choice. Fertil Steril. 1985;44:307–12.
3. Givens VM, Lipscomb GH. Diagnosis of Ectopic Pregnancy. Clin Obstet Gynecol. 2012;2:387–94.
4. Kooi S, Kock HC. Surgical treatment for tubal pregnancies. Surg Gynecol Obstet. 1993;176:519.
5. Seifer DB, Gutman JN, Doyle Jones EE, Diamond MP, DeCherney AH. Persistent ectopic pregnancy following laparoscopic linear salpingectomy. Obstet Gynecol. 1990;76:1121–5.

Ovarian Torsion

Robert J. Wilmoth and John Williamson

Indications

Symptomatic adnexal mass.
Ovarian torsion confirmed at operation for abdominal pain.

Preoperative Preparation

As in much of medicine, the eventual diagnosis begins with the history and physical examination. Approximately 90 % of patients with adnexal torsion present with moderate to severe pelvic pain and are subsequently discovered to have an adnexal mass. Many patients also report nausea with or without vomiting. Symptoms may be constant or intermittent. Fever and abnormal genital tract bleeding have classically been associated with adnexal torsion although only a minority of patients manifest these symptoms. Adnexal torsion in the absence of an adnexal mass does occur, particularly among the pediatric population. The abdominal examination typically reveals tenderness to palpation on the affected side. Rebound tenderness and guarding may or may not be present and likely are influenced by the duration and severity of vascular congestion, adnexal enlargement, and ischemia. Laceration of the ovarian cortex or the fallopian tube serosa may precipitate accompanying intraperitoneal hemorrhage and thereby increase the likelihood of peritoneal signs. An adnexal mass may or may not be palpable via bimanual pelvic examination. The size of the mass, the body habitus of the patient, and the experience of the examiner influence the sensitivity and specificity of the pelvic exam.

R.J. Wilmoth, M.D., F.A.C.S. (✉)
Department of Surgery, Clinical Medicine,
Lincoln Memorial University, Harrogate, TN 37752, USA
e-mail: Robert.wilmoth@lmunet.edu

J. Williamson, M.D., F.A.C.O.G.
Department of OB/GYN, Clinical Medicine,
Lincoln Memorial University, Harrogate, TN 37752, USA

As for all reproductive-age females with abdominal or pelvic pain, the laboratory evaluation should begin with a pregnancy test. An initial screen with a qualitative urine or serum screen for human chorionic gonadotropin (hCG) is sufficient. If the initial qualitative screen is positive then quantitative hCG assessment is indicated since there is considerable overlap in the clinical presentation of ectopic pregnancy and adnexal torsion. It is important to remember that a normal intrauterine pregnancy can coexist with adnexal torsion. In fact, pregnancy may increase a woman's risk of adnexal torsion since ovarian enlargement (usually due to a functional ovarian cyst) is the most common proximate cause for adnexal torsion. Determining the location and viability of a potential fetus is of utmost importance. Consultation with an obstetrician/gynecologist is recommended if there is any uncertainty in this regard. A complete blood count may provide additional information. Leukocytosis is commonly reported among patients with adnexal torsion and is theorized to be secondary to ischemic necrosis of the affected tissue. However, absence of a leukocytosis does not exclude the diagnosis of adnexal torsion. Anemia may or may not accompany adnexal torsion and, if present, suggests concomitant intraperitoneal hemorrhage. Serum chemistries are unlikely to be affected by adnexal torsion. Coagulation studies are expected to remain unchanged unless the degree of intraperitoneal hemorrhage is sufficient to create a consumptive coagulopathy.

Transvaginal pelvic ultrasound is the recommended imaging study for most patients. The presence of a unilateral adnexal mass associated with the symptom complex described above is an indication for surgical evaluation. Most adnexal masses associated with torsion are ≥ 5 cm. Doppler studies may reveal diminished or absent venous flow. Arterial flow can also be compromised as pressure increases due to vascular congestion. It should be noted, however, that the presence of arterial and/or venous flow does not exclude the diagnosis of adnexal torsion. The presence of free fluid in the posterior cul-de-sac suggests intraperitoneal hemorrhage has occurred. Transabdominal pelvic ultrasound may provide additional information not visible via transvaginal imaging. CT and/or MRI imaging of the

A.L. Halverson and D.C. Borgstrom (eds.), *Advanced Surgical Techniques for Rural Surgeons*,
DOI 10.1007/978-1-4939-1495-1_29, © Springer Science+Business Media New York 2015

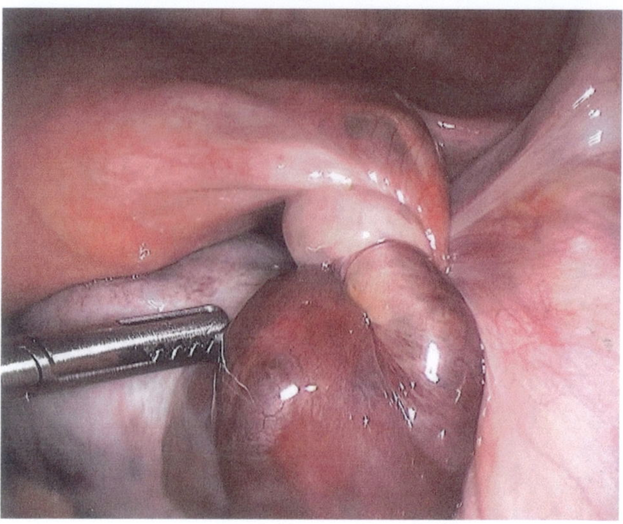

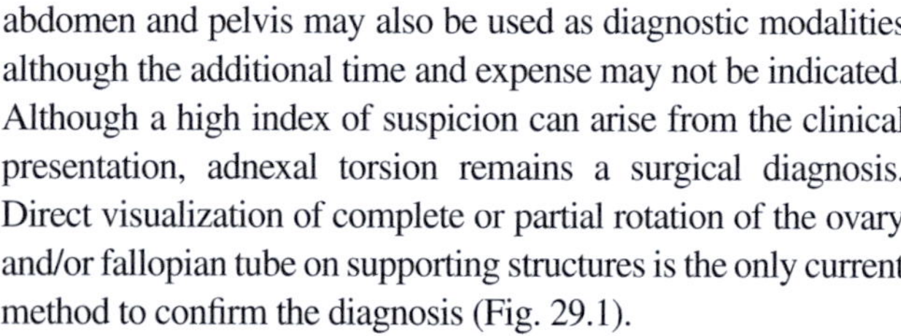

Fig. 29.1 Initial view of a right adnexa demonstrating torsion

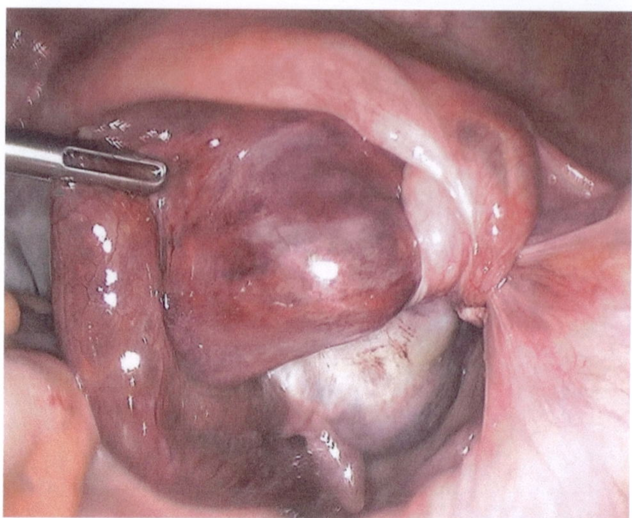

Fig. 29.2 Atraumatic graspers are used to detorse the ovary

abdomen and pelvis may also be used as diagnostic modalities although the additional time and expense may not be indicated. Although a high index of suspicion can arise from the clinical presentation, adnexal torsion remains a surgical diagnosis. Direct visualization of complete or partial rotation of the ovary and/or fallopian tube on supporting structures is the only current method to confirm the diagnosis (Fig. 29.1).

In preparation for surgical exploration patients should receive broad spectrum systemic antibiotics. Patients should be positioned in the dorsal lithotomy position. A foley catheter should be inserted prior to incision. It is important to have a uterine manipulator available.

Operative Strategy

One should visualize and explore the pelvis and adnexal structures bilaterally. Additionally, other potential causes of abdominal pain should be evaluated including appendicitis, diverticulitis, and Meckel's diverticulum. Once the diagnosis is confirmed, use atraumatic graspers to detorse the ovary in question to assess for viability with an emphasis on adnexal preservation, especially nulliparous females. Both oophoropexy and shortening of the infundibular ligament have been proposed as strategies to prevent recurrence.

Operative Technique

The authors advocate a laparoscopic approach, though open laparotomy may be performed based on the skill of the operator. Patient is positioned in dorsal lithotomy and uterine manipulator is placed.

Incisions

A vertically oriented infra-umbilical 11 mm incision is created and the abdomen is entered using an open technique. In the case of a pregnant patient, a supraumbilical incision may be preferable based on the size and position of the gravid uterus. The vertical orientation allows for extension to accommodate removal of a large adnexa if necessary due to edema and necrosis or underlying mass. Pneumoperitoneum to 14 mmHg is obtained, and additional 5 mm trocars are placed in the right and left lower quadrants under direct visualization.

Exposure

The patient is positioned in trendelenburg and the uterus is elevated out of the pelvis using the manipulator. Any remaining bowel in the pelvis is maneuvered out of the pelvis taking care not to induce serosal injury. The appendix, sigmoid colon, and terminal ileum are all examined. Both adnexa are inspected and the torsion is untwisted by manipulating the adnexa with atraumatic graspers in a hand over hand technique (Fig. 29.2). Showering of clot located within the ovarian vein was once felt to pose such risk as the preclude ovarian salvage, however, as experience with ovarian salvage has gained momentum, the risk of this posing clinical significance is much lower than originally thought. Once the torsion has been released, allowing blood flow to restore, monitor the ovary for viability. If the ovary is salvageable, preparation should be made for oophoropexy. If it is obviously necrotic, make preparations for oophorectomy.

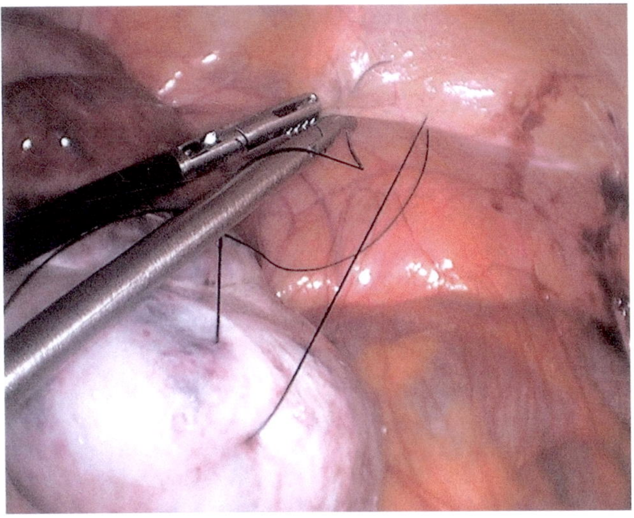

Fig. 29.3 Intracorporeal oophoropexy to pelvic sidewall

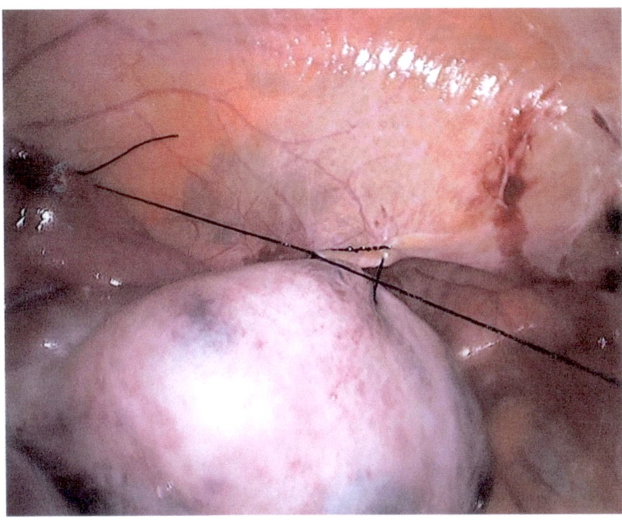

Fig. 29.4 Completed oophoropexy

Evaluation for Underlying Ovarian Pathology

Once the viability of the ovary has been determined as salvageable, the ovary should be carefully inspected for an underlying etiology predisposing to the torsion. Possible contributing factors include dermoid cysts, simple cysts, corpus luteum cysts in the case of pregnancy, and ovarian neoplasm. Management of these associated conditions should be based on clinical suspicion for malignancy as avoidance of spillage of malignant cells into the pelvis is of utmost importance. For benign conditions, preservation of as much functional ovarian tissue as possible should be employed. Cysts or teratomas can often be excised utilizing either ultrasonic or bipolar energy device. If a corpus luteum cannot be preserved prior to 10 weeks gestation, initiation of progesterone replacement should be performed. Any removed structures should be placed into an endoscopic retrieval bag to prevent spillage of contents during removal.

Oophoropexy

There is no consensus on technique of oophoropexy. It has been described by suturing the ovary to the posterior uterus, lateral pelvic sidewall (Fig. 29.3), and round ligament. Shortening of the infundibulopelvic ligament via a running suture has also been described as an adjunct to the oophoropexy. The authors prefer utilizing absorbable suture on a tapered needle such as 3–0 vicryl on an SH needle to facilitate intracorporeal suturing (Fig. 29.4). In nulliparous patients, trying to maintain the anatomic relationship of the ovary and fallopian tube is preferable to try to preserve fertility, rather than oophoropexy in a non-anatomic location.

Oophorectomy

If untwisting the ovary does not result in a decrease in edema and cyanosis or there are obvious changes consistent with irreversible ischemia, preparations for salpingo-oophorectomy should be made. We employ the use of either an ultrasonic or bipolar energy device to divide the fallopian tube at its junction with the uterus as well as the infundibulopelvic ligament, which contains the ovarian vessels. Take care to identify and preserve the course of the ureter as its position can sometimes be altered during the course of the torsion.

In cases of ovarian loss due to torsion, strong consideration of contralateral oophoropexy should be considered, especially in those patients who desire to preserve fertility.

Potential Pitfalls

Delay in diagnosis.

Failure to consider diagnosis in evaluation of abdominal pain in any age female.

Failure to counsel preoperatively the possibility of removal of adnexal structures and implications for future fertility.

Failure to consider contralateral oophoropexy.

Control of the ovarian vessels can be difficult especially in light of the engorgement associated with the ovarian vein. If there is question of the ability to control utilizing an energy device, intracorporeal suture ligation can alternatively be employed. We discourage against the use of a vascular stapling device as the possibility of inadvertently pulling the ureter up into the stapling device and resultant injury.

Postoperative Care

Routine postoperative care is employed. Patients can often be discharged home within 24 h of the operation. For any lesions of the ovary that were not excised, follow-up ultrasound should be performed.

Common Complications

Complications are rare and usually related to bleeding. Recurrent torsion of the same ovary and contralateral torsion have been reported. Ureteral injury is a rare complication that can be avoided by prudent dissection and identification during the operation.

When to Transfer

Ovarian torsion represents a true emergency in that the viability of the ovary is directly related to speed at which intervention occurs. Transfer to a larger hospital is associated with a prolonged period of ischemia. If your hospital does not contain obstetric facilities, patients presenting during the third trimester should be considered for transfer due to risk of preterm delivery. In preparation for transfer, any preoperative imaging studies should be prepared and transferred with patient to prevent any delays for re-imaging procedures.

Suggested Reading

1. Baker TE, Copas PR. Adnexal torsion. A clinical dilemma. J Reprod Med. 1995;40(6):447–9.
2. Bayer AI, Wiskind AK. Adnexal torsion: can the adnexa be saved. Am J Obstet Gynecol. 1994;171:1506–11.
3. Chang HC, Bhatt S, Dogra VS. Pearls and pitfalls in diagnosis of ovarian torsion. Radiographics. 2008;28(5):1355–68.
4. Hibbard LT. Adnexal torsion. Am J Obstet Gynecol. 1985;152:456–61.
5. Rossi BV, Ference EH, Zurakowski D, Scholz S, Feins NR, Chow JS, Laufer MR. The clinical presentation and surgical management of adnexal torsion in the pediatric and adolescent population. J Pediatr Adolesc Gynecol. 2012;25(2):109–13.
6. Shalev E, Peleg D. Laparoscopic treatment of adnexial torsion. Surg Gynecol Obstet. 1993;176:448–50.
7. Zweizig S, Perron J, Grubb D, Mishell DR. Conservative management of adnexal torsion. Am J Obstet Gynecol. 1993;168:1791–5.

Jennifer J. Lucas

Indications

Suprapubic tube placement is indicated in when bladder catheterization is indicated and not technically possible due to urethral obstruction. In many cases suprapubic catheter placement may be avoided by applying established techniques for difficult urethral catheterization.

If an initial attempt at Foley catheter insertion is, it is worthwhile to enquire if 12 mL of lidocaine jelly were gently injected per urethra prior to the catheter placement attempt. Remarkably often, the addition of this one step in Foley catheter placement can make the procedure a success. If the patient is in urinary retention and is a male over 50 years old, then using an 18 Fr Coude catheter is the best option, since the Coude tip will provide better purchase to slide the catheter past an obstructing prostatic urethra. The Coude tip should always be facing upward while the catheter is being placed. The balloon port on the Coude catheter is oriented in the same direction as the curve of the catheter tip. Keeping the balloon port facing upwards assures correct upward positioning of the catheter tip. If catheter placement fails using these techniques, then the decision must be made to either transfer the patient to a hospital where a urologist is available or perform suprapubic catheter placement.

Preoperative Preparation

Once the urethra is deemed impassable, then it should be confirmed that the patient has adequate bladder volume by using ultrasound. An ultrasound bladder scanner can be used. This technique does not give an image, but instead provides the bladder volume in mL. Abdominal ultrasonography is even more useful, if easily available, because it provides an image of the bladder to confirm urinary retention and enables the surgeon to visualize the bladder during actual suprapubic catheter placement. Suprapubic catheter placement *is not safe unless at least 350 mL* of fluid is present in the bladder, since bowel perforation during the blind placement of the trocar can easily occur if the bladder is not distended.

If the patient has a history of previous abdominal/pelvic surgery, then imaging such as a CT scan is required to make sure that the bowel does not lie anterior to the bladder. Morbid obesity is another relative contraindication for percutaneous suprapubic tube placement, since critical landmarks are obscured?

An undescended bladder is an absolute contraindication for suprapubic catheter placement in order to avoid bowel injury. If the urinary retention is significant and causing severe pain in the presence of an impassible urethra, then suprapubic catheter placement should be attempted. If the patient is not in pain and a coagulopathy is present, attempts should be made to correct this prior to attempting suprapubic catheter placement. If an active urinary tract infection is present and the patient is not in pain, infusing an IV antibiotic with good gram-negative coverage at least 30 min prior to suprapubic catheter placement is preferred.

Operative Technique

There are slight variations among the major brands of suprapubic tube placement kits. It is essential that the instructions and parts of a particular kit be reviewed prior to catheter placement. Use of a kit will facilitate placement.

The lower abdomen is prepped and draped in standard sterile fashion with the patient in the supine position. Local anesthetic is used to infiltrate the site. A spinal needle is then advanced through the skin at the midline, about two finger breadths cephalad to the symphysis pubis. The needle should be advanced straight down to the floor, aspirating while advancing. When urine is aspirated, the surgeon then has a

J.J. Lucas, M.D. (✉)
Department of Surgery, Bassett Medical Center,
One Atwell Road, Cooperstown, NY 13326, USA
e-mail: jennifer.lucas@bassett.org

A.L. Halverson and D.C. Borgstrom (eds.), *Advanced Surgical Techniques for Rural Surgeons*,
DOI 10.1007/978-1-4939-1495-1_30, © Springer Science+Business Media New York 2015

good idea of the proper position, angle, and depth for the trocar. A 1 cm horizontal skin incision should be made at the same site where the spinal needle successfully aspirated urine. The trocar should then be advanced through the skin incision, at the same angle and to approximately the same depth as the spinal needle. The obturator should then be removed. At this point, urine will flow out of the sheath. Quickly place the catheter through the sheath before the bladder completely drains. Next, the balloon is inflated to 12 mL using sterile water. The sheath can then be peeled off the indwelling suprapubic catheter. The catheter should then be sutured to the skin. The catheter should then be placed to gravity drainage.

Potential Complications

As mentioned earlier, bowel perforation is an uncommon but serious complication of percutaneous suprapubic catheter placement. Its diagnosis is confirmed with imaging if the patient shows signs and symptoms worrisome for peritonitis. Prompt surgical repair is required in these cases.

A certain amount of hematuria is always expected with suprapubic catheter placement. Rarely is the hematuria significant. If, however, the hematuria is such that the SP tube appears to have clotted off, then attempt to irrigate the SP tube with sterile normal saline and a Toomey syringe. If this fails and the patient is beginning to feel uncomfortable from the urinary retention, then the patient should be transferred to a medical center where a urologist is available.

When to Transfer

Unsuccessful suprapubic tube placement.
Suprapubic tube is clotted.

Jennifer J. Lucas and Carlos E. Bermejo

Indications

During major pelvic surgery, ureteral injury is always a concern. Pelvic abscesses, sigmoid colectomy for recurrent diverticulitis, and colectomy for ulcerative colitis are only some examples of surgeries where inflammation and loss of normal anatomic planes make a ureteral injury even more difficult to avoid. Preoperative ureteral catheter placement is a relatively straightforward procedure that allows for tactile recognition of the ureter during open pelvic surgery. Lighted stents may be used in open as well as laparoscopic surgery. These give the ureter a faint glow, providing visual identification of the ureter intraoperatively.

Preoperative Preparation

Ureteral Catheter Placement

If the surgeon is planning for ureteral catheter placement, it is imperative that a preoperative urine culture be obtained showing no growth, preferably in the 2 weeks prior to surgery.

Ureteral catheter placement is performed with the anesthetized patient in the dorsal lithotomy position with the genitalia prepped and draped in standard sterile fashion. Fluoroscopy is useful to guide catheter placement and is considered essential by some to safely insert the catheter. The surgeon will need the following:

- 21 Fr rigid cystoscope with 30° lens in place
- −0.038 Floppy-tipped guide wire
- 5 Fr open-ended ureteral catheter

- Edelman urethral drainage catheter specially designed for this purpose
- Silk suture to secure ureteral catheters to the Edelman catheter

Operative Technique

When the cystoscope is assembled, focused, and white-balanced, sterile lubricant is generously placed over the entire nose of the cystoscope. Surgical lubricant *must* be placed on the nose of the cystoscope prior to *each* pass through the urethra. Omission of this step can lead to trauma and eventual urethral stricture, which is the most common complication of transurethral surgery.

In the male patient, the glans penis is then firmly grasped with the nondominant hand, and the dominant hand gently advances the scope into the urethra. Sterile water or sterile normal saline may be used, but fluid must be running through the scope as it is being passed through the urethra. Always keep the nose of the scope in the center of the urethral lumen. If a urethral stricture is found, it is safest to abort catheter placement altogether. Attempts to force the scope past a urethral stricture can result in complete obliteration of the urethral lumen. This can render subsequent Foley catheter placement impossible, which necessitate suprapubic tube placement.

The verumontanum signals the arrival of the cystoscope in the prostatic urethra. The surgeon will need to drop the hand holding the scope at this point to remain in the center of the lumen, since the prostatic urethra curves upward toward the umbilicus. Once the cystoscope passes into the bladder, the water may be stopped. If the bladder is filled with urine, the scope can gently be taken apart between the sheath and the bridge, leaving the sheath in the bladder. The bladder can be quickly drained in this fashion, and the bladder then refilled with sterile water (or normal saline) for better visibility. In the female patient, the shorter urethra is technically easier to navigate. The nondominant hand separates the

J.J. Lucas, M.D. (✉) • C.E. Bermejo, M.D.
Department of Surgery, Bassett Medical Center,
One Atwell Road, Cooperstown, NY 13326, USA
e-mail: jennifer.lucas@bassett.org

A.L. Halverson and D.C. Borgstrom (eds.), *Advanced Surgical Techniques for Rural Surgeons*,
DOI 10.1007/978-1-4939-1495-1_31, © Springer Science+Business Media New York 2015

labia, while the dominant hand guides the scope through the urethral meatus and urethra.

The ureteral orifices are located on the floor of the bladder, in the trigonal ridge. If the male patient has a very large intravesical prostate, it can be extremely difficult to visualize the ureteral orifices. If the ureteral orifices are not readily visible, then do not proceed with ureteral catheter placement.

Once the ureteral orifices are localized, the floppy tipped-guide wire can be advanced through the working port of the cystoscope and into the ureteral orifice. Always confirm that the technician has handed the wire to the surgeon in such a way that the floppy tipped portion of the wire is advanced first into the ureteral orifice. The other end of the wire is very stiff, and if it is advanced first into the ureteral orifice, it can cause ureteral perforation and/or significant renal trauma.

Fluoroscopy with a C-arm may be used to follow the advancement of the wire up the ureter. If the wire does not advance easily, then it is safest to abort the procedure because ureteral perforation is always possible. When the wire reaches the renal pelvis, it will curl, confirming its proper positioning. Once the guide wire is appropriately curling in the renal pelvis, it is time to advance the open-ended ureteral catheter over the wire using Seldinger technique. Advance the ureteral catheter over the wire. It will easily fit through the working port and sheath of the cystoscope. Using fluoroscopic guidance, advance the catheter to the point where the wire begins to curl. Then, remove the wire, leaving the ureteral catheter in place. In order to remove the scope without inadvertently taking out the ureteral catheter, it is best to completely take apart the scope between the bridge and sheath, grasping the catheter to stabilize it.

The same procedure may be performed on the contralateral ureter if desired. Since ureteral catheter placement is not without complications, unilateral catheter placement is safest in procedures where there is no concern for the contralateral ureteral. (A good example of this would be sigmoid colectomy, where in most cases only a left ureteral catheter would be required.)

Once catheter placement is complete, the Edelman urethral catheter is placed, and the ureteral catheters are secured to the Edelman catheter with suture, then placed through the side ports of the Edelman catheter for drainage.

Potential Pitfalls

Urethral trauma.
   Failure to visualize ureteral orifice.
   Ureteral perforation.
   Hydronephrosis due to ureteral spasm.
   The ureteral catheters should be removed immediately postoperatively, prior to awakening the patient.

Common Complications

Complications of the procedure include ureteral perforation, renal injury, urinary tract infection, and urethral stricture. Even straightforward cases can occasionally be complicated by immediate postoperative hydronephrosis and flank discomfort caused by obstruction due to ureteral inflammation. For these reasons, it is prudent to limit ureteral catheter placement to the ureter crossing the expected surgical field. Also, if any step of the procedure is not advancing smoothly, it is safest to abort the catheter placement and do without.

Carlos E. Bermejo and Jennifer J. Lucas

Indications

When a testicular torsion is encountered, detorsion of the affected testicle is considered a urologic emergency. Once testicular pain starts, there is a 6 h window to detorse the testicle and reinstate blood flow, otherwise, atrophy or loss of the affected testicle is imminent. Testicular torsion can occur at any age, with a peak incidence in the first week of life, and a second peak at puberty.

Preoperative Preparation

Patients with a testicular torsion will present with acute pain. The differential diagnosis of testicular torsion is broad. Retroperitoneal and intra-abdominal pathology should be considered. Primarily, it should be differentiated from epididymitis. Doppler ultrasound is the gold standard for imaging of an acute scrotum. In testicular torsion, the lack of blood flow or presence of sharply diminished blood flow on a Doppler ultrasound confirms the diagnosis of testicular torsion. In epididymitis, Doppler ultrasound could reveal increased blood flow to the epididymis and testis.

Operative Strategy

Once the diagnosis of testicular torsion has been confirmed, time is of the essence to detorse the testicle to preserve testicular viability. To buy time, an attempt can be made to detorse the affected testicle manually prior to taking the patient to the OR for scrotal exploration. This can be done by turning the affected testicle laterally. This is often effective

because in two-thirds of cases, the testicle is rotated medially. If successful, the patient will have relief of pain. Manual detorsion may be a successful one up to 50 % of attempts. Even if manual detorsion appears successful, scrotal exploration is required to confirm testicular viability and to perform testicular fixation if the testicle remains viable. Intraoperative testicular fixation is imperative, since torsion recurrence rates are quite high. If the affected testis appears necrotic, then orchiectomy may be required. It is important that the patient and family be aware prior to surgery that loss of the testis is a definite possibility.

Operative Technique

A midline scrotal incision is made along the scrotal raphe (Fig. 32.1). This incision is carried down through the skin, dartos fascia, and tunica vaginalis of the affected testicle (Fig. 32.2). When entering the tunica vaginalis care should be taken not to injure the testicle.

The affected testicle is then brought out of the scrotum. Generally, there is a 360° twist in the spermatic cord (Fig. 32.3). The testis is then untwisted, which usually involves lateral turning of the testis. Notice the horizontal axis without a lower pole fixation, Bell clapper deformity, a transverse orientation of the testicle, which is seen in cases of testicular torsion (Fig. 32.4). Observe the testis during reperfusion. Intraoperative Doppler ultrasound can be used directly on the testis. If the testicle remains dark in color, and no blood flow is noted, then a small incision in the tunica albuginea may be made. If the testis does not bleed, then an orchiectomy must be performed. If an orchiectomy is to be performed, the spermatic cord should be divided in two sections, separating the vas from the vascular pedicle, and both should be suture ligated. If there is good flow documented with Doppler ultrasound after detorsion, and the color of the testicle returns to normal, then orchiectomy will likely not be required. The next step is to proceed with testicular fixation. A three-point fixation should be performed to prevent the

C.E. Bermejo, M.D. (✉) • J.J. Lucas, M.D.
Department of Surgery, Bassett Medical Center,
One Atwell Road, Cooperstown, NY 13326, USA
e-mail: carlos.bermejo@bassett.org

A.L. Halverson and D.C. Borgstrom (eds.), *Advanced Surgical Techniques for Rural Surgeons*,
DOI 10.1007/978-1-4939-1495-1_32, © Springer Science+Business Media New York 2015

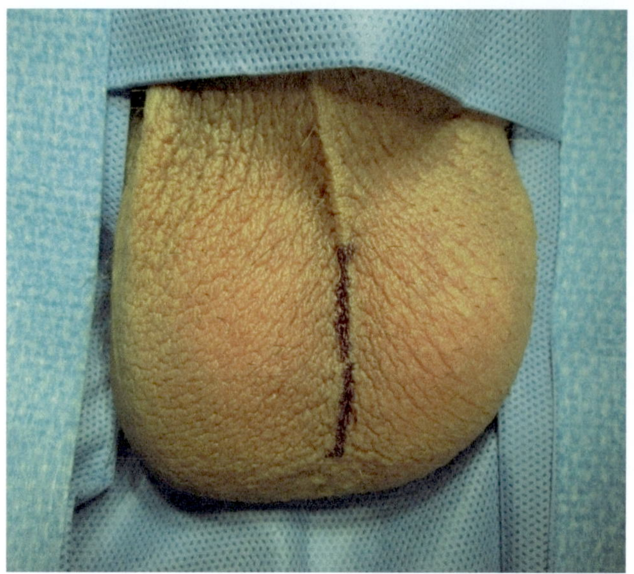

Fig. 32.1 Median raphe incision

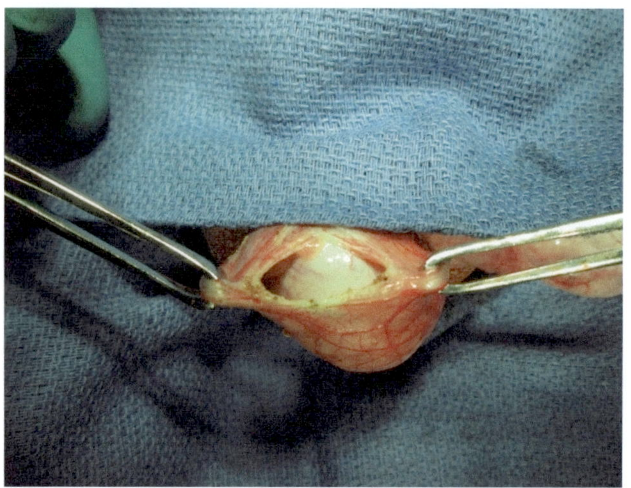

Fig. 32.2 Entry into the tunica vaginalis

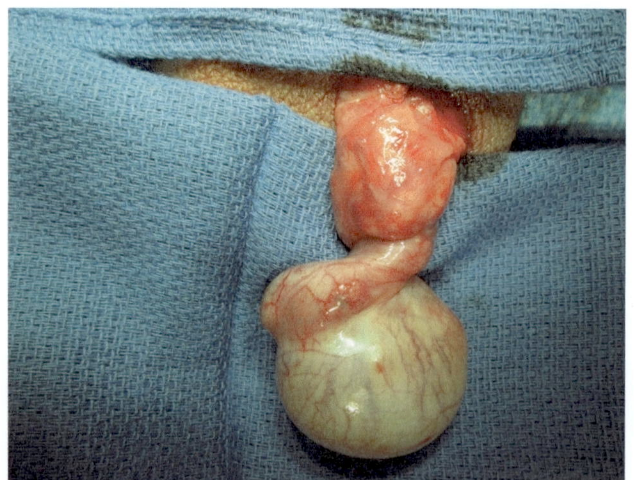

Fig. 32.3 360° twist of the spermatic cord

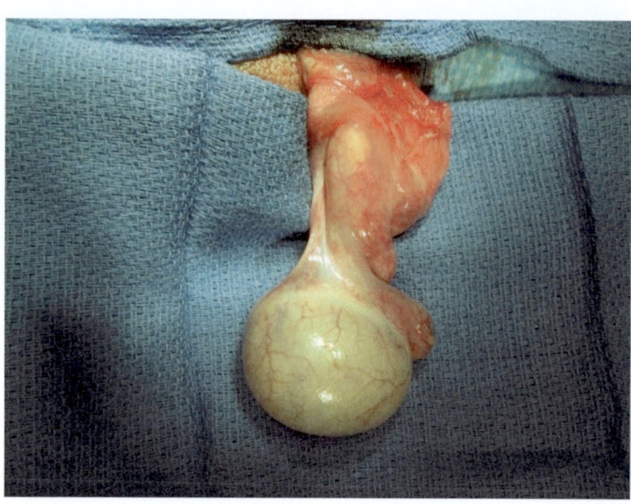

Fig. 32.4 Transverse orientation of the testicle, the "bell clapper deformity"

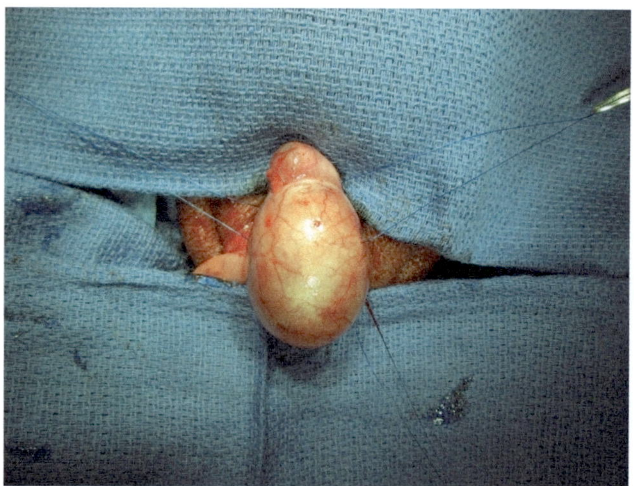

Fig. 32.5 Three-point fixation of the testicle

recurrence of torsion. The fixation should be performed using a 3-0 absorbable or nonabsorbable suture. The suture should be placed through the tunica albuginea and dartos muscle, being careful to avoid piercing the skin.

The sutures should be placed medially and laterally, away from the epididymis, and away from the incision to avoid problems with closure (Figs. 32.5, 32.6, and 32.7). The contralateral testis should be fixed in the same manner. Prior to tying down the sutures insert the testicle back into the scrotum and then tie the sutures (Fig. 32.8). This maneuver will make it easier to tie the sutures at the time of fixating the testicle to the scrotal wall.

The incision closure should be performed with a 3-0 absorbable synthetic suture, such as vicryl. The dartos muscle should be closed with running suture (Figs. 32.9 and 32.10). The tunica vaginalis does not need to be closed. For

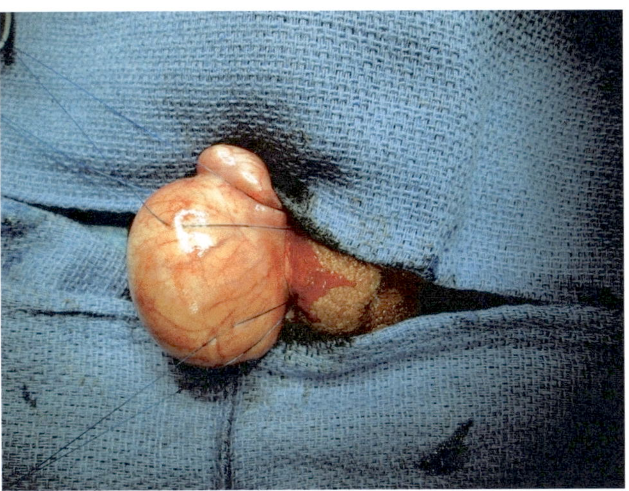

Fig. 32.6   Testicle sutured into the scrotum

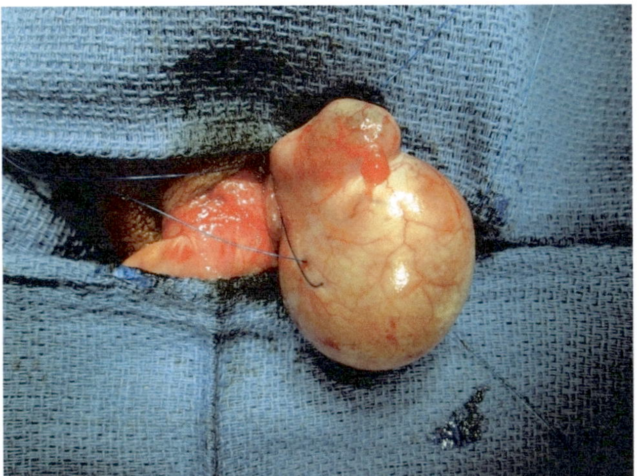

Fig. 32.7   Lateral testicular fixation

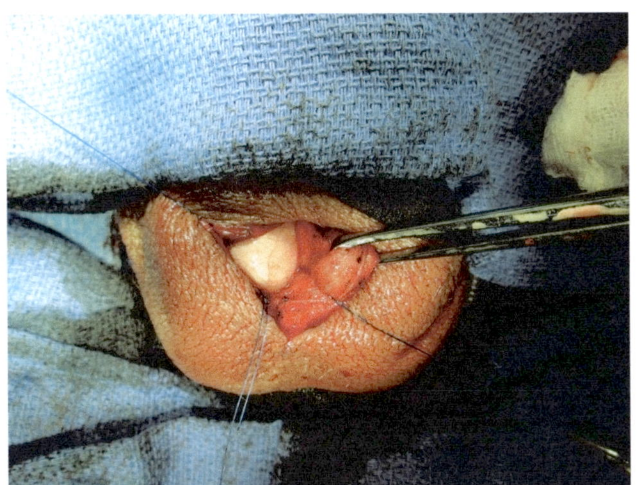

Fig. 32.8   Testicle returned to the scrotum before tying fixation sutures

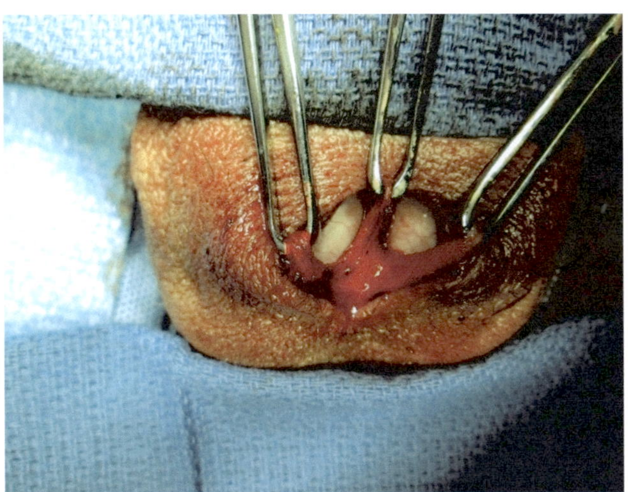

Fig. 32.9   Allis clamps on dartos muscle

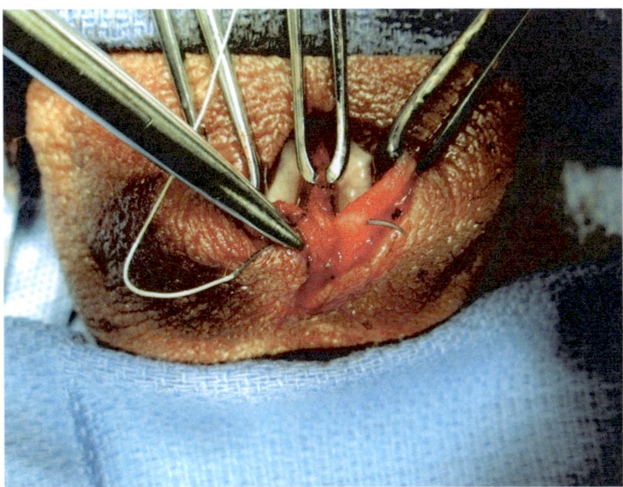

Fig. 32.10   Closure of dartos muscle

the skin closure, 3-0 or 4-0 synthetic absorbable suture should be used. A sterile dressing should then be placed, followed by gauze fluffs and a scrotal support.

Postoperative Care

The patient can be discharged to home the same day of surgery. The dressing should be removed in 48 h. The patient should follow up in 10–14 days for a wound check.

Potential Problems

Hematoma
Retorsion
Infertility

Timothy Whitaker

Indications

The reason for this procedure is to provide for permanent sterility. Vasectomy can be reversed but only through a technically difficult procedure that has a failure rate of 10–20 %.

Preoperative Preparation

This procedure needs to be discussed with the patient and this discussion may need to involve the patient's active sexual partner. It is imperative that the surgeon has a thorough discussion with the patient and document this discussion including the permanency of the procedure, the instructions that this cannot be relied on as the sole source of contraception until approximately 20 or more ejaculations and a semen analysis confirming the lack of sperm. At the same time as the procedure discussion, postoperative plans for wound care, activity, resuming sexual activity can be addressed. A complete medication review needs to be done preoperatively to address issues with anticoagulants. Failure to address this preoperatively may lead to a large postoperative hematoma.

A consideration that needs to be addressed before the procedure is the type of anesthesia to be used for this procedure. This can be done with local anesthetic or a combination of local anesthetic and sedation. The choice will be based on the surgeon's preference and the availability of services in surgical procedure room. On the day of the procedure the patient may be given a preoperative dose of oral anxiolytic or the like if the surgeon so chooses. The procedure

T. Whitaker, B.S., M.D., F.A.C.S. (✉)
Department of General Surgery, Bassett Healthcare,
One Atwell Road, Cooperstown, NY 13326, USA
e-mail: Timothy.Whitaker@Bassett.org

will need to be in a comfortable setting with the patient in the reclined or supine position. The operative environment needs to be warm to prevent significant cremasteric contraction, thereby making identification of the vas deferens slightly more difficult.

Operative Strategy

Gain direct visual access to the vas deferens on each side of the scrotum. Excise a portion of the vas. Ligate the open ends of the vas with or without cauterization of these ligated ends. The closure will use the anatomic tissue to separate the transected ends of the vas into different planes.

Use of the proper equipment and set up will provide a more comfortable experience for the patient and a more expeditious procedure for the surgeon. Figure 33.1 shows a type of vasectomy clamp that will provide excellent control of the vas throughout the procedure.

Operative Technique

With the patient in a comfortable reclined or supine position undressed from the waist down. A gauze 4×4 will be wrapped loosely around the head of the penis and used to apply traction to the penis cephalad. This gauze will be held in place with a clamp attached to patient's gown or shirt (Fig. 33.2).

The scrotum is prepped with hibiclens or betadine and pulled through the hole in a fenestrated sterile drape.

The vas deferens is palpated in the upper one-third of the scrotum on the lateral aspect. The skin over this area is anesthetized with local anesthetic.

Once adequate anesthesia is obtained the vas deferens is held in place with a pair of ring vasectomy clamps, above and below the area to be incised (Fig. 33.3).

The skin is incised with a 15 blade scalpel between these 2 clamps or the skin can be punctured and spread

A.L. Halverson and D.C. Borgstrom (eds.), *Advanced Surgical Techniques for Rural Surgeons*,
DOI 10.1007/978-1-4939-1495-1_33, © Springer Science+Business Media New York 2015

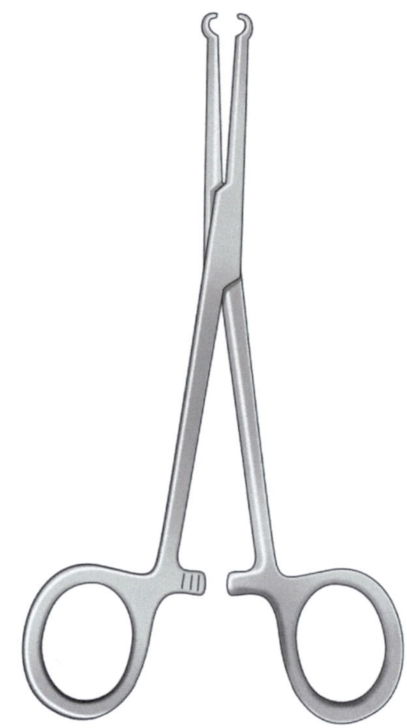

Fig. 33.1 Vasectomy clamp

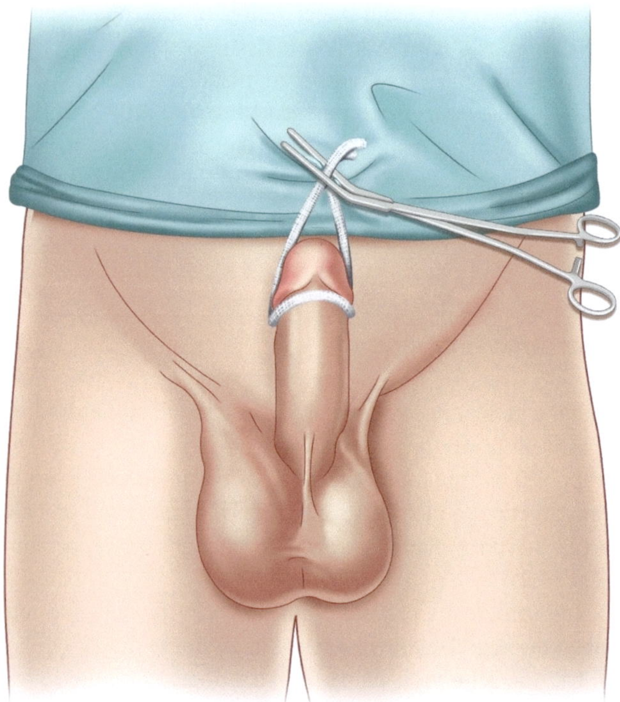

Fig. 33.2 The penis can be retracted with a rolled gauze and a clamp attached to the patient's shirt to provide better exposure of the scrotum

apart with a sharp mosquito like clamp for a "no scalpel technique."

Dissection is carried down through the subcutaneous tissue including the dartos muscle layer and the vas is identified by direct visualization.

Two Vicryl sutures are placed around the vas about 2 cm apart. These sutures are used to ligate both ends of the vas. A hemostat is placed on each of the sutures for traction (Fig. 33.4).

The vas is then excised between these two ligatures. Care should be taken to remove at least 1.5 cm of the vas. The ligated ends of the vas are then cauterized. The sutures can then be cut and the ligated cauterized ends allowed to retract back into the tissue (Fig. 33.5).

At this point the surrounding tissue can be closed over one end of the vas with a Vicryl suture to create a physical tissue barrier to prevent recanalization (Fig. 33.6).

Excellent hemostasis is a must. The tissues are then reapproximated in layers with absorbable suture. The skin can be dressed with skin glue or steri strips.

The procedure is then repeated on the opposite side.

Potential Pitfalls

Injury to the testicular artery and veins. This can be avoided by careful dissection and thorough identification of the vas before ligation and excision.

Postoperative Care

The key to postoperative care is to prevent swelling and hematoma formation. The patient is instructed to wear an athletic supporter daily for 5 days. Ice packs are to be applied to the incisions 3–4 times per day over the first 2 days after the procedure. The patient is cautioned to not perform any excessive straining for 5 days post-op. The patient may resume sexual relations 5 days post-op. Again it needs to be stressed to the patient that the vasectomy is not to be the only form of birth control until a semen sample shows no sperm. The patient is given a labeled collection bottle to return semen samples to the office 10 weeks postprocedure.

Complications

Bleeding and hematoma formation.

Pain that may require short-term narcotic use.

Fig. 33.3 The vas is held between the two clamps through the skin before the incision is made

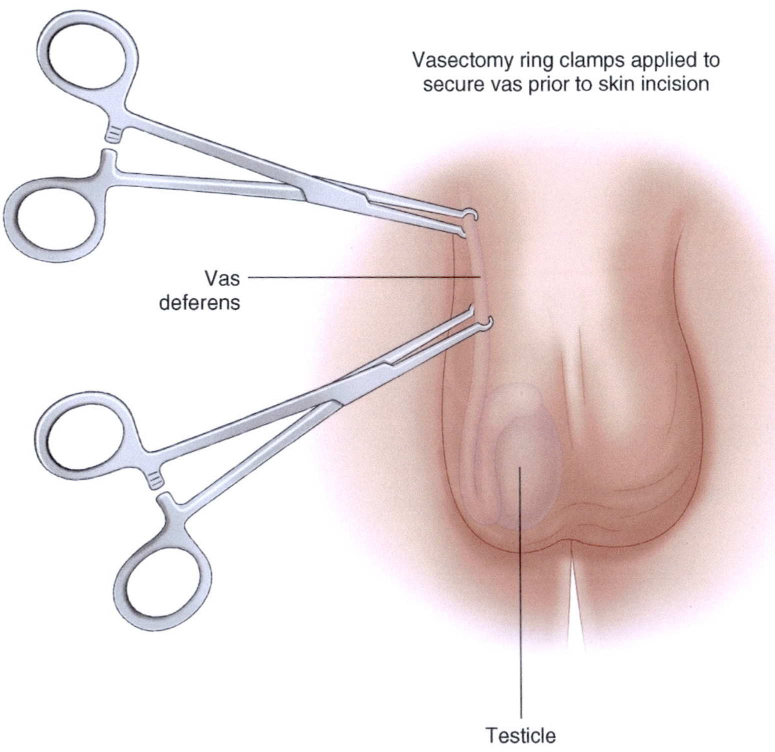

Fig. 33.4 This figure shows the vas exposed with the clamps now holding directly onto the vas to allow easy passage of the Vicryl ties around each end for ligation

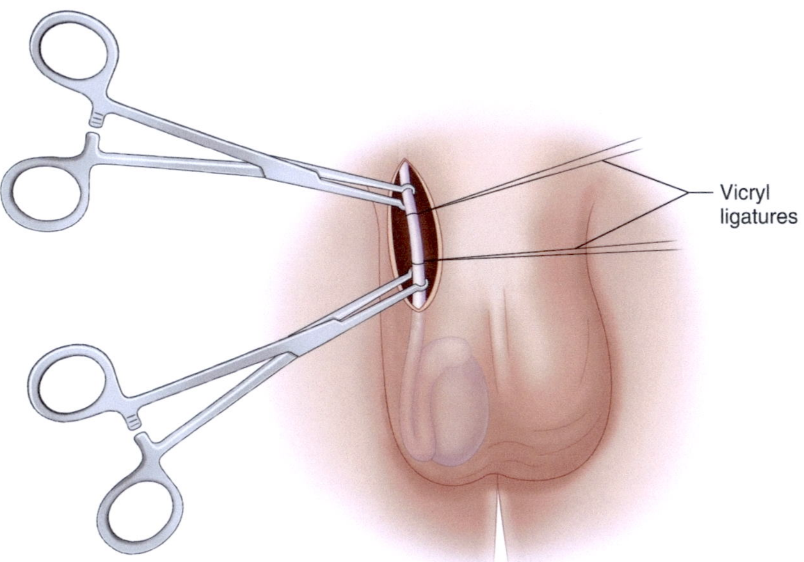

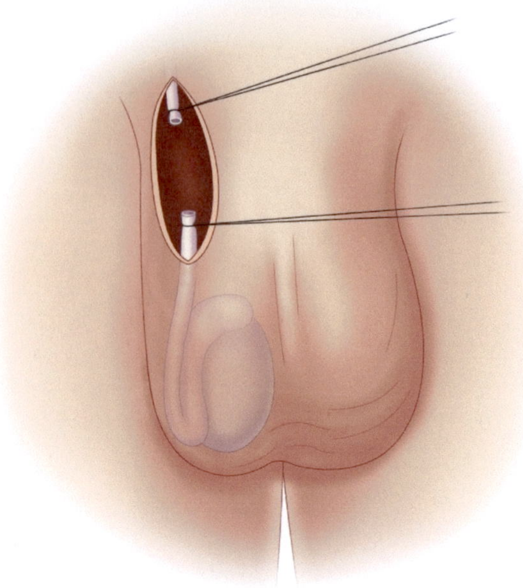

Fig. 33.5 The ligated vas is shown after excision of the intervening portion still with the Vicryl ties in place but with the clamps removed

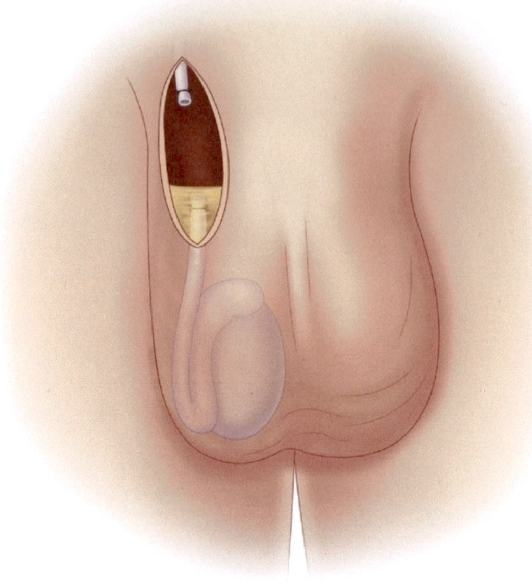

Fig. 33.6 The ligated ends are allowed to retract into the surrounding tissue, which can be closed over one end to prevent recanalization

When to Transfer

This is an elective office-based procedure that with proper preprocedure planning should allow for referral to a urologist for identified issues that may complicate the intended procedure.

Suggested Reading

1. Awsare NS, Krishnan J. Complications of vasectomy. Ann R Coll Surg Engl. 2005;87(6):406–10.
2. Griffin T, Oher R, Nowakowski K, Lloyd M, Maddern G. How little is enough? The evidence for post-vasectomy testing. J Urol. 2005;174(1):29–36.
3. Holt SK, Salinas CA, Stanford JL. Vasectomy and the risk of prostate cancer. J Urol. 2008;180(6):2565–7.
4. Sandlow J, Winfield HN, Goldstein M. Surgery of the scrotum and seminal vesicles. In: Wein A, Kavoussi L, Novick A, et al., editors. Campbell-Walsh urology. 9th ed. Philadelphia: Saunders; 2000.
5. Vasectomy (No-Incision and Standard) Surgery Details. http://www.flinturology.com/vasectomy.shtml

Part IX

Pediatric Surgery

Perioperative Management in Infants and Children

Brett Howard and Don K. Nakayama

Introduction

Infants and children who require surgical care will come to the attention in rural hospitals and clinics. Whether the surgeon chooses to provide care depends on his or her training and the capabilities of the facility and staff. Guidelines for treatment and transfer of pediatric surgical patients are under development by the American Pediatric Surgical Association. They will help surgeons in rural and remote areas develop the necessary resources to responsibly care for infants and children at their practice locations.

Pediatric patients will arrive and require some level of evaluation and treatment regardless of whether they receive definitive care or are transferred. The basic priorities of initial resuscitation remain the same: Airway, breathing, and circulation. Attention to these priorities and early stabilization will lead to better overall outcomes if proper steps are taken when the child is first seen and not delayed until after transfer to a referral hospital.

Vital Signs

The first essential step is to measure vital signs immediately upon admission. Table 34.1 lists normal vital signs by age group in a pattern intended to be easy to remember. Major pediatric age groups are newborn (under 28 days), infant (under 1 year), toddlers (1–3 years), and older children (over 6 years). Respiratory rates are more rapid in newborns (40/min) and infants (30) because of their higher basic metabolism by weight and the mechanical disadvantages of having small lungs and very compliant chest walls. As the respiratory system matures breathing rates slow (20 in toddlers) reaching adult levels in adolescents (rates in the "teens").

High metabolic rates associated with small size, demands of growth, and combating heat loss also account for high resting heart rates in the newborn (140/min) and infant age groups (120). The small size of infant hearts limit stroke volume, so any adjustments in cardiac output must come from changes in heart rate. Bradycardia (under 100 beats per minute) in infants is always ominous. Heart rates below 100 usually are due to hypoxemia and demand immediate attention. Supplemental oxygen must be administered and if the heart rate remains low external cardiac massage is mandatory. Small children have resting rates of 100, a number that may be concerning to practitioners used to slower adult values typical of adolescents (under 80).

Normal blood pressures among newborns (60 mmHg systolic) and infants (80) reflect the limited cardiac performance of the infant heart. A corollary is that any decrease in systolic blood pressure is a preterminal sign and immediate measures must be taken to support the blood pressure either with volume, pharmacological intervention, or external cardiac massage. Normal blood pressures increase with older children (100) and reach adult values in adolescents (120).

Body temperature, however, is the same in all age groups, 37 °C. In newborns and infants a skin temperature from the axilla is routine, and a slightly lower value expected (36.0–36.5°). Oral temperatures are hard to obtain and rectal values unnecessary (and potentially dangerous). Newborns and infants are especially prone to hypothermia because they have large surface area relative to body size, depend on brown fat metabolism for thermogenesis, and are unable to shiver to generate heat. Young patients should be wrapped in warm blankets before and after being seen and placed under warming blankets and radiant heat lamps when being examined or receiving active therapy.

B. Howard, M.D.
Department of Surgery, Mercer University School of Medicine, Medical Center of Central Georgia, 777 Hemlock Street, Macon, GA 31201, USA

D.K. Nakayama, M.D., M.B.A., F.A.C.S. (✉)
Department of Surgery, West Virginia University School of Medicine, Health Sciences Center, 1 Medical Center Drive, Morgantown, WV 26506, USA
e-mail: dknakayama@hsc.wvu.edu; nakayama.don@gmail.com

A.L. Halverson and D.C. Borgstrom (eds.), *Advanced Surgical Techniques for Rural Surgeons*, DOI 10.1007/978-1-4939-1495-1_34, © Springer Science+Business Media New York 2015

Table 34.1 Vital signs in infants and children

Age group	RR (breaths per min)	HR (beats per min)	BP (systolic; mmHg)
Newborn (birth to 28 days)	40	140	60
Infant (under 1 year)	30	120	80
Child (approx 3–6 years)	20	100	100
Adolescent	Teens	80	120

Any deviation from normal values requires constant electrocardiographic and respiratory monitoring, pulse oximetry, and periodic measurement of blood pressure. Admission or transfer to a higher level of care is required for persistent tachycardia or tachypnea, periodic breathing (periods of cessation of breathing efforts lasting seconds and not associated with other changes in heart rate), apnea (no breathing effort of 15 s or more, or any cessation of breathing effort associated with bradycardia), bradycardia, low blood pressure, and change in sensorium (persistent agitation, irritability, restlessness, stupor, or coma).

Airway and Breathing

Signs that an infant has respiratory distress can be subtle but demand the administration of supplemental oxygen and transfer to a higher level of care. Infants exhibit tachypnea, pallor, nasal flaring, and air hunger. Hypoxemia may become manifest as irritability and restlessness, so caution demands an evaluation with a pulse oximetry before sedatives or analgesics are considered. Retractions of the chest wall and soft tissues of the lower neck and upper chest reflect increased work of breathing. As the infant tires or begins to decompensate periods of apnea occur. Bradycardia, a late sign, indicates hypoxemia and impending cardiac arrest. Cyanosis is also a late sign and may not be seen because the patient may decompensate before desaturated hemoglobin levels reach 5 g/dL, the concentration associated with the color.

Infant airways tend to obstruct. Their large head and prominent occiput flex the neck and collapse the upper airway, easily opened by head tilt and jaw lift maneuvers (Fig. 34.1). Any parent knows that young children always have food and a variety of other foreign material near or in their mouths, always are eating, and frequently have a respiratory infection. Suction equipment must be close at hand. Early placement of a nasogastric tube is a necessary step in airway control to decompress the stomach and prevent aspiration. A common error is using a feeding tube that is too small for adequate decompression. Infants require at least a 10 French tube.

Supplies necessary for airway control must be at hand when seeing children with emergency conditions, including laryngoscopes and tubes of sizes appropriate for infants and

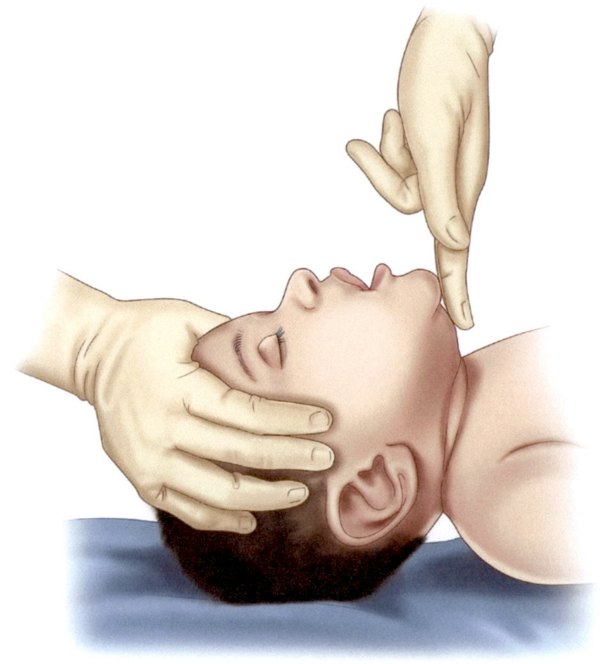

Fig. 34.1 Head tilt and chin lift in an infant. These are the first maneuvers to open the airway in infants and small children

small children. A useful memory aid is that the patient's little finger approximates the appropriate size of the endotracheal tube. Supplies must be inventoried and checked regularly to assure they remain in working order, especially items like laryngoscopes that have batteries and require illumination. Practice dummies of the infant head and neck allow practice intubation and fairly accurately reproduce the anatomic features that make the procedure a challenge. The orifice itself is small. The larynx lies high in the neck, obscured by the epiglottis, which is rigid and shaped like an "omega" rather than a broad based "U." The maneuver to visualize the larynx is to lift the tip of the epiglottis with the tip of a straight laryngoscope blade (Fig. 34.2). If the larynx cannot be seen the usual error is that the laryngoscope is too distally placed.

A surgical airway may be mandatory in massive upper airway injuries where there is bleeding or soft tissue trauma. If the patient is exchanging air the best initial maneuver is to provide supplemental oxygen and move to the operating room where light, equipment, and trained assistance are at hand. The most experienced anesthesiologist or anesthetist then attempts orotracheal intubation without paralytics or anesthesia. If standard airway control is unsuccessful after multiple attempts then the most experienced surgeon performs a tracheotomy using an incision with which he or she is most comfortable. In such a situation the incision must be of adequate size to provide immediate access to the trachea and control bleeding. Use a standard pediatric endotracheal tube—in such a situation a standard tracheotomy appliance is too short and the stay collars are cumbersome.

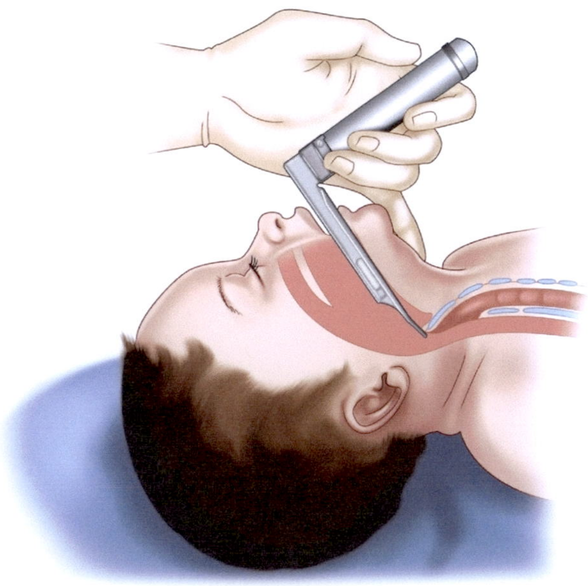

Infant

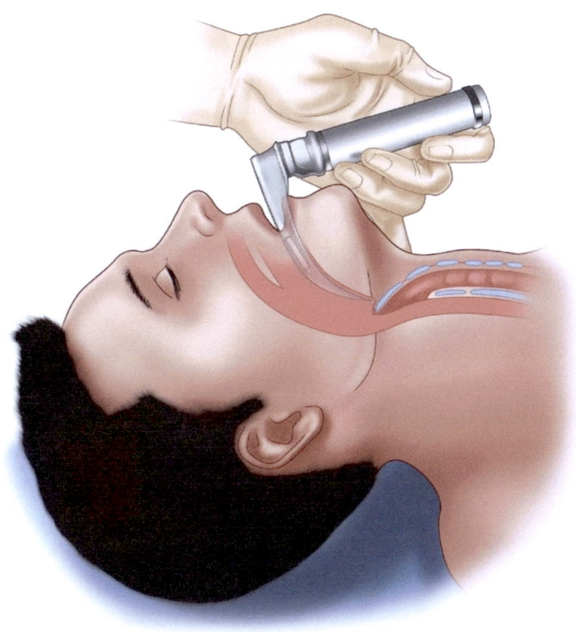

Adult

Fig. 34.2 The view at direct laryngoscopy in an infant (*left*) and an adult (*right*). The tip of a straight laryngoscope blade lifts the epiglottis in the infant, while a curved scope used in adults pulls the vallecula, anterior to the epiglottis upward to visualize the adult larynx

Circulation

Many signs of shock in infancy and childhood are similar to those that signal respiratory distress, so intravenous therapy is part of the initial resuscitation of a patient exhibiting tachypnea, tachycardia, pallor, and change in sensorium

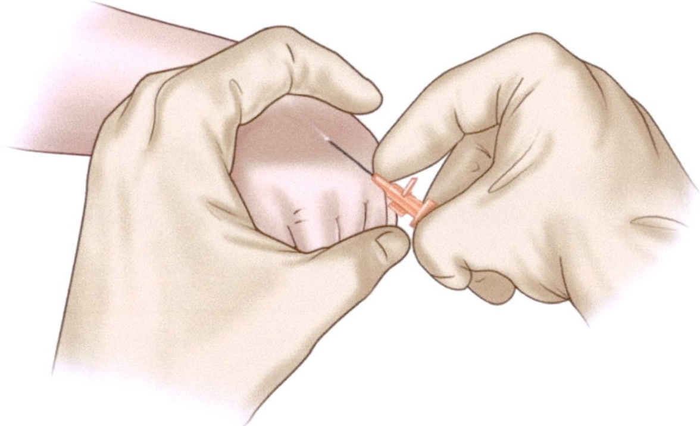

Fig. 34.3 Placement of a peripheral intravenous cannula in a vein in the dorsum of the wrist. Flexion of the wrist stabilizes the vein, the practitioner's index finger obstructing the vein distally to distend it for venipuncture

(restlessness, irritability, stupor). Delayed capillary refill and skin mottling reflect peripheral vasoconstriction that may be from hypovolemia but also being in a cold environment. As noted, active warming devices are mandatory in the treatment of infants and small children (radiant warmers, forced air warmers), and patients need to be kept covered when not undergoing active evaluation and therapy. The short, fat necks in infants and young children make neck vein distention useless as a sign of elevated central venous pressure. Young infants whose fontanelle is still open may have a depressed area if dehydrated and alternatively a bulging fontanelle if central pressures are elevated.

Urinary output (UO) is an important measure of adequacy of hydration, but young infants have limited capacity to concentrate urine and eliminate excess volume, so renal indices used to guide resuscitation in adults require caution when applied in infants. Very low (less than 0.5 mL/kg/h) and very high (more than 2 mL/kg/h) UO values should be avoided. UO of 1 mL/kg/h is an appropriate target.

Intravenous access may be a major challenge in management. Infants and children have the same sites familiar in older patients: antecubital fossa, greater saphenous vein at the ankle. The back and volar aspects of the wrist are relatively free of subcutaneous fat making candidate veins more easily seen (Fig. 34.3). Scalp veins require removal of hair, so anxious parents must be reassured of the necessity of the preliminary step. A wide gum band is used as tourniquet to distend scalp veins, with a short piece of tape to facilitate its quick removal once the catheter is in place. A 24 gauge catheter is adequate for resuscitation in infants, but 22 gauge access is necessary for resuscitation from shock and blood transfusion.

Placement of central venous catheters in children generally requires sedation. Young children and infants have short, fat necks that obscure landmarks generally used in internal jugular vein catheterization. The landmark for subclavian

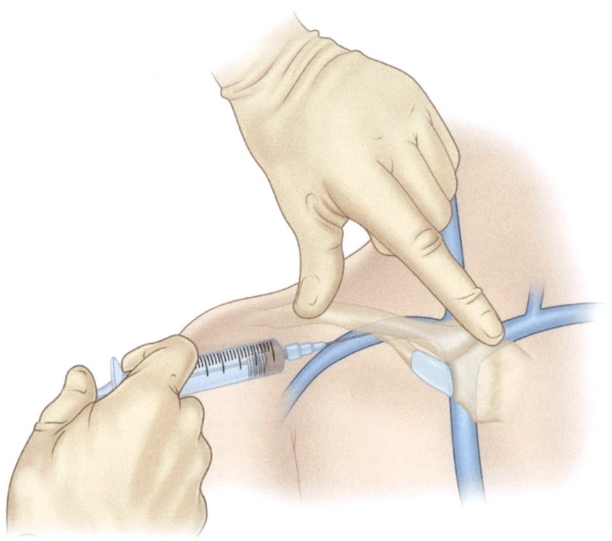

Fig. 34.4 Landmarks for subclavian venipuncture in an infant. The clavicle is divided into a medial and lateral half, and the needle is directed in a slightly cephalad direction from directly horizontal. This is in contrast to adult subclavian venipuncture, where the needle passes between the medial and middle thirds of the clavicle, and in a more cephalad direction

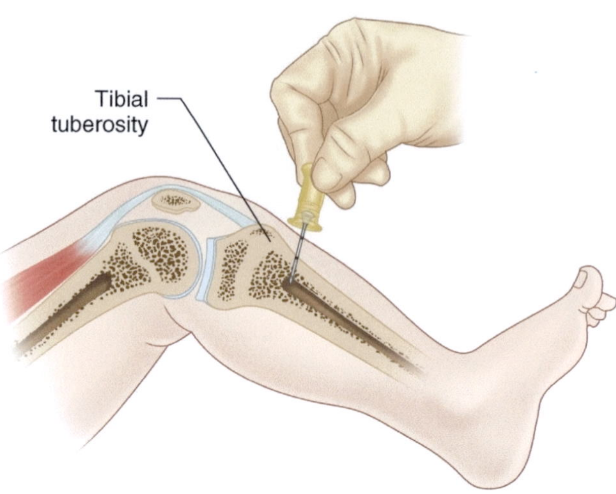

Fig. 34.5 Landmarks for intraosseous needle placement. A large hollow bore needle is inserted into the anterior aspect of the tibia, about 1 in. below the tibial plateau, at a 60° angle from vertical

venipuncture in younger children (just medial to the midpoint of the length of the clavicle) is lateral to the site generally used in adults (junction between the middle and medial thirds of the clavicle), with the angle of the needle more transverse and less cephalad in direction (Fig. 34.4). The diameter of the vein is small and distances are short, so care is necessary to keep the open tip of the catheter within the vein while advancing the catheter or cannulating. Especially in dehydrated infants, the only sign that the tip of the needle is within the vein may be a flash of blood returning into the catheter as it is withdrawn across the lumen of the vessel, rather than advanced into it.

An intraosseous needle placed in the tibia is an acceptable alternative (Fig. 34.5). Like any unusual procedure practitioners must practice placing the needles available in the facility using animal bones under simulated conditions. The landmark for insertion is 1 in. below the tibial plateau, the needle at a 60° angle. An attached syringe maintains suction as the needle is advanced, the appearance of bloody marrow the signal that the tip is in proper position, confirmed by free infusion of saline by gravity.

Inability to secure an I.V. in a patient requiring resuscitation or parenteral medication is an indication for transfer. Patients who have spent weeks in an NICU as a prematurely born infant (premie graduate) may have few obvious sites. Especially if such patients have had previous surgical operations early transfer may be the best approach for stable patients.

Patients with surgical emergencies have some degree of dehydration from a number of causes, including inability to take liquids by mouth, vomiting, and internal third space losses from obstruction or inflammation. The patient receives an initial infusion of 20 mL/kg of balanced electrolyte solution over 10–20 min, either normal saline (0.9 % NaCl) or lactated Ringer's solution. A second such infusion is necessary if signs of hypovolemia continue.

Infusions at 150 % of basal maintenances then continue until normal vital signs and urine output (1 mL/kg/h) are achieved. Generally a crystalloid solution of 0.45 % NaCl (one-half normal saline) is started until initial serum electrolyte levels are determined. Potassium chloride additives to give a final concentration of 20 mEq/L are started after an adequate urine output is established. Glucose is a mandatory component of all intravenous infusions in infancy because of the risk of hypoglycemia if the baby cannot take oral feedings. Dextrose concentration at 5 % is generally adequate, but newborns may require 10 % concentrations to keep serum glucose values above 100 mg/dL. Bedside determinations of glucose levels are necessary in all infants receiving solely intravenous fluids for hydration.

Blood volume is 80 mL/kg. Practitioners treating infants and children must determine the total blood volume and keep in mind the small volumes that may result in clinically significant hypovolemia. For example, a 4 kg baby has a blood volume of 320 mL, just less than a can of cola. Hypovolemia becomes significant at 20 mL/kg (25 % of blood volume), so 80 mL—a little more than one-fourth the volume of a standard soft drink can (355 mL)—represents significant blood loss. Practitioners must be alert to ongoing blood losses from injury but also volumes drawn for laboratory analysis and blood bank cross match requirements.

Preoperative Care

Pediatric patients who will be undergoing surgery in a rural practice require the same degree of stabilization before surgery as adult patients. Margins for error are narrower, so extra attention must be paid to any respiratory and circulatory issues that arise. Anesthesia personnel must feel comfortable with their ability to manage small airways and perform endotracheal intubation confidently and reliably. Adequate intravenous access is essential, and an initial infusion of 20 mL/kg of balanced salt solution begins to address dehydration that nearly always accompanies a sick patient with acute surgical disease. Time spent establishing adequate intravenous access and beginning fluid resuscitation, correcting acid–base and electrolyte imbalances, and establishing an adequate urine output is almost always time well spent.

Fasting requirements must be strictly observed, with standard proscriptions against any food, formula, or liquids for at least 6 h before induction of anesthesia. To prevent excessive dehydration among infants pediatric anesthesiologists allow clear liquids (Pedialyte, dilute apple juice, and water—not orange juice or breast milk) up to 2 h before operation.

The indications for preoperative antibiotics are the same for pediatric surgical patients as adults. All drugs are given on a per-kilogram basis, so rechecking doses with a standard pediatric drug handbook, or consulting the hospital pharmacist, are mandatory. Dosing intervals are nearly always different and must be double checked because of developmental differences in renal function and hepatic metabolism.

Intraoperative Care

Extra care must be taken to identify the operative site with parents and to confirm the correct side on routine procedures such as inguinal hernia and hydrocele repairs. Bulges present on an awake child standing in an office exam room disappear when he or she is under anesthesia.

Skin preparation solutions cannot be left to pool in skin creases and under the patient, as chemical irritation may result from prolonged contact. Povidone-iodine solutions (Betadine) are used in infants. Chlorhexidine preparations (Chlor-prep) are acceptable in older children.

Vapor anesthetics and neuromuscular blocking agents interfere with brown fat metabolism and nonshivering thermogenesis, so extra measures are necessary to maintain normal body temperatures. The ambient temperature in the operating room must be set at a level that maintains normothermia of the patient, often at the expense of the comfort of the operating room team members. The baby lies on a forced air convective warming blanket (Bair-Hugger) and under radiant warming lights. Drapes are impervious to moisture and exposed skin surfaces covered with plastic (Io-ban) to assure that the patient's skin remains dry to prevent evaporative heat loss.

Time spent away from critical care areas must be kept to a minimum. The operative team must be ready to begin as soon as anesthesia starts to avoid long delays between induction and the start of the procedure. Similarly operations must be well planned with all available instruments, equipment, and supplies at hand to assure procedures are performed efficiently, directly, and without unnecessary intraoperative delays. After surgery intubated patients often are transported back to the intensive care area under mechanical ventilation with an endotracheal tube so that the airway remains controlled during transfer.

Postoperative Care

Emergence from anesthesia may be unpredictable because of the larger proportion of cardiac output that goes to the infant brain, the relative immaturity of the blood–brain barrier, differences in volumes of distribution for inhalational anesthetics, and different uptake in fat stores in the infant body. Extubation depends upon the ability to make regular deep breaths and in infants, suggested by flexion of the hips.

Observation in the postanesthesia care unit must be of a sufficient duration to confirm that breathing continues without interruption, vital signs are normal without variation, pain control is adequate, and liquids can be ingested without vomiting. Before the patient receives anything to drink the surgeon must check the operative site to assure that an acute complication has not occurred that will require an immediate return to the operating room: Bleeding from the incision, a suture coming loose, or dehiscence.

Postoperative instructions are best reviewed during the preoperative visit and listed on paper given to the patient's family at that time. Instructions are then reiterated when the surgeon meets the patient and parents just before surgery, and once more after the procedure is completed. Instructions are best kept simple and direct. Bathing is allowed after 2 days, and anytime the site is soiled, with plain soap and water. Prolonged immersion, such as recreational swimming, is not allowed until 1 week after surgery. Infants are given acetaminophen (Tylenol, 10–15 mg/kg every 4 h), older children ibuprofen (Motrin, 10 mg/kg every 6 h) beginning immediately upon reaching home and then around the clock while awake. Break through pain is treated with oxycodone and acetaminophen (Lortab, 7.5 mg oxycodone and 500 mg acetaminophen per 15 mL elixir, each dose in mL equal to one-half the patient's age in years, every 4 h). There are no restrictions on activity for infants and young children. More vigorous activity and juvenile athletics are restricted according to standard guidelines.

Suggested Reading

1. American Pediatric Surgical Association. Optimal resources for children's surgical care in the United States. An outline to organize surgical care for infants and children, with an emphasis on regionalization of specialty care. http://community.eapsa.org/Resources/ViewDocument/?DocumentKey=d8c93de4-f17e-425c-b526-00965bb64da9. Accessed 7 Aug 2013.
2. Marquez TT, Antonoff MB, Saltzman DA. Physiology of the newborn. In: Holcomb III GW, Murphy JP, Ostlie DJ, editors. Ashcraft's pediatric surgery. 5th ed. Philadelphia: Elsevier Saunders; 2010. p. 3–18. (Chapter 1) This is an excellent basic reference for most pediatric surgical conditions. It is appropriate for libraries in all hospitals of any size.
3. Nakayama DK. Management of the surgical newborn: physiological foundations and practical considerations. J Pediatr Urol. 2010; 6:232–8. A review of classical physiological features in newborn infants that form the basis of surgical care.

Tracy L. Nolan, Brett Howard, and Don K. Nakayama

Indications

The name hypertrophic pyloric stenosis (HPS) comes from hypertrophy of the muscularis of the pylorus, the thickening creating a narrowing that causes a gastric outlet obstruction. The condition affects infants in the first weeks of life, symptoms starting between the ages of 1 and 6 weeks of life. Feedings typically proceed normally at birth, but the baby develops progressive feeding intolerance with worsening postprandial nonbilious vomiting that can be forceful and thus projectile. The baby may lose weight from dehydration or malnutrition. Bilious vomiting—any green tinge to the vomitus—indicates another cause for the symptom, and a contrast study of the upper gastrointestinal tract (UGI) must be urgently done to rule out malrotation of the small intestine and volvulus.

History of nonbilious vomiting in the first weeks of life suggests the diagnosis. While palpation of the enlarged pylorus in the epigastrium or right upper quadrant on physical exam is diagnostic, nearly all cases today are found by ultrasound (US) or UGI. An US exam of the epigastrium visualizes the pylorus and shows whether it opens with a small oral feeding or remains closed. Threshold measurements of pyloric muscle thickness (more than 3 mm) and channel length (more than 17 mm) help confirm the diagnosis. UGI opacifies the narrowed pyloric channel, only a small wisp of contrast traversing the pylorus, sometimes in two parallel channels that gives the appearance of a train track.

T.L. Nolan, M.D. • B. Howard, M.D.
Department of Surgery, Mercer University School of Medicine, Medical Center of Central Georgia, Macon, GA 31201, USA

D.K. Nakayama, M.D., M.B.A., F.A.C.S. (✉)
Department of Surgery, West Virginia University School of Medicine, Health Sciences Center, 1 Medical Center Drive, Morgantown, WV 26506, USA
e-mail: dknakayama@hsc.wvu.edu; nakayama.don@gmail.com

Preoperative Preparation

Gastric outlet obstruction requires decompression with a gastric tube placed either through the nose (NG) or the mouth. Drainage by gravity or moderate suction should continue through induction of anesthesia. The tube must be large enough—at least 10 French—to decompress the stomach of gas and fluid. Infant feeding tubes, typically 6 French or smaller, do not serve the purpose. Replogle tubes, designed for infants, have all of its holes within an inch of the tip. A sump port allows air to entrain back into the stomach and prevent collapse of gastric lining onto the suction openings.

The length of the tube to be inserted must be measured to assure that it is not inserted too far, risking unintentional gastric perforation. A useful guide used by experienced pediatric nurses before placing a gastric tube is to first place it alongside the child's mouth, hold it against the ear, extend the tip to the epigastrium, and note the length. The tube then is placed to that depth and secured.

Infants with HPS all have dehydration that can be severe. Abnormal loss of gastric juice creates hypokalemic, hypochloremic metabolic alkalosis. Renal mechanisms to absorb sodium and excretion of potassium and hydrogen ion in response to hypovolemia make hypokalemia worse and may create an acidic urine even in the presence of alkalosis (paradoxical aciduria).

Intravenous fluid resuscitation and correction of electrolyte and acid–base disturbances before surgery thus are mandatory. Babies with signs of severe dehydration—loss of weight below birth weight, tachycardia (above 160 beats per minute), severe metabolic alkalosis with a serum CO_2 content of greater than 32 mEq/L—may require initial treatment with balanced electrolyte solution, such as lactated Ringer's solution (LR), to restore euvolemia. On occasion an infant may arrive in shock—hypotension with a systolic blood pressure of less than 50 mmHg, tachycardia above 180, and stupor—and require rapid administration of LR as a 20 mL/kg bolus over 20 min. Infants in the first weeks of life have

A.L. Halverson and D.C. Borgstrom (eds.), *Advanced Surgical Techniques for Rural Surgeons*, DOI 10.1007/978-1-4939-1495-1_35, © Springer Science+Business Media New York 2015

limited capacity to eliminate fluid and concentrate urine, so in all other circumstances it is safest to restore fluid and correct electrolyte imbalances gradually.

Nearly all infants with HPS respond to a solution of 5 % dextrose in 0.45 % sodium chloride (D5/0.45 NaCl) administered at one-and-half times maintenance fluid rates. Under basal conditions infants require 100 mL per kg every 24 h, so a baby being prepared for surgery then will receive 150 mL/kg/24 h. This translates to 4 mL/kg/h for routine maintenance intravenous fluids in infants, making the initial fluid order for HPS patients D5/0.45 NaCl at 6 mL/kg/h. Potassium should initially be withheld until the patient urinates. Once the baby voids, potassium at 20 mEq/L is added to correct potassium deficits. Correction of electrolytes should be verified before proceeding with surgery. The baby is considered ready for operation if vital signs are normal, the serum sodium is above 132 mEq/L, potassium above 3.2, and CO_2 content less than 30 mEq/L.

Pyloromyotomy is a clean procedure and does not require preoperative antibiotics.

An anesthesiologist or anesthetist experienced with small infants administers general endotracheal anesthesia.

Operative Technique

A transverse incision in the right upper quadrant gives direct access to the pylorus. A number of other approaches have been described, including one through the umbilicus and laparoscopic techniques. The incision begins about half a centimeter to the right of the midline, just above the midpoint between the xiphoid and the umbilicus and extends about an inch directly laterally (Fig. 35.1). The incision should be below the edge of the liver and should be large enough to allow delivery of the pylorus. A prudent surgeon avoids retracting the liver in small infants, as the capsule is fragile. Bleeding from a capsular tear or subcapsular hematoma, once started, is exceedingly difficult to stop.

The filmy omentum is carefully swept inferiorly. The stomach is reasonably sturdy but the epiploic vessels may be avulsed from the greater curve by vigorous retraction. Once a Babcock clamp or Singley forcep pulls the stomach into the field it should be removed from the organ completely. Any further manipulation should be manual, aided by a gauze sponge to allow a firm but gentle grasp to coax the pylorus into view. An experienced surgeon recognizes that tearing of the serosa is a sign that the incision has to be enlarged.

A shallow longitudinal incision is made just through the serosa. The duodenum is closest to the serosa immediately adjacent to the pylorus, so it is prudent to begin the incision 2 mm proximal to its junction with the stomach (Fig. 35.2). The incision extends well onto the antrum, a distance of about 2 cm. There is a path for the incision free

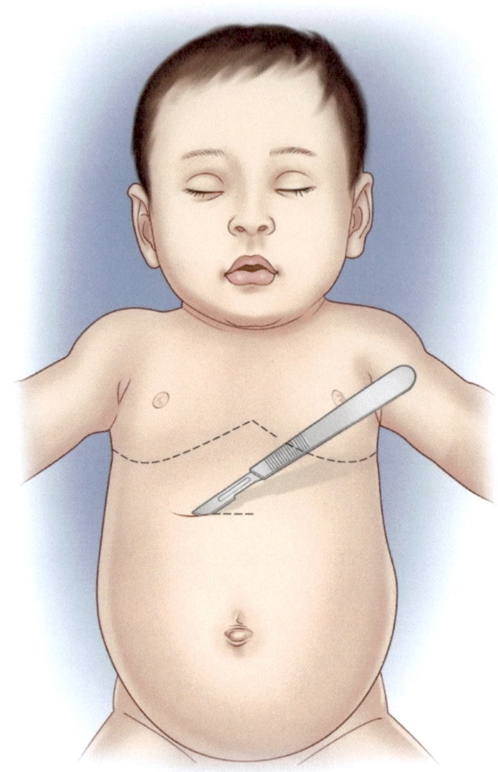

Fig. 35.1 A number 15 blade is used to make a transverse incision just above the midway point between the xiphoid and umbilicus. The incision should be below the liver edge, identified by palpation

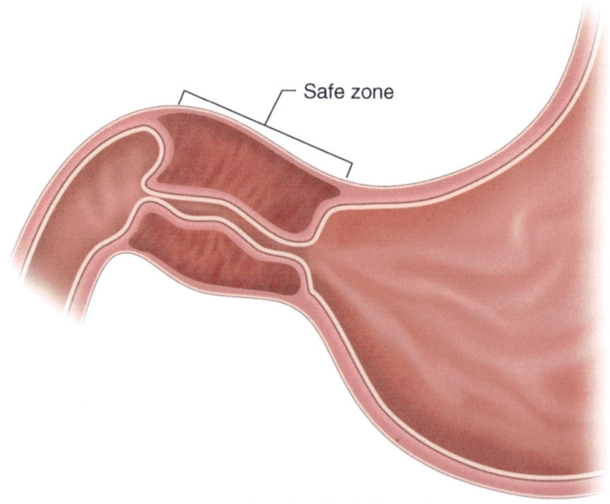

Fig. 35.2 The margin of the duodenal lumen at left has a superficial position. An incision placed too far distally may unintentionally enter the lumen at that point. The "safe zone" therefore begins 2 mm proximal to the duodenal–gastric junction

Fig. 35.3 The incision in the serosa of the pylorus starts distally about 2 mm proximal to the duodenal junction and extends in an avascular path between visible vessels from the superior and inferior margins. It extends well onto the antrum, a total distance of about 2 cm

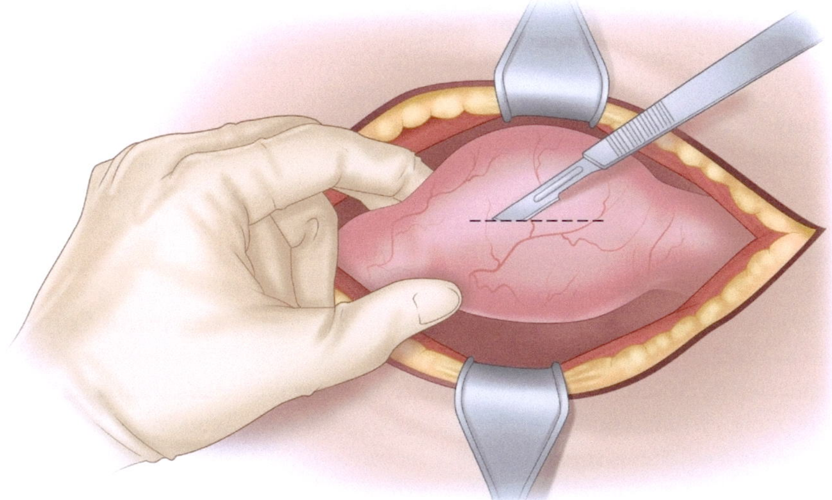

Fig. 35.4 Bluntly splitting the layer of hypertrophied muscle reaches the avascular submucosal plane. The tips of a curved Mosquito clamp points upward away from the submucosa to avoid damaging it. A constant spread of the upper and lower aspects of the muscularis completes the pyloromyotomy, allowing them to be rocked independently when grasped

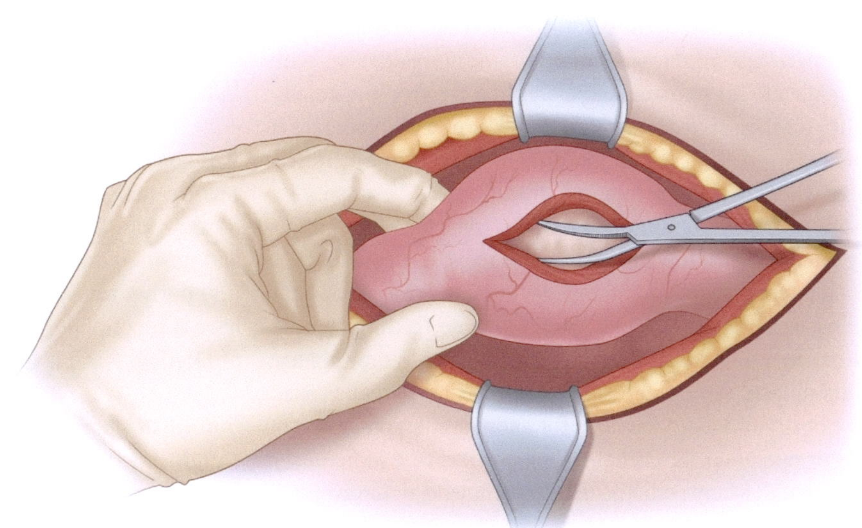

of visible vessels over the anterior aspect of the pylorus and antrum (Fig. 35.3). Bleeding is scant and generally does not require cautery.

An instrument is placed into the incision and used to break the fibers of the hypertrophied muscle. A "gritty" sensation may be felt through the instrument. A blunt scalpel handle or the serrated edge of one jaw of a clamp is appropriate to begin splitting the muscle. Once the muscle begins to divide the muscularis is split to the level of the submucosa (Fig. 35.4). Appropriate instruments for this task include a pyloric muscle spreader—a simple blunt-tipped instrument with serrations on the outside aspect of the jaws to hold the exposed muscle edges; a Mosquito clamp, tips directed

upward so that the mucosa is not perforated; or continued blunt splitting using the scalpel handle. The muscle is split until the pale pyloric submucosal layer is seen over the length of the incision, indicating complete division of the muscle fibers. An adequate pyloromyotomy is confirmed by assuring that the superior and inferior edges of the myotomy move independently.

The surgeon checks for mucosal perforation by milking the duodenum back toward the pylorus and observing for bubbles or bile leaking from the edge of the incision. The same is done with the stomach on the antral aspect of the incision. A small leak can be repaired with a fine absorbable suture (5-0) reinforced by a slip of omentum. A large disruption, or one found at reoperation, requires complete closure of the pylorus and a repeat pyloromyotomy at another unoperated surface of the pylorus, typically after rotating the structure 90 or 180°. Closure and transfer to a children's specialty hospital may be the most prudent approach for a major iatrogenic perforation.

Potential Pitfalls

Cardiovascular collapse at induction of anesthesia may complicate inadequate preoperative resuscitation and correction of hypokalemia. Severely dehydrated infants may require 24 h or more of fluid correction. Such cases may be best transferred to a children's specialty facility for care.

The major technical pitfall is mucosal perforation at the duodenal–pyloric junction. The intraoperative management of this technical error is discussed earlier. If not recognized at the time of operation, the infant becomes rapidly ill from generalized peritonitis, with fever, persistent tachycardia, abdominal tenderness, and rigidity. Resuscitation and administration of intravenous antibiotics must begin immediately, with arrangements for immediate transfer to a children's specialty facility for intensive care and surgery. Closure of the defect is mandatory—if the baby is more than an hour or so from a center where definitive care and operation can be done then closure of the perforation and transfer for later pyloromyotomy after stabilization and recovery is the safest course.

Inadequate pyloromyotomy is signaled by persistent feeding intolerance. Patients should tolerate feedings by the first or second feeding. One or two episodes of vomiting are commonplace. A contrast study confirms persistent gastric outlet obstruction and the need for another attempt.

After operation intravenous narcotics must be judiciously administered. Many pediatric texts recommend an intravenous dose of morphine sulfate of 0.1 mg/kg. Most experienced centers use oral sucrose solution and acetaminophen (10 mg/kg every 4 h) immediately after surgery, supplemented by morphine sulfate at 0.05 mg/kg every 2 h. Babies who require more than two doses of morphine at this level are transferred to a nursing unit that can provide constant monitoring of heart and respiratory rates. Hypoventilation (respiratory acidosis) is the compensatory response to uncorrected metabolic alkalosis, and thus may complicate postoperative care.

Postoperative Care

Many experienced practitioners have forgone complicated feeding ladders of gradual increases in concentration and volume of formula after pyloromyotomy. The simplest regimen is to withhold feeding for 6 h after surgery, and begin feedings ad libitum every 2 h. Patients may vomit once or twice after surgery; this should not be a reason to withhold feedings. Persistent vomiting is best managed by careful placement of a gastric tube (to a proper depth, see above) and gentle irrigation of the stomach with warm saline. Feedings may resume 2 h later. Persistent vomiting is an indication for a barium swallow to check for persistent gastric outlet obstruction. Once the infant is tolerating two ounces without emesis, intravenous fluids can be discontinued and the patient discharged.

Common Complications

Before surgery: Dehydration, metabolic alkalosis, hypokalemia, hyponatremia. Cardiac arrest at induction of anesthesia.

Operative: Duodenal perforation, inadequate pyloromyotomy.

Postoperative: Postoperative apnea, postintubation stridor. Delayed recognition of duodenal or gastric perforation and peritonitis.

When to Transfer

Any baby with pyloric stenosis, or suspected of having pyloric stenosis, should have a gastric tube placed from the nose or mouth. The tube should be aspirated to remove gas and gastric contents and be open to air or connected to suction during transport. If possible transferred patients should have a functioning intravenous cannula in place an infusion of D5/0.45 NaCl at 150 mL/kg/24 h (6 mL/kg/h).

Before surgery: Severe dehydration—infants below birth weight, systolic blood pressure below 50 mmHg, heart rate above 180; severe hypokalemic metabolic alkalosis (serum CO_2 content above 32); any infant needing fluid resuscitation and electrolyte correction for which the nursing unit is unprepared.

After surgery: Any case complicated by duodenal or gastric perforation, or suspected of having this complication; clinical or radiographic evidence of an inadequate pyloromyotomy.

Suggested Reading

1. Aspelund G, Langer JC. Current management of hypertrophic pyloric stenosis. Semin Pediatr Surg. 2007;16:27–33. An overall review of all aspects of care, including imaging, preoperative care, various surgical approaches, postoperative feeding regimens, complications, and medical management in lieu of surgery.
2. Koontz CS. In: Holcomb GW III, Murphy JP, Ostlie DJ, editors. Ashcraft's pediatric surgery. 5th ed. Philadelphia: Elsevier Saunders; 2010. p. 391–9. (Chapter 30) This is an excellent basic reference for most pediatric surgical conditions. It is appropriate for libraries in all hospitals of any size.

Index

A.L. Halverson and D.C. Borgstrom (eds.), *Advanced Surgical Techniques for Rural Surgeons*,
DOI 10.1007/978-1-4939-1495-1, © Springer Science+Business Media New York 2015